Essential Epidemiology
An Introduction for Students and Health Professionals

This is an accessible, easily readable and modern introduction to epidemiology for students of medicine and public health. It combines a strong public health perspective and rationale with modern methodological insights in a coherent and straightforward way. It emphasises the fundamental principles common to all areas of epidemiology and, unlike many other texts, integrates both public health and clinical epidemiology and the study of infectious and chronic diseases. It aims to give health professionals a good understanding of the methods and potential problems underlying epidemiological data and reports but also provides a thorough introduction for would-be epidemiologists. The 'nuts and bolts' of epidemiology are embedded in the wider health perspective, and the concluding chapter explores future possibilities and emphasises the integration of the various strands of the discipline. The basic messages are reinforced through numerous examples and questions, with answers provided.

Penny Webb
Queensland Institute of Medical Research

Chris Bain
School of Population Health, University of Queensland

Sandi Pirozzo
formerly School of Population Health, University of Queensland

Essential
Epidemiology

An Introduction for Students
and Health Professionals

Penny Webb, Chris Bain
and Sandi Pirozzo

...ntre

224...
e.mtw-tr.in... ...s.net

be returned/renewed by the last date shown

CAMBRIDGE UNIVERSITY PRESS
Cambridge, New York, Melbourne, Madrid, Cape Town, Singapore, São Paulo

CAMBRIDGE UNIVERSITY PRESS
The Edinburgh Building, Cambridge CB2 2RU, UK

Published in the United States of America by Cambridge University Press, New York

www.cambridge.org
Information on this title: www.cambridge.org/9780521546613

First published 2005
Reprinted with corrections 2006

Printed in the United Kingdom at the University Press, Cambridge

A catalog record for this book is available from the British Library

Library of Congress Cataloging in Publication data

Webb, Penny, 1963–
Essential epidemiology: an introduction for students and health
professionals / Penny Webb, Chris Bain, Sandi Pirozzo.
     p.;   cm.
Includes bibliographical references and index.
ISBN 0 521 54661 3 (pbk.)
1. Epidemiology. I. Bain, Chris, 1947– II. Pirozzo, Sandi, 1951– III. Title.
[DNLM: 1. Epidemiologic Research Design. 2. Epidemiologic Methods.
3. Public Health. WA 105 W367e 2005]
RA651.W385 2005
614.4–dc22   2004057005

ISBN-13: 978 0 521 83745 6 hardback
ISBN-10: 0 521 83745 6 hardback
ISBN-13: 978 0 521 54661 3 paperback
ISBN-10: 0 521 54661 3 paperback

Cambridge University Press has no responsibility for the persistence or accuracy of
URLs for external or third-party internet websites referred to in this book, and does not
guarantee that any content on such websites is, or will remain, accurate or appropriate.

Every effort has been made in preparing this book to provide accurate and up-to-date
information which is in accord with accepted standards and practice at the time of
publication. Although case histories are drawn from actual cases, every effort has been
made to disguise the identities of the individuals involved. Nevertheless, the authors,
editors and publisher can make no warranties that the information contained herein is
totally free from error, not least because clinical standards are constantly changing
through research and regulation. The authors, editors and publisher therefore disclaim all
liability for direct or consequential damages resulting from the use of material contained
in this book. Readers are strongly advised to pay careful attention to information provided
by the manufacturer of any drugs or equipment that they plan to use.

Contents

Professor Adrian Sleigh
National Centre for Epidemiology and Population Health,
Australian National University

Preface

This book has grown out of our collective experience of teaching introductory epidemiology both in the classroom and to distance students enrolled in public health and health studies programmes in the School of Population Health (formerly the Department of Social and Preventive Medicine), University of Queensland. It began life as a detailed set of course notes that we wrote because we could not find a single epidemiology text that covered all of the areas we felt were important in sufficient detail. As the notes were to be used primarily by distance students, we tried hard to make them accessible with lots of examples, minimal jargon and equations, and by engaging readers in 'doing' epidemiology along the way. Feedback from students and colleagues convinced us that the notes were both approachable and practical. We have built on this, and offer this text as a practical introduction to epidemiology for those who need an understanding of health data they meet in their everyday working lives, as well as for those who wish to pursue a career in epidemiology.

Chapter 1 is a general introduction that both answers the question 'what is epidemiology and what can it do?' and presents the main concepts that are the focus of the rest of the book. Chapters 2–8 cover the basic principles and underlying theory of epidemiology in a very 'hands-on' way, leading to Chapters 9–11, which integrate this information in a practical look at how we read and interpret epidemiological reports, think about assessing causality and finally synthesise a mass of information in a single review. Chapters 12–14 then look at some specific applications of epidemiology and Chapter 15 concludes with a fresh look at what epidemiology is and what it can do to help address the health concerns facing the world today.

Symbols

The following symbols are used to define key elements within the text. We strongly believe that the best way to learn anything is by actually doing it and so have included questions within the text for those who like to test their understanding as they go. Because we also know how frustrating it is to have to search for answers, we have provided these immediately following the questions for those in a hurry to proceed.

We have used numerous real-life examples from all around the world to illustrate the key points and to provide additional insights in some areas. Extra examples that provide added interest and complement the main message in the text are given in boxes featuring this symbol.

Many books present clinical epidemiology as a separate discipline from public health epidemiology – a distinction that is strengthened by the fact that clinical epidemiologists have developed their own names for many standard epidemiological terms. In practice all epidemiology is based on the same underlying principles, so we have integrated the two approaches throughout the book but have also highlighted specific examples more relevant to the clinical situation. (Please note that this book does not offer a comprehensive coverage of clinical epidemiology; rather we aim to show the similarity of the two areas where they overlap.)

We have deliberately tried to keep the main text free of unnecessary detail and equations but have included some epidemiological 'extras'. This material is not essential to the continuity of the core text but provides some additional information for those who like to see where things have come from or want a more detailed perspective.

Acknowledgements

If we were to name everyone who had contributed in some way to this book the list would be endless. We would, however, like to acknowledge some of the great teachers (and their books) from whom we have learned most of what we know, and the books we have relied heavily on for our teaching. These include Brian MacMahon (*Epidemiology: Principles and Methods,* MacMahon and Pugh, 1970), Olli Miettinen, Charlie Hennekens (*Epidemiology in Medicine*, Hennekens and Buring, 1987), Ken Rothman (*Modern Epidemiology*, 1986), *Foundations of Epidemiology* (Lillienfeld and Lillienfeld, 1980), and *Epidemiology* (Gordis, 1996). We would also like to thank our colleagues and friends, especially the Fellows from the NHMRC Capacity Grant in Longitudinal Study Methods in the School of Population Health, University of Queensland, and the staff and students from the Cancer and Population Studies Group at the Queensland Institute of Medical Research who willingly read drafts of the text and whose constructive feedback helped shape the final version. Particular thanks go to Adrian Sleigh (Australian National University) who authored Chapters 4 and 12 and also contributed to Chapter 15, Susan Jordan (QIMR) who helped with pulling everything together and Christine Howes (Bristol, UK) who drew all otherwise non-attributed illustrations. Finally, we would like to acknowledge the School of Population Health, University of Queensland, which provided the intellectual environment that led to this book as well as financial support to cover the costs of preparing the final draft.

Epidemiology is . . .

> **Box 1.1 Epidemiology is . . .**
>
> 'The science of epidemics' (*Concise Oxford Dictionary*, 1964)
> 'The science of the occurrence of illness' (Miettinen, 1978)
> 'The study of the **distribution** and **determinants** of disease in humans'
>   (MacMahon and Pugh, 1970)
> 'The study of the distribution and determinants of **health-related states or
>   events** in specified populations, and the **application of this study to
>   control of health problems**' (Last, 2001)

So what is epidemiology anyway? The *Concise Oxford Dictionary* (1964) defined it accurately, but not very helpfully, as 'the science of epidemics'. In 1970, MacMahon and Pugh came up with something a bit more concrete: 'the study of the *distribution* and *determinants* of disease'. Their definition succinctly identifies the two core strands of traditional epidemiology: *who* is developing a disease (and *where* and *when*), and *why* are they developing it? In his *Dictionary of Epidemiology*, Last (2001) takes this two steps further by broadening the scope to include health in general, not just disease, as well as highlighting the direct role of epidemiology in disease control.

Epidemiology, therefore, is about measuring health, identifying the causes of ill-health and intervening to improve health; but what do we mean by 'health'? Back in 1948, the World Health Organization (WHO, 1948) defined it as '. . . a state of physical, mental and social well-being'. Now, while this view is clearly what we hope for as individuals, the inclusion of 'mental and social well-being' would until recently have induced despair in epidemiologists. In practice what we usually measure is *ill-health* or disease: more disease equals poorer health, and this focus is reflected in the content of most routine reports of health data and in many of the health measures that we will consider here. However, methods that do attempt to capture these more elusive components of health are now emerging. Instead of simply measuring 'life expectancy', the WHO now uses 'health adjusted life expectancy' (HALE) to make international comparisons of the effectiveness of health systems. In doing so they are recognising that it is not longevity per se that we seek, but a long and healthy life. We will discuss this and other measures in more detail in Chapter 2.

Perhaps epidemiology's most fundamental role is to provide a logic and structure for the analysis of health problems both great and small. It also emphasises the sound use of numbers – we have to count and we have to think. We have to think about what is worth counting and how best to count it, about what is practical and, importantly, about how well we (or others) finally measured whatever it was we set out to measure, and what it all means. Accurate measurement of health is clearly the cornerstone of the discipline, but we believe the special value of epidemiology flows from a way of thought that is open, alert to the potential for error, willing to consider alternative explanations and, finally, constructively critical and pragmatic.

We offer this book as an aid to such thought. It does not aim to turn you into a practising epidemiologist overnight but will give clear directions if that is where you decide to go. Its primary goal is to help you interpret the mass of epidemiological literature and the various types of data that you may come across. We hope that you will see, by reading and by doing, that the fundamental concepts and tools of epidemiology are relatively simple, although the tasks of integrating, synthesising and interpreting health information are more challenging. Before adding more generalities, let us do some public health epidemiology.

A case of food poisoning

Epidemiology is a bit like detective work in that we try to find out why and how disease occurs. Our first example illustrates this. After an outbreak of food poisoning at a youth camp, the local public health unit was called in to identify the cause (Hook *et al.*, 1996). They first asked everyone at the camp what they had eaten prior to the outbreak and some results of this investigation are shown in Table 1.1. (Note that everyone is recorded as either having eaten or not eaten each food; and that most people will have eaten more than one of the foods.)

Looking at the numbers in Table 1.1, it is difficult to see which of the foods might have been responsible for the outbreak. More people became ill after eating potato fries than after eating cold chicken (184 versus 155) – but then more people ate the fries (422 versus 202). How then can we best compare the two foods? One simple way to do this is to calculate the *percentage* of people who became ill among those who ate (or did not eat) each type of food. For example, 156 out of 343 people who ate hot chicken became ill and

$$156 \div 343 = 0.45 = 45\%$$

Table 1.1 Numbers of people who became ill after eating various foods at a youth camp.

Food	People who ate the food		People who didn't eat the food	
	Total	Number ill	Total	Number ill
Friday dinner				
Hot chicken	343	156	231	74
Peas	390	175	184	55
Potato fries	422	184	152	46
Saturday lunch				
Cold chicken	202	155	372	75
Salad	385	171	189	59
Saturday dinner				
Fruit salad	324	146	250	84

(Adapted from Hook *et al.*, 1996, with permission.)

So 45% of people who ate hot chicken became sick. This is known as the **attack rate** for hot chicken, i.e. 45% of hot-chicken eaters were 'attacked' by food poisoning.

Calculate the attack rates for the other foods. Which food has the highest attack rate?

Although cold chicken has the highest attack rate (77%), not everyone who ate it (or, more precisely, who *reported* eating it) became ill and 20% or one in five people who did *not* eat cold chicken still became ill. This is par for the course; no matter what the cause of concern, it is rare that everyone who is exposed to it will show the effects (disease). What can help here is to work out how much *more likely* people who ate a particular food were to become ill than those who did not eat it. For example, 45% of people who ate hot chicken became ill, compared with 32% of people who did not eat hot chicken. Hot-chicken eaters were therefore 1.4 times (45% ÷ 32% = 1.4) more likely to become ill than people who did not eat hot chicken. This measure gives us the risk of sickness in hot-chicken eaters *relative* to non-eaters, hence its name – **relative risk**.

Calculate the relative risk of developing food poisoning associated with each of the other food items. Which food is associated with the highest relative risk of sickness?

We can now conclude that the food item most likely to have been responsible for the outbreak was the cold chicken – people who ate this were almost four times more likely to become ill than those who did not. This is quite a strong relative

Table 1.2 Numbers of people who became ill after eating various foods at a youth camp and attack rates and relative risks for each food.

Food	People who ate the food			People who didn't eat the food			Relative risk
	Total	Number ill	Attack rate (%)	Total	Number ill	Attack rate (%)	
Friday dinner							
Hot chicken	343	156	45	231	74	32	1.4
Peas	390	175	45	184	55	30	1.5
Potato fries	422	184	44	152	46	30	1.4
Saturday lunch							
Cold chicken	202	155	77	372	75	20	3.8
Salad	385	171	44	189	59	31	1.4
Saturday dinner							
Fruit salad	324	146	45	250	84	34	1.3

(Adapted from Hook *et al.*, 1996 with permission.)

risk; in comparison, eating any of the other foods was associated with no more than one and a half times the risk of disease. The relevant data, including the attack rates and relative risks, are summarised in Table 1.2, which is much more informative than the raw numbers of Table 1.1.

In identifying the cause of the outbreak you have just solved an epidemiological problem. The 'attack rates' and 'relative risks' that you used are fairly simple to calculate and are two very useful epidemiological measures. We will discuss them further in Chapters 2 and 5 and they will appear throughout the book.

Subdisciplines of epidemiology

The outbreak investigation above is an example of what might be called *public health epidemiology*, or *infectious disease epidemiology*, with the first name reflecting the broad field of application and the second the nature of both the aetiological (causal) agent and the disease. It is quite common now to specify such sub-fields of epidemiology, which range on the one hand from *nutritional* through *social* to *environmental epidemiology*, and on the other from *cancer* to *injury* or *perinatal epidemiology*: the former grouping being exposure-oriented and the latter focused on the particular disease or outcome. Nonetheless, the core methods and techniques of epidemiology remain common to all subdisciplines, so the contents of this book are relevant to all. Setting sub-speciality boundaries largely reflects the explosion of knowledge in these areas, although some areas do present special challenges. For example, capturing a person's usual diet is remarkably challenging and the subsequent data analysis equally so; epidemiologists coming fresh to the field of nutritional epidemiology will need to develop experience and expertise in that specific area.

It is of some interest to know a bit more about a few of the special epidemiologies. *Occupational epidemiology* has the longest history of all, with influential early observations of diseases linked to occupations such as mining appearing in the sixteenth century, and a systematic treatise on occupational diseases was published by Ramazzini back in 1700 (Rosen, 1958). Occupational health research in general, and epidemiology in particular, continue to contribute to enhancing workplace health today. Seminal contributions in the field include identification of the pulmonary (lung) hazards of asbestos for miners and construction workers (Selikoff *et al.*, 1965) and the work practices that led to an epidemic of a rare fatal cancer in workers in the polyvinyl chloride industry (Makk *et al.*, 1974). Company records of job tasks can provide measures of past exposure among employees, allowing researchers to look back in time and link, for example, past asbestos exposure to subsequent deaths in the workforce. (This type of study is a *retrospective cohort design* – see Chapter 6. It is only possible when there are good records of both exposure and outcome, usually death, and for this reason has proved particularly useful in occupational studies where such records often do exist.)

Far more modern are the subdisciplines of *molecular epidemiology* and *clinical epidemiology*. The first aims to weld the population perspective of epidemiology with the exploding insights into how variations in genes and their products affect the growth, form and function of cells and tissues. It thus has the potential for defining proximal biological consequences of exposures and linking these to disease risk; and additionally provides good biological markers of some of these exposures (e.g. changes to DNA following exposure to tobacco smoke). In contrast, clinical epidemiology does not involve exotic techniques but differs from other branches of epidemiology in its focus on enhancing clinical decisions to benefit *individual patients*, rather than improving the health of *populations*. For this reason, clinical epidemiology is sometimes regarded as a completely separate discipline. The situation is not helped by the fact that clinical epidemiology has developed its own names for many standard epidemiological measures. The foundations are, however, identical to those of public health epidemiology and we will discuss the two in parallel, highlighting any differences in language or approach along the way.

On epidemics

If we take the word 'epidemiology' itself, its origins from '*epidemic*' are clear. If we talk about an epidemic we immediately conjure up pictures of an acute outbreak of infectious disease but, both for practical and for etymological reasons,

Fig. 1.1 Time trends in lung cancer mortality rates (age-standardised to the 1970 US population) for white males (-----) and females (——). (Drawn from Devesa *et al.*, 1999.)

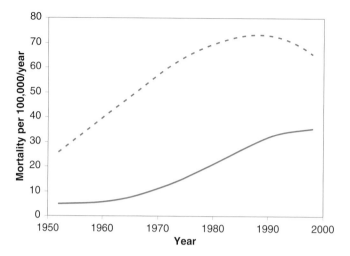

it seems reasonable to use the term to describe a notable excess of any disease over time. Many developed countries could, for example, be described as undergoing an epidemic of lung cancer over the last few decades (Figure 1.1). Notably the pattern of lung cancer over time differs for men and women; rates in men rose sharply between 1950 and 1980 but have been falling for some years now, while those of women rose later and have not yet peaked – a consequence of their later adoption of the smoking habit. To describe this excessive occurrence of disease (or death) as an 'epidemic' captures some of the urgency the numbers demand.

The derivation of the word 'epidemiology' itself is from the Greek *epi*, upon, *demos*, the people, and *logia*, study. Literally, therefore, it means the 'study (of what is) upon the people'. Such study suggests a simple set of questions that have long lain at the heart of epidemiology.

- **What** disease/condition is present in excess?
- **Who** is ill?
- **Where** do they live?
- **When** did they become ill?
- **Why** did they become ill?

The first question reflects the need for a sound, common definition of a disease so that like is compared with like. Epidemiology is all about comparison – without some reference of what is usual, how can we identify excess? The next three questions form the mantra of descriptive epidemiology: '*person, place and time*'. As Figure 1.2 shows, an 'epidemic of premature mortality' has occurred over the past decade among young and middle-aged men in Russia. This description captures the essence of the problem and prompts the next question: what has caused this epidemic? What has changed in the circumstances of younger Russian men to reverse the pattern of falling mortality in the early 1980s and cause it almost to double in less than 10 years? Other data show that there were no such mortality

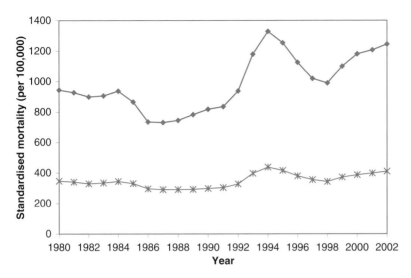

Fig. 1.2 Changes in all-cause mortality at ages 0–64 years in the Russian Federation during 1980–2002 (◆ men, ✳ women). (Data adapted from the European Health For All Database. Copenhagen, WHO Regional Office for Europe, www.euro.who.int/HFADB, accessed 8 April 2004.)

changes in Western Europe, nor among older Russian men or infants, nor (to the same extent) in Russian women. This simple graph captures a public health disaster for Russia and prompts urgent causal speculation: a slumping economy, social disruption, depression, excess consumption of alcohol, poor nutrition and violence have probably all contributed. Solving and responding to the final question, *Why did this happen?*, is critical for public health progress, but there is clearly no simple panacea. The example simply highlights the central importance of paying close attention to descriptive data that provide a 'community diagnosis' or take the public health 'pulse' of a nation. Much can be gleaned from apparently simple data to give a quite precise description of the health event or state of interest, as the following exercise shows.

An historical epidemic

Table 1.3 shows some data that relate to an actual human experience. It tells you how many people there were in various age, sex and socioeconomic groups and what percentage of these people died during the 'epidemic'. The challenge is to use these data to describe the event systematically in terms of **whom** this happened to (we have no data on place or time) and then to think about the sort of event that might have induced such a pattern.

The following questions are designed to help you identify key features of the data.

1. What is distinctive about this isolated population with regard to
   • the numbers of men and women (sex distribution),
   • the numbers of adults and children (age distribution) and
   • the numbers in each socioeconomic group (socioeconomic distribution)?

Table 1.3 An historical event.

SES[a]	Adult males		Adult females		Children (both sexes)		Total population	
	Total	% Dead	Total	% Dead	Total	% Dead	Total	% Dead
High	175	67.4	144	2.8	6	—	325	37.5
Medium	168	91.7	93	14.0	24	—	285	58.6
Low	462	83.8	165	53.9	79	65.8	706	74.8
Other	885	78.3	23	13.0	0	—	908	76.6
Total	1,690	80.0	425	25.6	109	47.7	2,224	68.0

[a] SES, socioeconomic status.
(*Source:* http://www.anesi.com, accessed 2 March 2004; for full details see reference list.)

2. What strikes you about the percentage of people who died (the 'death rate')? Is this different for (a) adults and children, (b) men and women, (c) high and low socioeconomic status (SES) and (d) any particular combinations of the above?

3. How many times more likely were
   • men to die than women and
   • those of low SES to die than those of high SES?

4. To what historical event might these data refer?

Table 1.3 displays more complicated data than Table 1.2, since you had to consider the joint effects of three factors (sex, socioeconomic status and age) on mortality. The sequence of questions aims to underline a sound general principle in describing such tables, i.e. to look at overall patterns first, then move on to more detail (see Box 1.2). We all see things in different ways, but until you develop your own style this approach is one that can help you avoid becoming lost in the array of possible relationships. You need first to grasp the size of the *whole group* under study and how many died; then check the overall patterns (numbers and mortality rates) across each 'exposure' separately (sex, SES, age). These are sometimes called the 'marginal' rates based on row and column totals, e.g. first look at the rates for all adult males, ignoring their SES, or for all people of high SES, ignoring their age and sex. Only then consider the more complex 'inner' set of joint effects such as the influence of SES on mortality among women.

In tackling this and the previous problem you have already done some serious epidemiology: you have *described* data, *interpreted* the patterns you observed and used *epidemiological measures* to help do this. We will build on this throughout the book, but first let's step back a little and see what other lessons we can learn from the past.

Box 1.2 An historical event

Things to note about the population include

- the predominance of adult males ($1{,}690 \div 2{,}224 = 76\%$), the much smaller proportion of adult females (19%) and the very few children;
- the substantial excess of persons of low SES (men and children in particular); and
- the total population (2,224) is quite large – a village, small town, armed encampment . . . ?

Things to note about the 'death rates' include the following.

- The overall death rate is very high – more than two-thirds died.
  (Note: these death rates are essentially identical in form to the attack rates in Table 1.2.)
- Overall, death rates increased with decreasing SES.
- The death rate in men (80.0%) was much higher than that in women (25.6%); the death rate in children was between these two.
- In men, the death rate was high in all socioeconomic classes, although those of high SES fared better than the rest; in women, the death rate was always less than that for males of equivalent SES, but it increased strikingly from high to medium to low SES.
- The only children to die were of low SES.

Overall, the relative risk (RR) for men versus women is $80.0 \div 25.6 = 3.1$

The RR for low versus high SES is $74.8 \div 37.5 = 2.0$

The RR for women of low SES versus women of
   high SES is $53.9 \div 2.8 = 19.3$

The RR for men of low SES versus women of high SES is $83.8 \div 2.8 = 29.9$

A disaster has occurred, causing a high death rate that predominantly affected men (of all social classes) and, to a lesser extent, women and children of low social class. Overall there is a modest benefit of belonging to a higher social stratum, and among women this protection was exceptionally strong (a 19-fold higher risk of dying for low versus high SES).

Such substantial differences in risk reflect powerful preventive effects and in this instance it was a mix of social custom and the physical consequences of social stratification. The event was the sinking of the Titanic, where those of higher SES were situated on the upper decks and were therefore closer to the lifeboats. The males gallantly helped the females and children into the lifeboats first. Those of 'other' SES were the crew.

Box 1.3 On airs, waters and places

Whoever wishes to investigate medicine properly, should proceed thus: in the first place to consider the seasons of the year, and what effects each of them produces . . . Then the winds, the hot and the cold, especially such as are common to all countries, and then such as are peculiar to each locality. We must also consider the qualities of the waters . . . In the same manner, when one comes into a city to which he is a stranger, he ought to consider its situation, how it lies as to the winds and the rising of the sun; for its influence is not the same whether it lies to the north or the south, to the rising or to the setting sun. These things one ought to consider most attentively, and concerning the waters which the inhabitants use, whether they be marshy and soft, or hard, and running from elevated and rocky situations, and then if saltish and unfit for cooking; and the ground, whether it be naked and deficient in water, or wooded and well watered, and whether it lies in a hollow, confined situation, or is elevated and cold; and the mode in which the inhabitants live, and what are their pursuits, whether they are fond of drinking and eating to excess, and given to indolence, or are fond of exercise and labour . . .

(Extracted from Hippocrates of Cos, 400 BC.)

The beginnings[1]

Modern historical practice eschews the 'great man' approach, for good reason; but here we are seeking not insights into the social and economic forces which stimulated the emergence of epidemiology, but rather a sense of the nature and timing of early forays into population health that we might claim as epidemiological. As such, linking these to individuals adds some charm, and, if it helps embed the lessons they still have for us, all the better. Good epidemiological practice and reasoning started long ago.

Hippocrates of Cos (460–375 BC) was perhaps the first proto-epidemiologist (*proto* because he did not actually count anything). He recognised that both environmental and behavioural factors could affect health (see Box 1.3).

The Dark Ages and Middle Ages (AD 500–1500) have little to say to us, other than in the development of causal reasoning, which we will set aside until later in the book (Chapter 10). The introduction of more quantitative methods into epidemiology and, in fact, into biology and medicine in general, has been

---

[1] The material in this section is drawn from a mix of primary and secondary sources, with the latter including a number of texts, most helpful being those of Stolley and Lasky (1995) and Lilienfeld and Lilienfeld (1980).

Table 1.4 An historical example of a life-table.

Exact age (years)	Deaths	Survivors	Chance of living to that age (%)
0	—	100	
6	36	64	64
16	24	40	40
26	15	25	25
36	9	16	16
46	6	10	10
56	4	6	6
66	3	3	3
76	2	1	1
86	1	0	

(Adapted from Graunt, 1662.)

attributed to John Graunt (1620–1674), a haberdasher and early Fellow of the Royal Society in London, although his friend William Petty may well have been a seminal influence too. In 1662 Graunt published his *Natural and Political Observations Mentioned in a Following Index and Made Upon the Bills of Mortality*. He studied parish christening registers and the 'Bills of Mortality', and noted many features of birth and death data, including the higher numbers of both male births and deaths in comparison with females, the high rates of infant mortality and seasonal variations in mortality. He also provided a numerical account of the impact of the plague in London as well as making the first attempts to estimate the size of the population. In an attempt to define a 'law of mortality' he constructed the first life-table (Table 1.4). This summarised the health of a population in terms of the chance of an individual surviving to a particular age. Notice that at this time only three out of every hundred people reached the age of 66, and the majority of deaths occurred in early life. This technique was a forerunner of that used by life insurance companies for calculating insurance premiums today, as well as a fundamental approach to measuring a population's health.

During the nineteenth century the mainstream developments of the collection and uses of health statistics for what we now call descriptive epidemiology built on this start in England, and also derived from a brief flowering in France. Of particular influence as a teacher was Pierre Charles-Alexandre Louis (1787–1872), who conducted some of the earliest epidemiological studies of treatment effectiveness when he demonstrated that bloodletting did not aid recovery from disease. Among his students was William Farr (1807–1883), physician, statistician and director of the Office of the Registrar General for England and Wales from 1837, its second year of operation. Farr studied levels of mortality in different occupations and institutions and in married and single persons, as well as other facets of the distribution of disease. He published these and other findings in the *Annual Reports of the Registrar General*, and the present UK system of vital statistics stems directly from his work.

John Snow (1813–1858), a physician and contemporary of Farr, was better known at the time for giving chloroform to Queen Victoria during childbirth, but is now remembered for his pioneering work in elucidating the mode of transmission of cholera (Snow, 1855). This remains a classic and exciting example of epidemiological detection and some of Snow's personal account of it is given below and again later in the chapter.

Snow's initial observations were based on a series of reports of individual cases of cholera and, in every instance, he was able to link the case to contact with another infected person (or their goods), thereby demonstrating that the disease could spread from person to person. He then surmised, contrary to popular belief at the time, that cholera could be transmitted through polluted water, a view that was strengthened by his observations linking a terrible outbreak of cholera around Broad Street, London, in 1854, to the local water pump (Box 1.4).

Box 1.4 John Snow and the Broad Street Pump (1854)

Within two hundred and fifty yards of the spot where Cambridge Street joins Broad Street, there were upwards of five hundred fatal attacks of cholera in ten days . . . The mortality would undoubtedly have been much greater had it not been for the flight of the population . . . so that in less than six days from the commencement of the outbreak, the most afflicted streets were deserted by more than three-quarters of their inhabitants.

There were a few cases of cholera in the neighbourhood of Broad Street, Golden Square, in the latter part of August; and the so-called outbreak, which commenced in the night between the 31st of August and the 1st of September, was, as in all similar instances, only a violent increase of the malady. As soon as I became acquainted with the situation and extent of this eruption of cholera, I suspected some contamination of the water of the much-frequented street-pump in Broad Street . . . but on examining the water . . . I found so little impurity in it of an organic nature, that I hesitated to come to a conclusion. Further inquiry, however, showed me that there was no other circumstance or agent common to the circumscribed locality in which this sudden increase of cholera occurred, and not extending beyond it, except the water of the above mentioned pump.

(continued)

Box 1.4 *(continued)*

On proceeding to the spot, I found that nearly all the deaths had taken place within a short distance of the pump. There were only ten deaths in houses situated decidedly nearer to another street pump. In five of these cases the families of the deceased persons informed me that they always sent to the pump in Broad Street, as they preferred the water to that of the pump which was nearer. In three other cases, the deceased were children who went to school near the pump in Broad Street. Two of them were known to drink the water; and the parents of third think it probable that it did so. The other two deaths, beyond the district which this pump supplies, represent only the amount of mortality from cholera that was occurring before the irruption took place . . . (*Snow used a spot map to show the spread of cases in relation to this and other pumps*) I had an interview with the Board of Guardians of St James's parish, on the evening of Thursday, 7th September, and represented the above circumstances to them. In consequence of what I said, the handle of the pump was removed on the following day.

Snow was also able to explain why some groups of people within the area did not develop cholera:

The Workhouse in Poland Street is more than three-fourths surrounded by houses in which deaths from cholera occurred, yet out of five hundred and thirty-five inmates, only five died of cholera, . . . The workhouse has a pump well on the premises, . . . and the inmates never sent to Broad Street for water. If the mortality in the workhouse had been equal to that in the streets immediately surrounding it on three sides, upwards of one hundred persons would have died. (*Note Snow's comparison of the 'observed' number of cases with the number 'expected'.*)

There is a Brewery in Broad Street, near to the pump, and on perceiving that no brewery men were registered as having died of cholera, I called on Mr Huggins, the proprietor. He informed me that there were above seventy workmen employed in the brewery, and that none of them had suffered from cholera . . . The men are allowed a certain quantity of malt liquor, and Mr Huggins believes they do not drink water at all . . .

The limited district in which this outbreak of cholera occurred, contains a great variety in the quality of the streets and houses; Poland Street and Great Pulteney Street consisting in a great measure of private houses occupied by one family, whilst Husband Street and Peter Street are occupied by the poor Irish. The remaining streets are intermediate in point of respectability. The mortality appears to have fallen pretty equally amongst all classes, in proportion to their number.

Fig. 1.3 The Broad Street
cholera epidemic, 1854.
(Drawn from Snow, 1855.)

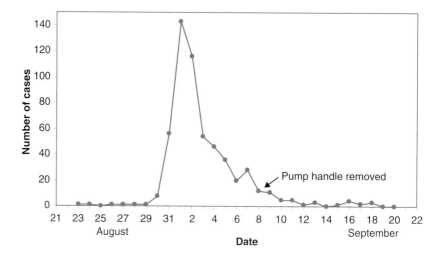

Fig. 1.3 The Broad Street cholera epidemic, 1854. (Drawn from Snow, 1855.)

Snow went to a lot of trouble to explain why some people developed cholera when they were believed *not* to have drunk the water from the Broad Street pump. He attributed these cases to the use of water from the pump in the local public houses, dining rooms and coffee shops. He was also able to explain why some groups of people within the area did not develop cholera when they lived in the affected area. If these low-risk groups (brewery workers, poorhouse dwellers) had been users of the nearby Broad Street pump, Snow's hypothesis would have been in tatters. His findings among the 'exceptions' of both sorts thus bolster his arguments considerably: for the most part he found convincing explanations for why some people apparently at risk did not fall ill, and so too for the small group not living near the pump who did contract cholera. His openness to collecting all the facts, not just those that obviously supported his contention, is a salutary reminder – effective public health action requires realistic information about the problem in hand.

In addition to mapping the distribution of cases by place, Snow tabulated the numbers of cases and deaths over time. His time data are displayed graphically showing what is called an 'epidemic curve' in Figure 1.3.

When did the epidemic start? When did it end? What role did Snow's dramatic removal of the pump handle on 8th September play in interrupting its course?

The epidemic curve shows that the rise above the preceding baseline began on 30 August, with a dramatic increase over the next two days. And although the fall from the peak starts shortly thereafter, case numbers are high for quite some days later, not getting close to the preceding baseline until two weeks from the commencement. The epidemic had waned substantially before Snow's intervention on 8 September, probably largely due to the flight of much of the populace. However, since the graph shows the total *number* of cases occurring and does not take into account the size of the population, the *rate* of disease (the number

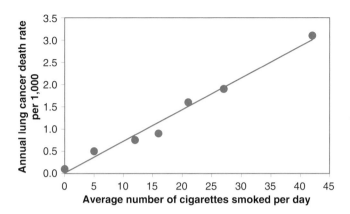

Fig. 1.4 Age-standardised death rates from lung cancer in relation to the number of cigarettes smoked per day, British Doctors Study, 1951–1961. (Doll and Hill, *BMJ*, 1964;1: 1399–1410, reproduced with permission from the BMJ Publishing Group.)

of new cases occurring among the smaller number of people remaining in the area) could still have been fairly high. Snow's action may therefore truly have contributed to containment of the outbreak.

The second half of the nineteenth century saw the expansion of epidemiology in the direct service of public health in the UK, with a similar trend in the USA starting early the next century. Infectious diseases remained the core interest until the early 1900s when Joseph Goldberger showed that pellagra was not infectious but of dietary origin and Wade Hampton Frost articulated the value of non-experimental epidemiology in discovering disease origins. Other pioneering work was undertaken prior to 1950, some of it entirely unnoticed until recently, but in that year the publication of two case–control studies of lung cancer, by Richard Doll (epidemiologist) and Austin Bradford Hill (statistician) in the UK and Ernest Wynder (medical student) and Evart Graham (surgeon) in the USA, publicly marked the start of modern epidemiology. Both papers (Doll and Hill, 1950; Wynder and Graham, 1950) showed that patients with lung cancer (*cases*) tended to smoke much more than people without lung cancer (*controls*).

Doll and Hill then tried to confirm the findings using a different, prospective design (a *cohort study*). They wrote to a large number of British doctors to find out how much they smoked and then 'followed' them (by mail and death records) over subsequent years to see what they died from. They again showed quite clearly that those who smoked cigarettes were much more likely to die of lung cancer than those who did not smoke, and the more they smoked the higher their risk (Figure 1.4). The British Doctors Study is still going on today and is now well beyond its ruby anniversary with over 40 years of data collection (Doll *et al.*, 2000). Unfortunately, in spite of this and other clear evidence of the harmful effects of smoking, it was many years before attempts to discourage people from smoking were made, and it is only recently that tobacco companies have begun to admit that their products cause disease.

Twenty years after those key case–control studies saw publication of the first comprehensive and widely influential disciplinary text: *Epidemiology: Principles and Methods* by Brian MacMahon and Thomas Pugh (1970). Highly readable and erudite, it remains a benchmark for successors.

What does epidemiology offer?

You will have discerned parts of the answer to this question from what you have already read and done in reaching this point. Here we recap and expand to bring the elements together more directly and fully, and thereby effectively map the content of the rest of the book. This section sketches the broad purposes of epidemiology and the next aims to illuminate these through some concrete examples.

A large part of public health is about identifying health problems within a community (who is becoming ill, where and when?), identifying what is causing the problems and then testing possible solutions to try to resolve or reduce the problem. Epidemiology is fundamental in providing the data needed to make public health judgements in each of these areas and the data come from studies of 'populations' (groups of people) of all sorts and sizes. Epidemiology largely deals with descriptions and comparisons of groups of people who vary widely in their genetic make-up, behaviour and environments. The great challenge for epidemiologists is to deal with such multiple influential health-modifiers in a systematic and logical way that produces information of practical value (to improving a community's health). How this challenge is met is what this book is all about.

Description of health status of populations

The observation and recording of health status makes it possible to identify sudden (and not-so-sudden) changes in the level of disease over time that might point to a need for action or further investigation. Similarly, differences between groups of people in one area, or between different geographical areas, can also give clues regarding the causes of disease (or health) in those groups. Such *descriptive statistics* are also important for health authorities and planners who need to know the nature and size of the health challenges faced by their communities.

Causation

Once a problem has been identified, we need to know what causes it, and probably the best-recognised use of epidemiology is in the search for the causes of disease. In some cases strong genetic factors have been identified, as for example with cystic fibrosis, a lung disease that occurs because of specific genetic defects. In other instances major environmental factors are crucial, such as asbestos in the development of lung mesothelioma (a rare form of lung cancer). In general, though, there is almost always some interaction between genetic and environmental factors in the causation of disease. Epidemiological tools are central to the identification of modifiable factors that will allow preventive interventions. (Note that in epidemiology and public health there remains some confusion over what is meant by *environmental factors*. We, and most others, take this to mean the sum of all non-genetic factors, including psychological, behavioural, social and cultural traits.)

Evaluation of interventions

Once we have identified a factor that causes disease, we then want to know whether we can reduce a population's exposure to this factor and so prevent the occurrence of disease – a 'primary' prevention programme (we will discuss prevention further in Chapter 13). Epidemiology has a core role to play in this process as well as in the evaluation of different treatments for a particular disease (an aspect of both mainstream and clinical epidemiology) and in assessing the effectiveness of health services.

Natural history and prognosis

Epidemiologists are also concerned with the *natural history*, or the course and outcome, of disease, both in individuals and in groups. *Prognosis* often implies the course of disease after treatment, but the terms tend to be used rather interchangeably. Such knowledge has obvious value for discussing treatment options with individual patients, as well as for planning and evaluating interventions. Of particular interest is whether sub-clinical disease is present for long before symptoms drive someone to seek medical attention. If this early disease can be detected and if treatment is thus more effective, this opens the way for screening programmes that aim to improve treatment outcomes. Lack of full knowledge of the natural history of prostate cancer is presently hampering control efforts severely. (We will discuss screening further in Chapter 14.)

What do epidemiologists do?

How then are these objectives of epidemiological research attained in practice? Let us look briefly at some more examples of what the practice of epidemiology can yield across some of its main dimensions.

Descriptive studies: person, place and time

By 'person'

In some countries there is concern over health differences between indigenous people and the rest of the population. Figure 1.5 shows Australian mortality data

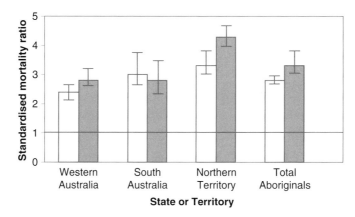

Fig. 1.5 Age-standardised mortality ratios in Aboriginal groups compared with the total population in selected Australian states, 1990–1992 (reproduced with permission from AIHW, 1994). The bars indicate how much higher mortality was among Aboriginal men (open bars) and women (solid bars) than in the total population. The vertical lines indicate 95% confidence intervals for these estimates (a measure of how certain the figures are).

comparing Aboriginal people with the whole country. The horizontal line at the level '1' indicates the overall death rate in Australia. The bars show how many times greater the death rate is in Aboriginal men and women in three Australian States and Territories (Western Australia, South Australia and the Northern Territory) than in all Australians.

How many times higher is the death rate in Aboriginal males in the Northern Territory than in Australia as a whole?

What is the obvious striking fact about relative mortality in Aboriginal people in general?

The death rate in Aboriginal men in the Northern Territory is just over three times that in the whole of Australia and the difference for women is even greater. The data presented indicate a much worse health situation for the indigenous peoples of Australia than for the country as a whole. (Note: these *standardised mortality ratios* are similar to the relative risk in the food poisoning example earlier. They show how many times more likely it was for an Aboriginal to die compared with the average Australian in 1990–1992. The process of *standardisation* also takes account of the fact that Aboriginal people are, on average, younger than the rest of the population. We will discuss these measures further in Chapter 2.)

By 'place'

How 'healthy' is any given country in relation to the rest of the world – are things better or worse there? Figure 1.6 shows cardiovascular disease mortality rates in males in different countries. You can readily see that men in the Netherlands,

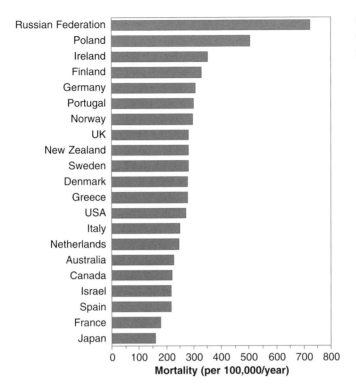

Fig. 1.6 Cardiovascular disease mortality for males, about 1996. (Drawn from AIHW, 2002.)

for example, are considerably better off than those in the UK, New Zealand and particularly Poland and Russia; but things could be better – as shown by the lower rates in Spain, France and Japan. What is it about Japanese men that makes them less likely to die of cardiovascular disease than Dutch men? If we can work this out then perhaps we could reduce cardiovascular mortality in the Netherlands to the level seen in Japan (provided that the differences are not purely genetic). By studying patterns of disease and relating them to variations in risk factors for the disease we can come up with possible reasons why some people or places have higher rates of disease than others or why disease rates have changed over time.

By 'time'

What emerges if we look at the changing patterns of mortality in a country over time? The graph in Figure 1.7 shows mortality trends for selected conditions and groups over two decades (1979–1998) in the USA.

What are the most notable features of Figure 1.7?

The picture we see is mixed, some good news, some concerning. The most obvious health success story is the consistent downward trend in deaths from heart attacks, with about 80 fewer people in every 100,000 (half as many) dying from

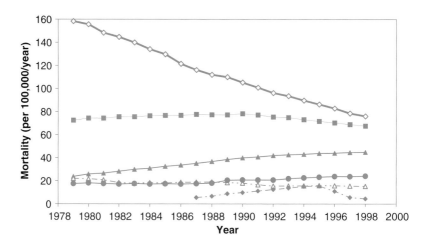

Fig. 1.7 Mortality rates, in the USA, 1979–1998, for heart attack (◇), lung cancer in males (■), lung cancer in females (▲), motor vehicle accidents (△), diabetes (●) and AIDS (◆). (Drawn from CDC Wonder (US DHHS), accessed February 2004.)

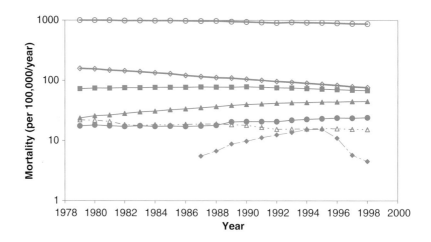

Fig. 1.8 Mortality rates in the USA (log scale), 1979–1998, for all causes (○), heart attack (◇), lung cancer in males (■), lung cancer in females (▲), motor vehicle accidents (△), diabetes (●) and AIDS (◆). (Drawn from CDC Wonder (US DHHS), accessed February 2004.)

them at the end of the period. A less dramatic decline is seen for motor vehicle accidents. Deaths from AIDS rose until 1995 and have fallen since (an epidemic where perhaps the worst is past, at least for the USA). The same is true for lung cancer in men, although on this scale it is not striking. Most worrying is the steady rise in lung cancer deaths among women.

However, these details don't give us the big picture. Some up, some down, some changing direction: what was happening to overall mortality in the USA during the period? Total mortality rates fell from about 1,000 to 870 per 100,000 per year, but we would not be able to fit this information onto the same graph without losing almost all the details we noted above. We could, of course, draw a separate graph showing the total death rate, but we can do both by changing the scale of the vertical axis, as in Figure 1.8.

Box 1.5 Smallpox

The elimination of smallpox had a major impact on the health of millions of people, especially in many of the poorest countries. Descriptive epidemiology played a major role by providing information about the distribution of cases (*jointly by person, place and time*) and levels of transmission, by mapping outbreaks and by evaluating control measures. In 1967, there were 10–15 million new cases and 2 million deaths from smallpox in 31 countries. By 1976, smallpox was being reported in only two countries and the last naturally occurring case was recorded in 1977. Elimination of this scourge was helped by simple but painstaking case-finding and counting.

Instead of a linear scale (1, 2, 3, 4, . . .), we have now used a 'log' (logarithmic) scale (1, 10, 100, 1,000, . . .) where the distance between 1 and 10 (a 10-fold difference) is the same as the distance between 10 and 100 (also a 10-fold difference) and so on. Now we can fit mortality rates as different as 4.5/100,000 (AIDS mortality in 1998) and 1,000/100,000 (all-cause mortality in 1979) on the same page. It also allows us to compare *relative* changes in mortality rates directly, with parallel slopes reflecting equal rates of change. The fall in heart attacks looks much less dramatic now: the drop is only about 2%–3% per year but, as Figure 1.7 showed, this led to a large absolute benefit, because the death rate was so high to start with. The rate of change for AIDS looks much steeper on a log scale because the percentage change is greater, but the absolute benefits are clearly much less. In public health we need to think on both relative and absolute scales: they tell us different things that are useful for different purposes. We will take this further later in the book.

Analytic studies

Ideas generated by such *descriptive* work can then be tested further in *analytic* studies, looking for associations between potential causal agents and diseases. This research is based on facts collected from groups of individuals, not large-scale population statistics. Are people with higher blood pressure more likely to develop coronary heart disease than those with normal blood pressure? Are people who smoke more likely to develop lung cancer than those who do not? Even more usefully, how *much* more likely is a smoker to develop lung cancer than a non-smoker? Does risk depend on the number of cigarettes smoked? That is, how *strong* is the effect of the exposure; and does it increase with higher levels of exposure? In the British Doctors Study mentioned earlier, Doll and Hill found that the risk of lung cancer increased steadily as people smoked more cigarettes (Figure 1.4). This adds weight to the idea that smoking cigarettes really does affect the chance that an individual will develop lung cancer.

Box 1.6 The Nurses' Health Study

This cohort study of 120,000 US nurses was started in 1976 by Frank Speizer of the Channing Laboratory, Harvard Medical School. The study was initially funded for five years to study whether the oral contraceptive pill caused breast cancer, but the nurses are still being followed almost 30 years later. Hundreds of scientific papers have been published, covering scores of diseases and exposures and investigating their inter-relationships. The study has been particularly influential in the field of diet and disease (nutritional epidemiology), owing to diet questionnaires that the nurses have been completing since 1980. As with other long-term follow-ups of cohorts, such as the British Doctors Study of Doll and Hill, its success is jointly dependent on the enthusiasm and commitment of researchers and participants. For the latter this has extended to providing blood, toenail clippings (for measurement of trace metals) and samples of tapwater over the years! This human side to epidemiology does not feature much in textbooks but is fundamental to successful fieldwork.

Once we have found an association, the challenge is then to evaluate this in order to determine whether something really **causes** disease or is linked to it only secondarily. If we find that people with a peptic ulcer drink a lot of milk, does this mean that drinking milk causes ulcers or simply that people with an ulcer drink milk to ease their pain? In Chapter 10 we will look more deeply at this challenge.

Intervention studies

Finally, epidemiologists evaluate new preventive measures, programmes or treatments that are designed to reduce ill health or promote good health. They also monitor the effectiveness of these 'intervention' programmes after they have been implemented: do they actually achieve the good they set out to do? These programmes can include evaluations of different health promotion strategies targeted at individuals or whole communities, or clinical trials of new drugs designed to cure disease. Does taking aspirin reduce your chance of having a heart attack? Which of several strategies is better at helping people give up smoking? Is one drug better than another for treating a heart attack?

A natural experiment

We will end this chapter with another example from John Snow's *On the Mode of Communication of Cholera* (1855) because, although this text is more than

Box 1.7 A grand experiment

Although the facts . . . afford very strong evidence of the powerful influence which the drinking water containing the sewage of a town exerts over the spread of cholera, when that disease is present, yet the question does not end here; for the intermixing of the water supply of the Southwark and Vauxhall Company with that of the Lambeth Company, over an extensive part of London, admitted of the subject being sifted in such a way as to yield the most incontrovertible proof on one side or the other . . . A few houses are supplied by one Company and a few by the other, according to the decision of the owner or occupier at that time when the Water Companies were in active competition . . . Each Company supplies both rich and poor, both large houses and small; there is no difference either in the condition or occupation of the persons receiving the water of the different Companies. Now it must be evident that, if the diminution of cholera, in the districts partly supplied with the improved water, depended on this supply, the houses receiving it would be the houses enjoying the whole benefit of the diminution of the malady, whilst the houses supplied with the water from Battersea Fields would suffer the same mortality as they would if the improved supply did not exist at all. As there is no difference whatever, either in the houses or the people receiving the supply of the two water Companies, or in any of the physical conditions with which they are surrounded, it is obvious that no experiment could have been devised which would more thoroughly test the effect of water supply on the progress of cholera than this which circumstances placed ready made before the observer.

The experiment, too, was on the grandest scale. No fewer than three hundred thousand people of both sexes, of every age and occupation, and of every rank and station, from gentlefolk down to the very poor, were divided into two groups without their choice, and, in most cases, without their knowledge; one group being supplied with water containing the sewage of London, and amongst it, whatever might have come from the cholera patients, the other group having water quite free from such impurity.

To turn this grand experiment to account, all that was required was to learn the supply of water to each individual house where a fatal attack of cholera might occur . . .

The epidemic of 1854

When the cholera returned to London in July of the present year . . . I resolved to spare no exertion . . . to ascertain the exact effect of the water supply on the progress of the epidemic, in the places where all the circumstances were

(continued)

Box 1.7 *(continued)*

so happily adapted for the inquiry . . . I accordingly asked permission at the General Register Office to be supplied with the addresses of persons dying of cholera, in those districts where the supply of the two Companies is intermingled in the manner I have stated above . . . I commenced my inquiry about the middle of August with two sub-districts of Lambeth . . . There were forty-four deaths in these sub-districts down to 12th August, and I found that thirty-eight of the houses in which these deaths occurred were supplied with water by the Southwark and Vauxhall Company, four houses were supplied by the Lambeth Company, and two had pump-wells on the premises and no supply from either of the Companies.

As soon as I had ascertained these particulars, I communicated them to Dr Farr, who was much struck with the result, and at his suggestion the Registrars of all the south districts of London were requested to make a return of the water supply of the house in which the attack took place, in all cases of death from cholera. This order was to take place after the 26th of August, and I resolved to carry my inquiry down to that date, so that the facts might be ascertained for the whole course of the epidemic.

The inquiry was necessarily attended with a good deal of trouble. There were very few instances in which I could at once get the information I required. Even when the water rates were paid by the residents, they can seldom remember the name of the Water Company till they have looked for the receipt. In the case of working people who pay weekly rents, the rates are invariably paid by the landlord or his agent, who often lives at a distance, and the residents know nothing about the matter. It would, indeed, have been almost impossible for me to complete the inquiry, if I had not found that I could distinguish the water of the two companies with perfect certainty by a chemical test. The test I employed was founded on the great difference in the quantity of chloride sodium [salt] contained in the two kinds of water, at the time I made the inquiry . . .

According to a return which was made to Parliament, the Southwark and Vauxhall Company supplied 40,046 houses from January 1st to December 31st, 1853, and the Lambeth Company supplied 26,107 houses during the same period; consequently, as 286 fatal attacks of cholera took place, in the first four weeks of the epidemic, in houses supplied by the former Company, and only 14 in houses supplied by the latter, the proportion of fatal attacks to each 10,000 houses was as follows. Southwark and Vauxhall 71, Lambeth 5. **The cholera was therefore fourteen times as fatal at this period amongst persons having the impure water of the Southwark and Vauxhall Company as amongst those having the purer water from Thames Ditton.**

(Excerpted from Snow, 1855.)

150 years old, the methods he used and his combination of flair, skill, logic and dogged persistence remain the cornerstones of modern epidemiology. His work also exemplifies, in more detail than modern papers, the logical dissection of evidence about disease patterns to identify practical preventive strategies – which is still the key function of epidemiology – and it gives an excellent sense of the role and utility of epidemiology in practical public health.

In the early 1850s, London was cholera-free for a number of years and during that period one of the major water supply companies (the Lambeth Company) moved their waterworks out of London, thereby obtaining water free of the sewage of the city. During the next major cholera outbreak in 1853–1854 Snow was able to obtain information about the number of deaths occurring in the different sub-districts of London and he found that cholera mortality was lower in areas supplied by water from the Lambeth Company than in those supplied by the Southwark and Vauxhall water company which continued to take water from Battersea in the city. He did not stop there, but went on to conduct his 'Grand Experiment' (see Box 1.7).

Conclusions

Again we have a vivid picture of a master epidemiologist at work. Not satisfied that his hypothesis had been adequately tested, Snow identified the opportunity to conduct an even more rigorous test – his '*Grand Experiment*' – and in doing so he addressed the major epidemiological issues that still concern us today.

- He identified a situation in which people were unknowingly divided into two groups differing only in the source of their water, thereby creating what was effectively a *randomised trial* (we will look at the different types of epidemiological study in Chapter 6).
- In doing so, he realised the importance of ruling out other differences between the groups (e.g., sex, age, occupation, socioeconomic status) that could explain any mortality differences (a problem known as *confounding* that we will come back to in Chapter 8).
- He worked long and hard to acquire *accurate information* about both the water supply and the number of cholera deaths in each house – we will consider sources of data in Chapter 3 and will discuss the problem of error in Chapter 7.
- He *measured the occurrence of cholera* in the two groups of houses served by the different water companies – we will look further at measures such as these in Chapter 2.
- He calculated *how many times more common* cholera deaths were in those houses receiving the contaminated water – we will come back to this measure (again a r*elative risk*) in Chapter 5.

- He then integrated all of his information to reach the conclusion that cholera was indeed *caused* by contaminated water – Chapter 10.

He did not stop there, but went on to make a series of clear practical recommendations to prevent transmission of cholera in future – sensible measures including the need for cleanliness and sterilisation that are still practiced today.

Snow's work therefore sets the scene for the chapters to come but, before you move on, take a minute to stop and think. Imagine that someone asked you what epidemiology was and why it was useful. Could you now give them a satisfactory explanation in a few sentences?

REFERENCES

AIHW (Australian Institute of Health and Welfare). (1994). *Australia's Health 1994: The Fourth Biennial Health Report of the AIHW*. Canberra: AGPS.

(2002). *Australia's Health 2002*. Canberra: AIHW.

Concise Oxford Dictionary, 5th edn. (1964). Oxford: Oxford University Press.

Devesa, S. S., Grauman, D. J., Blot, W. J. *et al.* (1999). *Atlas of Cancer Mortality in the United States: 1950–1994*. Washington: US Government Print Office.

Doll, R., and Hill, A. B. (1950). Smoking and carcinoma of the lung. *British Medical Journal,* **2**: 739–748.

(1964). Mortality in relation to smoking: ten years' observations of British doctors. *British Medical Journal*, **1**: 1399–1410, 1460–1467.

Doll, R., Peto, R., Boreham, J. and Sutherland, I. (2000). Smoking and dementia in male British doctors: a prospective study. *British Medical Journal*, **320**: 1097–1102.

Graunt, J. (1662). *Natural and Political Observations Mentioned in a Following Index and Made Upon the Bills of Mortality*. London. (http://www.books-on-line.com)

Hippocrates. (400 BC). *On Airs, Waters, and Places*. Translated by Francis Adams. (http://classics.mit.edu)

Hook, D., Jalaludin, B. and Fitzsimmons, G. (1996). *Clostridium perfringens* food-borne outbreak: an epidemiological investigation. *Australian and New Zealand Journal of Public Health*, **20**: 119–122.

Last, J. M., Ed. (2001). *A Dictionary of Epidemiology*, 4th edn. New York: Oxford University Press.

Lilienfeld, A. M. and Lilienfeld, D. E. (1980). *Foundations of Epidemiology*, 2nd edn. New York: Oxford University Press.

MacMahon, B. and Pugh, T. F. (1970). *Epidemiology – Principles and Methods*. Boston: Little Brown.

Makk, L., Creech, J. L., Whelan, J. G. and Johnson, M. D. (1974). Liver damage and angiosarcoma in vinyl chloride workers – a systematic detection program. *Journal of the American Medical Association*, **230**: 64–68.

Miettinen, O. S. (1978). *Course Notes – Principles of Epidemiologic Research*. Harvard School of Public Health.

Rosen, G. (1958). *A History of Public Health*. New York: MD Publications.

Selikoff, I. J., Churg, J. and Hammond, E. C. (1965). Relation between exposure to asbestos and mesothelioma. *New England Journal of Medicine*, **272**: 560–565.

Snow, J. (1855). *On the Mode of Communication of Cholera*, 2nd edn. London: Churchill. (http://www.ph.ucla.edu/epi/snow/snowbook.html)

Stolley, P. D. and Lasky, T. (1995). *Investigating Disease Patterns: the Science of Epidemiology*. New York: Scientific American Library.

US DHHS (United States Department of Health and Human Services), Centers for Disease Control and Prevention (CDC), National Center for Health Statistics (NCHS), Office of Analysis, Epidemiology, and Health Promotion (OAEHP), Compressed Mortality File (CMF) compiled from CMF 1968–88, series 20, No. 2A 2000, CMF 1989–98, series 20, No. 2E 2003 and CMF 1999–2000, series 20, No. 2F 2003 on CDC WONDER On-line Database. (http://wonder.cdc.gov/)

WHO (World Health Organization). (1948). Text of the constitution of the World Health Organization. *Official Record World Health Organization* **2**: 100.

www.anesi.com/titanic.htm, Titanic disaster: official casualty figures and commentary.

Wynder, E. L. and Graham, E. A. (1950) Tobacco smoking as a possible etiologic factor in bronchiogenic carcinoma. A study of six hundred and eighty-four proved cases. *Journal of the American Medical Association*, **143**: 329–336.

How long is a piece of string? Measuring disease frequency

Box 2.1 Who drinks the most beer?

According to the Brewers Association of Japan, Americans drink the most beer in the world (23,000 million litres in 1999) closely followed by the Chinese (21,000 million litres). In contrast the Czech Republic ranked a lowly 14th in terms of total consumption (1,800 million litres) and Ireland didn't even make the top 25. This information may be useful for planning production, but do the Americans and Chinese really drink more beer than the rest of us? An alternative and possibly more informative way to look at these data is in terms of consumption *per capita*. When we do this, the USA falls to 12th position in the 'beer drinking league table' (84 litres per capita in 1999) and China falls way off the screen (a mere 16 litres per capita). The Czechs are now the champions (161 litres per capita) closely followed by the Irish (153 litres per capita). Australians, who tend to pride themselves on their beer drinking, might be disappointed with their ranking in ninth place.

(Source: www.brewers.or.jp, accessed 8 April 2004.)

Many different measures of health and disease are used to describe the health of populations. In this chapter we will introduce you to some of these so that you can use and interpret this information correctly. As you will see, this is not always as straightforward as it might seem.

What are we measuring?

Although we are primarily interested in 'health', this is a somewhat abstract concept. In practice, it is much easier to define ill-health or disease and this is what we usually measure. Lack of a particular disease does not necessarily imply 'health' but simply a lack of the disease of interest.

"DON'T WORRY. AFTER WE RUN SOME TESTS, WE'LL KNOW FOR SURE WHAT'S CAUSING YOUR HEADACHES."

Before we can start to measure disease, we have to have a very clear idea of what it is that we are trying to determine. In general, the diagnosis of disease is based on a combination of *symptoms*, subjective indications of disease reported by the person themselves; *signs*, objective indications of disease apparent to the physician; and additional *tests*. Criteria for making a diagnosis can be very simple: the presence of antibodies against an infectious agent can indicate infection, and diagnosis of most cancers is fairly straightforward on the basis of tissue histology (examination with a light microscope); but for some diseases the diagnostic criteria are much more complex, involving combinations of signs and symptoms.

For health data to be meaningful, diagnostic criteria leading to a case definition have to be clear, unambiguous and easy to use under a wide range of circumstances. It is important to remember that different case definitions can lead to very different pictures. As shown in Figure 2.1, a study in the United Arab Emirates showed that the prevalence of gestational diabetes (diabetes during pregnancy) in a group of 3,500 women was much higher using one set of criteria (Carpenter's criteria, 30.4%) than another (O'Sullivan's criteria, 20.2%) (Agarwal and Punnose, 2002). If you want to compare information from different reports the first thing to check is that you are comparing apples with apples – have they all measured the same thing using the same criteria? This can be a particular problem when trying to compare patterns of disease over time because changes in diagnostic criteria can lead to sudden increases or decreases in the number of cases recorded.

Fig. 2.1 Percentage of
population with gestational
diabetes according to two sets of
diagnostic criteria. (Drawn from
Agarwal and Punnose, 2002.)

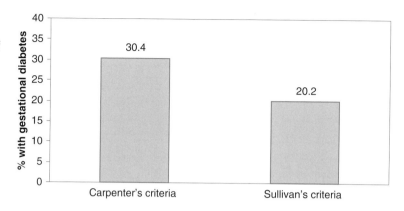

Fig. 2.1 Percentage of population with gestational diabetes according to two sets of diagnostic criteria. (Drawn from Agarwal and Punnose, 2002.)

Prevalence and incidence

Once we have defined what we mean by disease, we can then go on to study its occurrence and, more particularly, to measure how often it occurs. These measures form the basis of *descriptive epidemiology*.

In Table 2.1 we see the estimated number of people living with HIV/AIDS in the various regions of the world at the end of 2001, and the number of new cases of HIV infection during 2002. These data clearly show the huge burden borne by Sub-Saharan Africa, which has five times more cases than any other region, but what can they tell us about the relative importance of HIV/AIDS in other regions? The USA and Canada and East Asia/the Pacific and East Europe/Central Asia all had approximately one million people living with HIV/AIDS at the end of 2001. How can we describe and compare the burden of HIV/AIDS in these populations more fully?

What percentage of people in the USA and Canada had HIV/AIDS at the end of 2001?

What percentage of people in the USA and Canada became HIV-positive during 2002?

At the end of 2001, 950,000 of the 316,941,000 people in the USA and Canada or 0.3% of the population were living with HIV/AIDS. During 2002, another 45,000 people or 0.014% of the population became infected with HIV. Now 0.014% is a very small number. It simply tells us that there were 0.014 new HIV infections for every 100 people during 2002, so an alternative way to present the same information would be to multiply the numbers by 1,000 and say that there were 14 new infections in every 100,000 people (14/100,000 or 14/10^5).[1]

---

[1] If you are not familiar with this nomenclature, the superscript number is simply a shorthand way to say how many zeros the number has. So, 10^2 would be 100, 10^5 is 100,000 and 10^6 is one million (1,000,000).

Table 2.1 Estimates of the number of people living with HIV/AIDS and the number of new HIV infections around the world.

Region	Population (×1,000)	People living with HIV/AIDS (end of 2001)	New HIV infections (2002)
Sub-Saharan Africa	633,816	28,500,000	3,500,000
East Asia and Pacific	1,497,066	1,000,000	270,000
Australia and New Zealand	23,146	15,000	500
South and Southeast Asia	1,978,430	5,600,000	700,000
East Europe and Central Asia	393,245	1,000,000	250,000
West Europe	407,021	550,000	30,000
North Africa and the Middle East	349,142	500,000	83,000
USA and Canada	316,941	950,000	45,000
Caribbean	32,489	420,000	60,000
Latin America	488,031	1,500,000	150,000
Total	6,119,327	40,035,000	5,088,500

(*Data source:* UNAIDS, 2002a, 2002b, accessed via www.unaids.org, 16 October 2003.)

What you calculated above were, first, the **prevalence** of *existing* HIV/AIDS at the end of 2001 and, secondly, the **incidence** of *new* HIV infections in the USA and Canada during 2002. These measures give us two different ways of quantifying the amount of disease in a population. Table 2.2 shows the same information for each of the regions. These data confirm the high levels of HIV/AIDS in Sub-Saharan Africa and show us that, despite the relatively low number of cases in the Caribbean region, the small size of the population means that the prevalence and incidence there are also high. The data also show us that, although the actual *numbers* of cases in the USA and Canada and the East Asia/Pacific and East Europe/Central Asia regions are similar, the *prevalence* per 100 people (%) is much lower in East Asia/Pacific than in the other two regions.

Prevalence

The **prevalence** of a disease tells us what proportion of a population actually has the disease at a specific point in time: 0.3% or 300 of every 100,000 people in the USA and Canada had HIV/AIDS at the end of 2001. This is a snapshot of the situation at a single point in time and, for this reason, it is sometimes called the 'point' prevalence. (Note: you may also see references to 'period prevalence'. This measures the proportion of the population that had the disease *at any time during a specified period*. It is a complex measure that combines prevalence (everybody

Table 2.2 The prevalence of HIV/AIDS and incidence of HIV infection around the world in 2001–2002.

Region	Population (×1,000)	People living with HIV/AIDS (end of 2001)	Prevalence (%)	New HIV infections (2002)	Incidence (per 100,000 per year)
Sub-Saharan Africa	633,816	28,500,000	4.50	3,500,000	552.2
East Asia and Pacific	1,497,066	1,000,000	0.07	270,000	18.0
Australia and New Zealand	23,146	15,000	0.06	500	2.2
South and Southeast Asia	1,978,430	5,600,000	0.28	700,000	35.4
East Europe and Central Asia	393,245	1,000,000	0.25	250,000	63.6
West Europe	407,021	550,000	0.14	30,000	7.4
North Africa and the Middle East	349,142	500,000	0.14	83,000	23.8
USA and Canada	316,941	950,000	0.30	45,000	14.2
Caribbean	32,489	420,000	1.29	60,000	184.7
Latin America	488,031	1,500,000	0.31	150,000	30.7
Total	6,119,327	40,035,000	0.65	5,088,500	83.2

(*Data source:* UNAIDS, 2002a, 2002b, accessed via www.unaids.org, 16 October 2003.)

who had the disease at the start of the period) and incidence (all of the new cases of disease during the period).

Prevalence measures the amount of a disease in a population at a given point in time:

$$\text{Prevalence} = \frac{\text{Number of people with disease at a given point in time}}{\text{Total number of people in the population}} \qquad (2.1)$$

Prevalence measures are just one number (the number of people with disease) divided by another number (the total number of people in the population). They have no units, and are mostly reported simply as a proportion or a percentage (4.5% of Sub-Saharan Africans had HIV/AIDS at the end of 2001), but may also be shown as cases/population (60/100,000 Australians and New Zealanders had HIV/AIDS at the end of 2001). Although you will often see the term 'prevalence rate', this is not a true rate because a rate should include units of time. (An example of a true rate is the use of distance travelled *per hour*, i.e. kph or mph, to measure the speed of a car.) The time point at which people are counted should, however, always be reported when giving an estimate of prevalence. This is often a fixed point in calendar time, such as 31 December 2001, but it can also be a fixed point in life, for instance, birth or retirement. For example, if 1,000 babies were born alive in one hospital in a given year and, of these, five babies were born with

Box 2.2 A note about percentages

From experience we have found that people are sometimes confused by percentages because there is often more than one way in which they can be calculated and this can lead to problems with interpretation.

Imagine a study that gave the following results:

	Asthma	No asthma	Total
Non-smokers	40	360	400
Smokers	30	170	200
Total	70	530	600

There are two ways that we can look at these data. One way would be to calculate the percentages of (a) non-smokers and (b) smokers who have asthma – these are row percentages because we use the total of each row, the number of non-smokers or smokers, as the denominator (note: the *denominator* is the bottom half of a fraction and the *numerator* the top half):

	Asthma	No asthma	Total
Non-smokers	40 ÷ 400 = 10%	360 ÷ 400 = 90%	400 = 100%
Smokers	30 ÷ 200 = 15%	170 ÷ 200 = 85%	200 = 100%

This tells us that 10% of non-smokers and 15% of smokers have asthma.

Alternatively, we could use the same data to calculate the percentage of people with and without asthma who smoke – these are column percentages because now we use the total of each column, the number of people with or without asthma, as the denominator:

	Asthma	No asthma
Non-smokers	40÷70 = 57%	360 ÷ 530 = 68%
Smokers	30÷70 = 43%	170 ÷ 530 = 32%
Total	70 = 100%	530 = 100%

This tells us that 43% of people with asthma and only 32% of people without asthma are smokers.

It is very important to decide first which percentages are most relevant for a particular situation and then to calculate and interpret the percentages correctly. Saying that 43% of people with asthma are smokers (correct) is not the same as saying that 43% of smokers have asthma (incorrect; 15% of smokers have asthma).

congenital abnormalities, we would say that the prevalence of congenital abnormality *at birth* was 5/1,000 live births in that year. Prevalence can be expressed per 100 people (%; see Box 2.2) or per 1,000 (10^3), 10,000 (10^4) or 100,000 (10^5). It doesn't matter as long as it is clear which is being used.

In practice, all prevalent cases of disease will rarely be identified at one precise point in time; e.g., a blood pressure survey may take weeks or months to conduct, given limited numbers of researchers, amounts of equipment and availability of those being measured. The exact size of the population may also not be known on a given day and this might well be based on an estimate or projection from census data.

Incidence

The **incidence** of disease measures how quickly people are catching the disease. During 2002, 0.55% of people in Sub-Saharan Africa were newly diagnosed as HIV-positive or, in other words, the incidence of HIV infection was 552/100,000 per year (Table 2.2). (Note that the actual answer is 0.005 522 1 or 552.21 per 100,000. For simplicity we have *rounded* this to the nearest whole number, 552.[2]) This is the **incidence rate** for HIV and it differs from the prevalence because it considers only *new* infections that occurred in a one-year time period. Also, unlike measures of prevalence, the incidence rate is a true rate because it measures the number of new infections *per year*.

Incidence measures how quickly people are developing a disease:

$$\text{Incidence rate} = \frac{\text{Number of people who develop disease in one year}}{\text{Average number of people in the population in the same year}} \quad (2.2)$$

Population at risk

In the example above it is probably not unreasonable to assume that everyone might be at risk of contracting HIV, although, obviously, some groups will be more 'at risk' than others; but what if the disease of interest were something like cervical cancer? To use the whole population to calculate rates of cancer of the cervix (or neck of the uterus), would be inappropriate, because a man could never develop the disease. We would calculate a *sex-specific* rate by dividing the number of cases by the number of *females* in the population. However, many

---

[2] If the first number that is cut off is between 0 and 4 you round *down* – in this case the first number to go was a 2 so we rounded 552.21 *down* to 552. If, however, the number is between 5 and 9 you round up, so 552.7 would be rounded *up* to 553.

women will have had a hysterectomy and their uterus will have been removed. They are then no longer at risk of developing cervical cancer and so, strictly speaking, should not be included in counts of the population at risk. You should be aware that rates may be presented in different ways using different populations. We discussed above the importance of making sure that different reports used the same definition of disease (i.e., they counted the same thing in the numerator); it is also crucial to ensure that the denominators represent equivalent populations (e.g., they are similar in age, sex distribution, etc.).

The relationship between incidence and prevalence

If two diseases have the same incidence, but one lasts three times longer than the other, then, at any point in time, you are much more likely to find people suffering from the more long-lasting disease. Very crudely (and assuming that people do not move into or out of the area), the relationship between prevalence (P) and incidence (I) depends on how long the disease persists before cure or death (average duration of disease, D):

$$P \approx I \times D \tag{2.3}$$

where ≈ means approximately equal to.

For example, hepatitis A has a relatively high incidence: according to the US Centers for Disease Control and Prevention (CDC) there were approximately 93,000 new infections in the USA in 2001 (CDC National Center for Infectious Diseases, 2002). However, because it is an acute infection and people recover quickly, the prevalence of hepatitis A infection at any one point in time would be quite low. In contrast, hepatitis C infection is much less common (approximately 25,000 new infections in 2001) but once you are infected you are usually infected for life because there is currently no cure. This means that the prevalence of hepatitis C infection is much higher – in 2001 an estimated 2.7 million Americans were chronically infected.

If a new treatment were developed for a disease, what effect would this have on the prevalence and incidence of the disease?

If the new treatment meant that people were cured more quickly and so were ill for less time then the prevalence would fall. However, if the disease had previously been fatal and the new treatment meant that people lived longer with the disease then the prevalence would increase. In general, a new treatment will not affect the incidence of a disease. The only exception to this rule might be for an infectious disease: if people were ill and thus infectious for less time, they might pass the infection to fewer people and so the incidence would fall.

As you can see, the prevalence of a disease reflects a balance of several factors. If the incidence of a disease increases then the prevalence will also increase; if the

Box 2.3 More about the relationship among prevalence, incidence and duration

The relationship $P \approx I \times D$ is approximately true in what is called a *stationary* population where the number of people entering the population (immigration and birth) balances the number of people leaving (emigration and death). A second requirement is that the prevalence of disease must be low (less than about 10%). This is the case for many diseases, but a more general formula that does not require the disease to be rare is

$$\frac{P}{1 - P} \approx I \times D \tag{2.4}$$

where P is the prevalence of disease expressed as a proportion and $1 - P$ is the proportion of *non-diseased* people; e.g., if the prevalence (P) is 2% or 0.02 then $1 - P$ is 0.98.

duration of sickness changes then the prevalence will change (see Box 2.3). This means that the prevalence of a disease is generally not the best way to measure the underlying forces driving the occurrence of the disease – we must use the incidence rate for this. Nonetheless, prevalence is useful for measuring diseases that have a gradual onset and long duration such as type-2 diabetes and osteoarthritis, and the prevalence of congenital malformations at birth. It is of most direct value for describing the overall disease burden of a population and, consequently, for assessing health care needs and planning health services.

Measuring disease in epidemiological studies

There are three fundamental measures of disease occurrence: **prevalence** and two measures of incidence – the **incidence rate** and **cumulative incidence**. These can be calculated from routinely collected data (as in the HIV example above) or from results of studies conducted specifically to measure the incidence or prevalence of disease. We will come back to the use of routine data, and for now will concentrate on how we measure the occurrence of disease in an epidemiological study. To measure the *prevalence* of disease we need to conduct a *cross-sectional study* or *survey* in which a random sample (or cross-section) of the population is questioned to ascertain whether they had a particular condition at a particular point in time. To measure the *incidence* of disease we need to start with a group (or *cohort*) of people who are currently free of the disease of interest but who are 'at risk' of developing it. We then follow them over time to see who actually develops the disease (a *cohort study*; e.g., the British Doctors Study mentioned in Chapter 1).

When we conduct a study we can specify exactly who is in the study and usu-ally collect individual data for all (or most) of those people. We can identify who is 'at risk', calculate quite accurate measures of disease incidence (or prevalence) and also relate the occurrence of disease to its potential causes.

Consider, for example, a study conducted in a hypothetical primary school with 100 pupils. Imagine that, on the first day of the new term, nine children had a cold. Over the next week another seven children developed a cold.

What percentage of children had a cold on the first day of term?

What percentage of the children who didn't have a cold on the first day of term developed one during the next week?

The first measure that you calculated is the **prevalence** of the common cold in this group of children: 9 out of 100 children or 9% had a cold on the first day of term. The second measure is known as the **cumulative incidence** of colds: out of 91 children 'at risk' of developing a cold (i.e., they did not have one already), 7 or 7.7% developed one during the first week of term. The denominator (population at risk) is 91 in this case because 9 of the 100 children already had a cold and were not therefore 'at risk' of catching another at the same time. The cumulative inci-dence thus measures the proportion, or percentage, of people (children in this case) who were at risk of developing a cold and who did so during the period of the study (one week). Note that it is always important to specify the time period – a cumulative incidence of 5% in 1 year would be very different from a cumulative incidence of 5% in 20 years. The cumulative incidence is sometimes known as the **attack rate**, especially when it refers to a short time period, usually with respect to an outbreak of infectious diseases as in the food poisoning example in Chapter 1.

The above example was simple because the common cold is just that, very common, and we were only interested in the children for one week. Imagine that we were trying to measure the incidence of a much rarer disease such as cancer. We would obviously need a much larger group of people and we would need to follow them for much longer to see who developed the cancer. In this situation it is very difficult to keep track of people and we would inevitably lose some from the study group and not know what happened to them. Another problem is that people will die from other 'competing' causes and so they will no longer be at risk of developing the cancer. In this situation, calculations of the cumulative incidence may be inaccurate (or will become so over time) because we will not know exactly who has developed the disease. In practice, we can calculate cumu-lative incidence only when we have a clearly defined group of people who are all (or almost all) followed for the whole follow-up period.

When this is not the situation we use a different method to calculate inci-dence. Instead of counting the actual *number* of people at risk of disease, we count up the *length of time* they were at risk of disease. Imagine that we followed a group of 1,000 men for 5 years and that during this time 15 of them had a non-fatal heart attack. This gives us a cumulative incidence of 1.5% for the 5-year period. During this period the men have lived a total of $1,000 \times 5 = 5,000$ years of life or '*person-years*'. We could have obtained the same number of person-years by following a group of 5,000 men for 1 year each, or a group of 500 men for 10 years each. Alternatively, we could have followed some men for one year, some for two years, some for three years, etc., to arrive at the same total of 5,000. We are no longer so focussed on the actual number of people who were at risk of the disease, but rather on the total person-time (number of person-years) they were at risk. This gives us much greater flexibility. Assuming that we still saw 15 heart attacks during our 5,000 person-years (py), we could calculate the **incidence rate** (sometimes called the incidence density) as 15 per 5,000 *person-years* or, more usually, 3 per 1,000 or 300/100,000 person-years.

Cumulative incidence (**CI**) measures the *proportion of people* who develop disease during a specified period:

$$CI = \frac{\text{Number of people who develop disease in a specified period}}{\text{Number of people at risk of developing the disease}} \qquad (2.5)$$
$$\text{at the start of the period}$$

The incidence rate (**IR**) measures how *quickly* people are developing a disease:

$$IR = \frac{\text{Number of people who develop disease}}{\text{Number of \textit{person-years} when people were at risk}} \qquad (2.6)$$
$$\text{of developing the disease}$$

Note that, although Equation (2.6) looks slightly different from Equation (2.2), they are measuring the same thing. We will come back to this under 'Measuring disease occurrence using routine data'.

Example

Imagine that we identified a group of 10 healthy people on 1 January 1995 and that we decided to follow these people for seven years to see who developed a particular disease. Figure 2.2 shows the hypothetical experience of these people: four developed the disease of interest and three of them died, and another three were 'lost to follow-up' (e.g., they moved away or died of some other disease). Let us now look at how we would calculate the different measures of disease occurrence in this group.

Prevalence

Remember that prevalence tells us the proportion of the population who were sick at a particular point in time (Equation (2.1)). For example, on 1 January

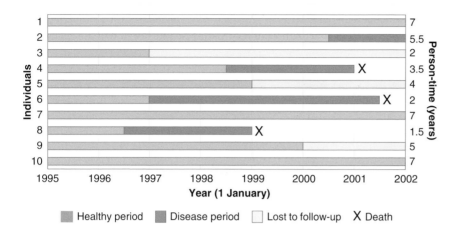

Fig. 2.2 A hypothetical follow-up study.

1998, two people were sick out of the nine people left in our group on that date (one was lost to follow-up), so

Prevalence = 2 ÷ 9 = 22%

What was the prevalence of the disease on 30 June 1999?

On 30 June 1999 two people were sick but there were only seven people left in the group on that date (one had died and two had been lost to follow-up), so

Prevalence = 2 ÷ 7 = 29%

Cumulative incidence

This tells us the proportion of a population 'at risk' of developing a disease who actually became ill during a specified time interval (Equation (2.5)). It is also the probability or average *risk* that an individual will develop the disease during the period: if 30% of people in a population develop a disease then each individual has a 30% chance of developing it themselves. (Note that this is the average risk for the population, the risk for any individual is either zero (they won't develop the disease) or one (they will)).

In this example, 4 of the 10 people who were at risk at the start of the study developed the disease, but three were lost to follow-up and we do not know whether they developed the disease. This means that we cannot accurately calculate the cumulative incidence at seven years, but a *minimum estimate* would be

CI = 4 ÷ 10 = 40% in seven years

This is assuming that none of those lost to follow-up developed the disease. If any of them had developed the disease then the true cumulative incidence would have been higher than 40%. The *maximum estimate* of the cumulative incidence would assume that all three of the missing people developed the disease:

CI = 7 ÷ 10 = 70% in seven years

Note that we could calculate an accurate cumulative incidence at two years – since we do have complete follow-up to that point:

CI = 1 ÷ 10 = 10% in two years

Incidence rates

Although we do not know what happened to three people in the group, we do know that they had not developed the disease before they were lost to follow up. We can use this information to help us calculate the incidence rate (Equation (2.6)). This is the number of new cases of disease (four) divided by the total amount of *person-time* at risk of developing the disease. An individual is at risk of developing the disease until the actual moment when they do develop it (in practice, when they are diagnosed) or until they are lost to follow-up. In this example, individual number one would contribute seven years of person-time; individual number two would contribute five and a half years; individual number three would contribute two years, and so on.

What is the total amount of person-time at risk?

What is the incidence rate for this disease per 100 person-years?

The total amount of person time is

7 + 5.5 + 2 + 3.5 + 4 + 2 + 7 + 1.5 + 5 + 7 = 44.5 person-years

So the incidence rate is

4 cases ÷ 44.5 person-years = 0.09 cases/person-year or 9 cases/100 person-years

Incidence rates versus cumulative incidence

The distinction between a measure of *cumulative incidence* and an *incidence rate* can be confusing. An analogy that we have found helpful is to think of these measures in terms of driving a car.

- The *incidence rate* is equivalent to the average *speed* of a car at a particular point in time, e.g., 60 km/hour.
- The *cumulative incidence* is analogous to the *distance* travelled by a car during a specified interval of time, e.g., 60 km in one hour.

The *distance* a car travels depends both on its average *speed* and on the length of time it travels for. If a car travels at an average speed of 60 km/hour then it will cover 30 km in 30 minutes, 60 km in one hour and so on. When we consider a time interval of one hour, the total distance travelled (60 km in one hour) looks

Box 2.4 The randomised clinical trial (RCT)

One type of study in which the study group is clearly defined and loss to follow-up is usually minimal is a **clinical trial** (see Chapter 6) and this means that the cumulative incidence is an appropriate and common measure of outcome in this type of study. However, the field of clinical epidemiology has developed its own terminology. As a result, you will find that in clinical trials what we have called the **cumulative incidence** is often called the **experimental event rate (EER)** when it describes the cumulative incidence in the intervention or treatment group and the **control event rate (CER)** in the control or placebo group.

For example, a group in the USA investigated whether four weeks of aspirin treatment would reduce the risk of blood clots in patients being treated with antibiotics for infective endocarditis (an infection of the lining of the heart that usually affects the heart valves). In total 115 patients were enrolled in the study and assigned at random to receive aspirin ($n = 60$) or placebo ($n = 55$). During the study, 17 patients in the aspirin group (EER or $CI_{Intervention} = 17 \div 60 = 28.3\%$) and 11 in the placebo group (CER or $CI_{Control} = 11 \div 55 = 20.0\%$) experienced blood clots (Table 2.3). The authors concluded that aspirin treatment did not reduce the risk of clots (Chan *et al.*, 2003).

Table 2.3 Results of an RCT evaluating aspirin use for infective endocarditis.

	Total patients	Number with blood clots	Event rate (cumulative incidence of blood clots) (%)
Aspirin	60	17	28.3
Placebo	55	11	20.0

very similar to the average speed because this is expressed per hour (60 km/hr). Distance and speed are, however, fundamentally different.

In the same way, the incidence rate describes the 'speed' at which new cases of disease are occurring, and therefore reflects what is sometimes called the underlying *force of morbidity*. Cumulative incidence is a measure of the proportion of a group who develop the disease over a particular time and is thus a function both of the underlying incidence rate and of the length of follow-up. If the incidence rate is 10 per 100,000/year then the cumulative incidence will be 10 cases in 100,000 (=0.0001 or 0.01%) in one year, 20 cases in 100,000 (=0.0002 or 0.02%) in two years and so on. As with the car example, when we consider a time interval of one year, a cumulative incidence expressed as 10 per 100,000 people *in one year* looks much like an incidence rate (10 per 100,000 *per year* or *person-years*) because we usually show incidence rates per year. It is important to recognise that, as with distance and speed, the measures are different. A good way to avoid confusion is to ensure that the cumulative incidence is expressed as a proportion (e.g., 0.0001) or percentage rather than 'per 100,000'.

Measuring disease occurrence using routine data

In practice most of our information about the occurrence of disease comes from routine statistics, collected at a regional, national or international level (we will discuss some of the sources of these data in Chapter 3), and in this format they comprise the core of many published reports. The data are not based on specific information about *individuals* but relate the number of cases of disease (or deaths) in a *population* to the size of that population (often an estimate from a census). This is a problem when we try to relate the occurrence of disease to potential causes. For example, if a region has a very high level of unemployment and also has a high incidence of suicide it might be tempting to jump to the conclusion that being unemployed drives people to commit suicide. However, we have no way of knowing from routine statistics whether it is the same people who are unemployed who are also those committing suicide. (This dilemma is often called the *ecological fallacy* and we will discuss it again in Chapter 6.)

A second drawback of routine data relates to the fact that in public health we often want to measure the *incidence* of disease – how quickly are people becoming ill? Mortality data are uninformative for many diseases that are common and troublesome, but not usually fatal – things like osteoarthritis, non-melanoma skin cancers, psoriasis and rubella (German measles) to name but a few. Even for those diseases from which a high proportion of cases die, mortality figures might not mirror the underlying incidence of disease, for example if a more effective treatment is introduced. Mortality data can also lag well behind changes in incidence, delaying identification of changes over time that may be important for planning or for providing clues as to the causes of the disease.

Unfortunately, it is often difficult to obtain reliable information about *incidence* because few illnesses are captured in routine statistics. Some diseases, such as HIV infection and cancer, are 'notifiable' in many countries and, therefore, all cases *should* be reported to a central body. (Unfortunately such reporting does not always occur in practice. When HIV/AIDS first came to world attention and again during the 2003 SARS (severe acute respiratory syndrome) outbreak, some countries suppressed the real numbers of cases for both political and economic reasons.) These examples are, however, the exceptions rather than the rule and such data are not routinely available for most diseases. As a result, many common measures that you will come across will be measures of death or *mortality rates* because death and cause of death are regularly and reliably recorded in many countries. Incidence and mortality rates have exactly the same form, but for incidence we count new cases of a disease whereas for mortality we count deaths.

Crude incidence and mortality rates

As you saw above, when we conduct an epidemiological study we calculate the incidence rate as the number of cases of disease divided by the total *person-time* at risk of disease (where this is summed over all of the individuals in the study). At the population level we may be dealing with millions of people and so it is clearly not feasible to calculate the person-time that each is at risk. Instead we usually work on the assumption that everyone is at risk for the whole of the year that we are interested in. The fundamental concept is the same – the essential distinction is that the 'routine rates' are based on population averages, whereas the 'epidemiological rates' are based on adding together carefully measured units of individual person-time to give a precise denominator. They are also presented slightly differently: routine incidence rates are usually described per 100,000 *people per year*, whereas in epidemiological studies using individual data they are usually shown per 100,000 *person-years*.

When we are working with routine data, therefore, an incidence rate is calculated by dividing the total number of new cases of a specific disease (or the number of deaths) in a specified period, usually one year, by the average number of people in the population during the same period (Equation (2.2)). This is then usually multiplied by 100,000 (10^5) and presented as a rate per 10^5 people per year. The size of the population will, inevitably, change over a period of a year, so ideally we would use the number of people in the population in the middle of the year, the 'mid-interval' population, for our calculations. Depending on the data available, this may be calculated as the average of the size of the population at the start and at the end of the period of interest, or estimated from census data. Incidence rates may be calculated for a broad disease group (e.g., cancer) or a more specific disease (e.g., breast cancer). Similarly, mortality rates may include deaths from all causes (sometimes called *all-cause* mortality) or only those from a specific cause. These basic rates are called 'crude' rates because they describe the overall incidence or death rate in a population without taking any other features of the population into account (in contrast to standardised rates – see below).

Table 2.4 shows crude mortality rates for ischaemic heart disease (IHD) in men in seven countries. We see that Germany, Australia and Canada have high mortality rates, with intermediate rates in Singapore and Spain and low rates in Japan and Brazil. This correctly describes the total burdens that the different health systems have to cope with, but does it give an accurate picture of the level of mortality from IHD in each country? If we were to take this information at face value we would conclude that the death rate for IHD is three to four times higher

Table 2.4 Crude mortality rates (per 100,000 per year) for ischaemic heart disease (IHD) in males from selected countries, 1995–1998.

Country	Crude IHD mortality rate (per 10^5 per year)
Germany	211
Australia	168
Canada	160
Singapore	118
Spain	116
Japan	50
Brazil	47

(*Data source:* Global Cardiovascular Infobase, www.cvdinfobase.ca, accessed 23 September 2003.)

Box 2.5 Cardiovascular diseases simplified

You will find that, when we use examples relating to cardiovascular diseases, the conditions often have different names and abbreviations. Cardiovascular diseases are grouped and described in many different ways, emphasising the need to be sure that you know what the numbers you are looking at represent. The following is a simplified summary of some commonly used terms:

MI: myocardial infarction: heart attack

IHD: ischaemic heart disease: heart attack (MI) or angina

CHD: coronary heart disease: essentially identical to IHD

CVD: cardiovascular disease: includes CHD, stroke and other cardiac and vascular diseases (note that CVD can also be used as an abbreviation for cerebrovascular disease, i.e., stroke and transient ischaemic attack, but we will not use it in this way)

in Western countries such as Germany, Australia and Canada than in countries like Japan and Brazil. Is that reasonable?

Age-specific incidence and mortality rates

A major disadvantage of crude rates is that they are just that – crude. They do not take into account the fact that different populations have different age structures

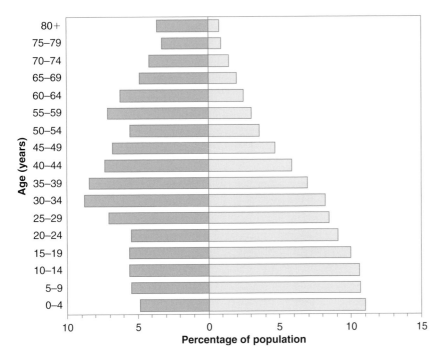

Fig. 2.3 Age distribution of the population in Brazil (1995, light bars) and Germany (1998, dark bars). (Drawn from Global Cardiovascular Infobase, www.cvdinfobase.ca, accessed 23 September 2003.)

and that the risk of becoming ill or dying varies with age. Many diseases are more common among older people and the older a person is, the greater their risk of dying. Developed countries like Germany have a high proportion of older people whereas less developed countries like Brazil have a much greater proportion of young people, at a relatively lower risk of dying. Their contrasting population structures are shown in Figure 2.3. In the example above it turns out that we are trying to compare countries with very different age structures, so a crude comparison of IHD mortality has little meaning if we are trying to assess the comparative 'cardiovascular health' of these countries (see also Box 2.5).

One obvious way to avoid this problem is to calculate separate rates for different age groups (*age-specific rates*). The rate in a particular age group can then be compared between countries. This process can be extended to calculate separate rates for other groups, for instance men and women (*sex-specific rates*), and for different racial or socioeconomic groups. Table 2.5 extends Table 2.4 to show selected age-specific mortality rates for the seven countries.

If we compare the age-specific rates we can see that in each country the rate is much higher in the older age group. We can also see that, while the crude rates for Singapore and Spain are similar, the age-specific rates are about twice as high in Singapore, which now has the highest rates of all the countries. Brazil has also moved up in the IHD rankings.

Table 2.5 Crude and age-specific mortality rates (per 100,000 per year) for ischaemic heart disease in males from selected countries, 1995–1998.

Country	Crude rate (per 10^5 per year)	Age-specific rates (per 10^5 per year)	
		45–54 years	55–64 years
Germany	211	76	245
Australia	168	68	222
Canada	160	73	239
Singapore	118	100	346
Spain	116	59	156
Japan	50	20	60
Brazil	47	64	183

(*Data source:* Global Cardiovascular Infobase, www.cvdinfobase.ca, accessed 23 September 2003.)

Standardised incidence and mortality rates

If age-specific rates are presented for a large number of different age groups, as well as for both sexes, we end up with a lot of numbers to compare and interpret (only two age groups are shown in Table 2.5 for simplicity). An alternative is to summarise or combine these age-specific rates using the process of **direct standardisation**. This involves calculating the overall incidence or mortality rate that you would have expected to find in a 'standard' population if it had the same age-specific rates as your study population. (The details of the calculations are shown in Appendix 1.) The same methods can also be used to standardise for sex because disease rates often differ markedly between men and women.

The age-standardised rates can then be compared across the populations (assuming that the disease is defined in the same way in each) because the problem of different age patterns has been removed (Table 2.6). You will notice that, in countries with an older population, the standardised rate is much lower than the crude rate, but that it is higher than the crude rate in Brazil, which has a much younger population. The age-standardised rates give a more accurate picture of the relative levels of IHD mortality in the seven countries than the crude rates did because they take into account the larger numbers of older people in the more developed countries.

A note about standard populations

It is important to add a word of caution at this stage. There are many different standard populations and, in practice, you can age-standardise to *any* population. You will often come across rates that have been standardised to the 'world'

Table 2.6 Crude and age-standardised mortality rates (per 100,000 per year) for ischaemic heart disease (IHD) in males from selected countries, 1995–1998.

Country	Crude IHD mortality rate (per 10^5 per year)	Age-standardised rate (per 10^5 per year)
Germany	211	121
Australia	168	111
Canada	160	108
Singapore	118	121
Spain	116	65
Japan	50	29
Brazil	47	60

(*Data source:* Global Cardiovascular Infobase, www.cvdinfobase.ca, accessed 23 September 2003.)

population which reflects the average age structure of the whole world. Other common standard populations reflect the typical age structure of 'developed' or 'developing' countries. If the aim is to compare rates in different groups within the same country then it is common practice to use the overall age structure of that country as the standard population. To some extent the choice is arbitrary, but it is important to note that, if you standardise to two very different populations, you will get very different standardised rates and the relationships between different populations may change. For this reason, it is always important to note what standard population has been used.

For example, when we standardised IHD mortality in Germany to the world standard population we found an age-standardised rate of $121/10^5$ per year. If we had standardised to the younger 'African' standard population, we would have found an age-standardised rate of only $60/10^5$ per year, whereas if we had standardised to the older 'European' standard population we would have found an age-standardised rate of $198/10^5$ per year. In this example we were comparing populations around the world, so it was appropriate to use the world standard population. If all the countries had been in Europe or Africa then the European or African standard populations might have been more appropriate.

The World Health Organization (WHO) has recently proposed a new world standard population that reflects the general ageing of populations around the world. (This and examples of other common standard populations are provided in Appendix 2.) However, what seems like a logical updating of information has major ramifications for anyone looking at time trends in the occurrence of disease because rates cannot be compared if they have been standardised to different populations.

Box 2.6   An over-night doubling of all-cause mortality rates in the USA?

Prior to 1999, various US health agencies had used different standard populations, including the 1940 population and the 1970 population, to report vital statistics. This made comparisons between data from different agencies problematic. In 1999 many of these agencies changed their standard population to the projected population in the year 2000 (the Year 2000 Population Standard). In comparison with the earlier populations, the Year 2000 population has fewer people under the age of 35 and more people in the middle and older age groups. Because the Year 2000 population is older and incidence and mortality rates of most diseases increase with age, rates standardised to this population tend to be much higher than those standardised to the 1940 and 1970 standards.

The change dramatically increased age-standardised rates in the USA. The all-cause mortality rate in 1979 was 577/100,000 per year (standardised to the 1940 population) and 1,011/100,000 per year (standardised to the Year 2000 standard population). The comparable difference for the all-cause mortality rate in 1995 was between 504/100,000 per year (1940 standard) and 919/100,000 per year (2000 standard). More reassuringly, in this example at least, the *relative* reduction in mortality between 1979 and 1995 was similar regardless of which standard population was used. Using the 1940 standard, the mortality rate appeared to fall from 577 to 504/100,000 per year, a drop of 13% over the period; using the Year 2000 standard, the rate fell from 1,011 to 919/100,000 per year, a drop of 9% (Anderson and Rosenberg, 1998).

Measuring cumulative incidence using routine statistics

Routine statistics may also be used to estimate cumulative incidence. This gives the probability or risk that someone will develop disease (or die) within a given time period, and this time period can be anything from a few days to a lifetime (a lifetime is commonly taken as ages 0 to 74 years). For example, men in Australia have a lifetime cumulative incidence of lung cancer of 4.8% or, in other words, 4.8% of Australian men will develop lung cancer before their 75th birthday. An alternative way to look at the same information is to say that the average *lifetime risk* of lung cancer in Australian men is '1 in 21' or, in other words, 1 in every 21 Australian men will develop lung cancer before their 75th birthday. Note that these measures assume that someone remains 'at risk' of lung cancer until their 75th birthday and they also do not take into account any other factors, such as smoking. (The methods for calculating cumulative incidence and lifetime risk for routine data are shown in Appendix 3.)

Other measures commonly used in public health

We will now consider a range of other measures that are used commonly in public health. They are expressed in a variety of ways – some are ratios, some are usually percentages, i.e., per 100 population, while others are shown per 1,000, 10,000 or 100,000 population. In some cases different people will use the same term to describe a slightly different measure. The definitions that we give are as in Last's *A Dictionary of Epidemiology* (Last, 2001) and are probably those most commonly used. Whenever you come across these rates it is advisable to check exactly what the numbers being compared are, and what the size of the reference population is – whether the rate refers to 100, 1,000 or 100,000 events or people.

Standardised incidence and mortality ratios

Figure 1.5 in Chapter 1 showed standardised mortality ratios (SMRs) for various Aboriginal populations in Australia. These come from an alternative way of stand-ardising rates called **indirect standardisation** (see Appendix 4). In this example the standardisation is for age but the same process is commonly used to adjust for sex and/or to compare data from different time periods. The actual number of deaths 'observed' in a population (e.g., Aboriginal men in Western Australia) is compared with the number of deaths that would have been 'expected' if the death rates in the Aboriginal population had been the same as those for the whole of Australia. The standardised mortality ratio (SMR) is calculated by dividing the observed number of deaths (O) by the expected number (E). This measure tells us how much more common death is in the Western Australian Aborigines than in the whole of Australia (about two times in this case). We can do exactly the same thing with incidence rates to calculate a standardised incidence or morbidity ratio. (Note that some people will use SMR to describe both standardised mortality and morbidity ratios, while others use SMR and SIR to distinguish between mortality and incidence. Standardised incidence ratios are commonly reported by cancer registries since they are one of the few groups who have access to reliable incidence data at the population level.) The SMR and SIR are similar to the relative risk that you met in Chapter 1. Remember also that Snow used observed and expected numbers of deaths to show that cholera mortality in the workhouse near the Broad Street pump was unexpectedly low.

Strictly speaking, SMRs and SIRs are *measures of association* because they compare disease incidence or mortality in one population with that in a refer-ence population and, as such, would fit more logically into Chapter 5. We have included them here because of the parallels between the processes of direct and indirect standardisation.

The proportional (or proportionate) mortality ratio (PMR)

This is a measure of the relative importance of a particular cause of death in a given population. A PMR looks like an SMR but it is used when there is insufficient information to calculate an SMR (usually because information is available only about those who have died, so it is not possible to calculate mortality rates). It is calculated by dividing the *proportion* of deaths due to a specific cause in a group of interest by the *proportion* of deaths due to the same cause in a comparison group. A PMR is commonly multiplied by 100, so a PMR of 100 means that the proportions of deaths due to a specific cause are the same in the study and comparison groups, and a PMR of 200 indicates that twice as many deaths in the study group are due to the specific cause. Proportional mortality ratios are most commonly used in occupational studies. For example, a study of deaths among electrical workers on construction sites in the USA found that 127 of the total of 31,068 deaths (0.4%) were due to electrocution. This value was almost 12 times higher (PMR = 1,180) than the proportion of such deaths that would be expected in the general US population (Robinson *et al.*, 1999). Proportional mortality ratios are not particularly useful measures and are usually calculated only when no population data are readily available and precise mortality rates cannot be calculated. Proportional mortality ratios cannot easily be compared across different populations.

The case–fatality ratio (CFR)

The CFR (often called the case–fatality *rate*, although, strictly speaking, it is not a rate, see Box 2.7) is the proportion of people with a given disease or condition who die from it in a given period. It is a common measure of the short-term severity of an acute disease and allows a direct assessment of the effectiveness of an intervention. For example, the CFR for myocardial infarction (heart attack) is usually measured over a period of 28 days. When deaths occur over a longer time period then it is more appropriate to consider the survival rate (see below). The CFR is usually expressed per 100 cases, i.e. as a percentage. As an example, the overall CFR in the 2003 SARS epidemic was estimated to be 14%–15%, i.e., approximately one in every seven people who contracted SARS died. However, this average ratio hides the fact that, while patients under the age of 25 were unlikely to die (CFR = 1%), approximately half of patients over the age of 65 died (CFR = 50%). (Note that the mortality from SARS occurred so quickly that the particular time period the CFR refers to is generally not specified.)

Survival rate and relative survival rate

As we discussed above, the CFR is an appropriate measure for short-term mortality (a month or so) but is less useful for conditions in which death may occur further down the track. For conditions such as cancer, mortality is often expressed

Box 2.7 Rates, ratios and proportions

A **ratio** is simply one number divided by another number. For example, the number of beers drunk in one year divided by the number of people in the population (beers per capita) or the number of cases observed divided by the number of cases expected.

A **proportion** is a special type of ratio in which everything or everyone in the numerator is also counted in the denominator. For example, the number of people who develop disease divided by the total number of people in the population (those with and without disease). A proportion can be expressed as a number between 0 and 1 or as a percentage between 0 and 100%. All proportions are ratios – not all ratios are proportions.

A **rate** should contain some measure of time, for example 60 km *per hour*, 17/100,000 *per year*.

As an example, the **case–fatality ratio** is a proportion and, therefore also a ratio, but is not a rate (although it is often described as such) because it does not contain units of time.

in terms of the proportion of patients who are still alive a specified number of years after diagnosis – the **survival rate**. This proportion is often adjusted to allow for the fact that, depending on the age group being considered, some people would have been expected to die anyway from causes other than their cancer and this is known as the **relative survival rate**. A relative survival rate of 100% thus indicates that mortality does not differ from that experienced by the general population. For example, in developed countries relative five-year survival rates for breast cancer are approximately 75%–80%, compared with rates of only about 15% for lung cancer.

Measures of mortality related to childbirth and early life

Table 2.7 shows a number of different measures that are commonly used to describe the patterns of mortality of mothers and infants before, during and after childbirth. These rates, especially the infant mortality rate, are often used as critical indicators of the general level of health in a community. (Note that, technically, these measures are *proportions* rather than true *rates* because they do not have units of time; they are, however, commonly described as rates and we will also use this terminology.)

The underlying concept of each rate is the same – it is the ratio of the actual number of deaths that occur in one year to the total population 'at risk of death' in the same year. Because it is not always possible to obtain an accurate figure for the number of people at risk, an approximation is sometimes used. For example,

Table 2.7 Measures of mortality related to childbirth and early life.

Measure	Deaths (numerator)	Population at risk (denominator)	Notes
Maternal mortality rate	Deaths among women from causes related to childbirth in 1 year (usually only deaths up to 42 days after birth, sometimes deaths up to 1 year after birth are included)	Number of live births in the same year	Strictly speaking, the denominator should be *all* pregnant women, but this information is not recorded directly.
Stillbirth or fetal death rate	Number of stillbirths in 1 year, where a still birth is usually a fetal death after 28 weeks gestation, although other time points may also be used (e.g. 20 weeks)	Live births plus fetal deaths in the same year	Sometimes calculated as the ratio of the number of fetal deaths to the number of live births (excluding fetal deaths). This is often called the *fetal death ratio*.
Perinatal mortality rate	Fetal deaths and deaths up to 7 days of life	Live births plus fetal deaths in the same year	May be calculated as the ratio of the number of deaths to the number of live births (excluding fetal deaths) and called the *perinatal death ratio*. May also include deaths up to 28 days of life.
Neonatal mortality rate	Deaths in children aged less than 28 days	Number of live births in the same year	Only live births are included in the denominator because only babies born alive are at risk of dying before the age of 28 days.
Post-neonatal mortality rate	Deaths in children aged from 28 days to 1 year	Number of live births in the same year	Strictly speaking, the denominator should exclude children who die before age 28 days because they are no longer at risk.
Infant mortality rate	Deaths in children up to 1 year of age	Number of live births in the same year	Probably the most widely used single indicator of the overall health of a community.
Child death rate	Deaths in children aged 1–4 years	Number of children aged 1–4 years in the population	An example of an age-specific mortality rate.

any woman who is pregnant is at risk of maternal death but the number of women who are pregnant in a given year is not routinely recorded, so in practice this is estimated by taking the number of live births in one year. It is also worth noting that the infant mortality rate is the number of infant deaths (age 0–1 year)

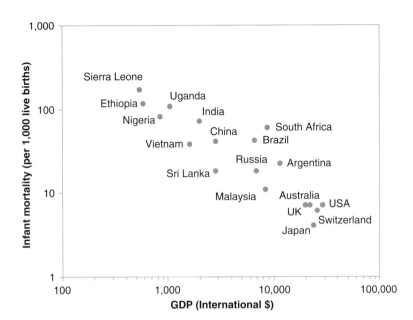

Fig. 2.4 Infant mortality rates in relation to GDP in 18 countries around the world. (Drawn from World Health Chart, WHC 2001 Public Beta 0.1, www.whc.ki.se, accessed 6 October 2003.)

relative to the number of live births in the same year. This means that the children in the numerator (deaths) are not the same as those in the denominator (births) because many of those who die will have been born in the previous year. This is not a problem if the birth rate is fairly stable.

For each rate we have given the most standard definition but, as you will see, there are some variations. For example, the *stillbirth* (or *fetal death*) *rate* should be calculated as the ratio of stillbirths to the number of live births *plus* the number of stillbirths. This is because all of these children (live plus stillbirths) were at risk of being stillborn although not all of them were. This measure is, however, sometimes presented as a *stillbirth* or *fetal death ratio* where only live births are counted in the denominator. The WHO in particular tends to use this variant. Because the number of live births will be less than the number of live births plus stillbirths, the fetal death or stillbirth ratio will always be slightly larger than the stillbirth rate. You will also notice that there is not always a standard definition of what constitutes a case (in this case a death). It just goes to reinforce how important it is to check exactly what the numbers refer to in order to make sure that you are always comparing like with like.

Figure 2.4 shows the enormous variation in infant mortality rates around the world, reflecting the great disadvantages under which many countries still labour. It also shows the very strong inverse correlation between GDP (gross domestic product) and infant mortality – the more wealthy a country the lower the infant mortality rate. In a poor country like Sierra Leone the rate is as high as 170 per 1,000 live births or, in other words, almost 2 in every 10 babies die before their first birthday, compared with only 4 per 1,000 live births in Japan.

It is important to remember that all of these measures just give an average picture for the whole population. Low average rates can often hide much higher rates in some subgroups of the population. This is particularly true in countries that include more than one ethnic group. For example, as you saw in Chapter 1, in Australia the indigenous Aboriginal population has mortality rates that are several times higher than those of Australians as a whole and in the USA in 2001 infant mortality was considerably higher among Black or African-American babies (13.3 per 1,000 live births) than among White babies (5.7 per 1,000) (NCHS, 2003).

Other measures of health status

Various other rather different mortality-related measures are also used to describe the health of populations. New and more sophisticated variations are continually being introduced as organisations such as the WHO attempt not only to measure disease, but also to take into account related conditions such as pain, disability and loss of income that are associated with ill-health. These measures bring us closer to measuring the overall 'health' of a population according to the WHO definition of health, as opposed to emphasising only disease or death as the more traditional measures described above do.

Life expectancy and healthy life expectancy

Life expectancy is the average number of years that an individual of a given age is expected to live *if current mortality rates continue*. It is thus largely hypothetical and is not a realistic measure of how long an individual will actually live, since it cannot take account of future changes in incidence and/or treatment of diseases. It can be presented as life expectancy at any age, but is used most commonly to describe life expectancy at birth. For example, a boy born in the Russian Federation in 2002 has a life expectancy of 58.4 years, compared with 78.4 years for a boy born in Japan (WHO, 2003).

A more recent modification used by the WHO is the concept of **health-adjusted** or **healthy life expectancy** (HALE) in recognition that increased life expectancy per se may be of little benefit if your health is poor during the additional years. Health-adjusted life expectancy is based on life expectancy at birth but includes an adjustment for time spent in poor health. It represents the equivalent number of years an individual can expect to live in full health. A health-adjusted life expectancy of 60 years might therefore represent an expectation of 50 years life in full health plus an additional 20 years at 50% or 30 years at 33% of full health. Another variation is **disability-adjusted life expectancy** (DALE), which estimates the numbers of years an individual can expect to live free of disability.

Table 2.8 shows data on life expectancy and healthy life expectancy for a number of different countries. Notice that healthy life expectancy is consistently 6–8

Table 2.8 Life expectancy and healthy life expectancy at birth in 2002 (years).

	Males			Females		
	Life expectancy at birth	Healthy life expectancy		Life expectancy at birth	Healthy life expectancy	
		At birth	At age 60		At birth	At age 60
Australia	77.9	70.9	16.9	83.0	74.3	19.5
India	60.1	53.3	10.8	62.0	53.6	11.4
Japan	78.4	72.3	17.5	85.3	77.7	21.7
Malawi	39.8	35.0	9.7	40.6	34.8	10.4
Russian Federation	58.4	52.8	10.1	72.1	64.3	14.2
Switzerland	77.7	71.1	17.1	83.3	75.3	20.4
UK	75.8	69.1	15.7	80.5	72.1	18.1
USA	74.6	67.2	15.3	79.8	71.3	17.9

(*Data source:* World Health Organization, 2003.)

years less than life expectancy for men and 7–10 years less for women. This difference is a function both of the expected number of years of life at less than full health and of the extent of disability. Because life expectancy at birth is partly dependent on mortality in the first year of life, it is inevitably much lower in developing countries, which tend to have much higher neonatal and infant mortality rates than developed countries. Once an individual has survived the first few years of life in a developing country, however, their chances of living to old age are then much greater and the difference between developed and developing countries becomes less marked. As an example, see the apparent paradox in Malawi. Healthy life expectancy at birth for a man in 2002 was only 35 years, due largely to the enormous toll that HIV/AIDS has taken on the countries in Sub-Saharan Africa; but, if a man made it to 60, he could then expect another 10 years of healthy life. Notice also that, while in most countries women can expect to live about 5 years longer than men, the recent increase in mortality rate among young Russian men (Figure 1.2) means that the difference in the Russian Federation is currently almost 14 years.

Years of potential life lost (YPLL)

This is a measure of premature mortality that takes into account not only the number of deaths that occur, but also the ages at which they occur. A death at a young age, therefore, counts much higher than a death in old age. It counts the years of (potential) life lost (YPLL or YLL) for each death that occurs before a specified age. This age is frequently taken to be 65 but, with increasing numbers of people now living active lives well beyond this age, some reports now consider deaths before 70 to be 'premature' deaths. The measure is calculated by counting the total number of deaths from a specific cause in each age group and then multiplying this by the average number of years of life lost as a result of each of these deaths. For example, taking 65 as the cut-off age, a death from coronary heart disease at age 60 would contribute only 5 years to the total YPLL, compared with 15 years for a death at age 50. Thus, although there are fewer deaths among younger people, each contributes a greater number of YPLL than the deaths in the elderly. Note that this measure does not take any account of deaths that occur above the specified cut-off age.

An alternative version of this measure called **expected years of life lost** counts up the years of life lost in each age group compared with the standard life expectancy for the population.

Quality- and disability-adjusted life years (QALYs and DALYs)

Like health-adjusted life expectancy, various other measures also attempt to measure not only years of life but also the quality of that life. These are sometimes described generically as **health-adjusted life years** (HALYs) and the most common are quality- and disability-adjusted life years. **Quality-adjusted life years** weight each year of life by the perceived quality of that life from a value of one for perfect health down to zero for death. One QALY would thus represent a year of life in perfect health while 0.5 QALY could represent 6 months lived in perfect health or 12 months with 50% disability (or ill-health). Measurements of QALYs have often been used to compare the effects of different treatments. For example, the QALYs gained from a radical treatment that increases life expectancy by 10 years but is associated with major side-effects might be lower than those from a less effective drug that increases life expectancy by only 8 years but does not have any major side-effects.

In contrast, **disability-adjusted life years** estimate loss of healthy life. They are calculated as the sum of the years lost due to premature death and healthy years lost through disability. As for QALYs, the extent of disability is weighted from zero to one, although the weights go in the opposite direction – from zero for a year spent in perfect health to one for a year lost to death. (Note that the actual calculations are somewhat more complicated than this because they also take age into account and consider that productive years lost in mid-life are more important than years lost at very young or old ages.) One DALY can be thought of as one lost year of healthy life. Thus, if a person lives with a moderate disability for 10 years, this might equate to five DALYs or the loss of 5 years of healthy life. Measurements of DALYs have often been used to estimate the burden of various diseases in different countries, as for example in the World Health Reports produced by the WHO (WHO, 2003), and to identify priorities for health intervention. A recent variation on this theme that we liked comes from the field of

Fig. 2.5 Years of potential life lost (YPLL) and disability-adjusted life-years (DALYs) for AIDS, breast cancer and injury in relation to research expenditure by the US National Institutes of Health in 1996. (Drawn from Gross *et al.*, 1999.)

Box 2.8 Suicide rates: are we winning or losing?

Suicide is a major cause of premature mortality in many countries, but is the situation becoming better or worse? Data from the UK show that
• between 1981 and 1998, suicide rates in men and women aged 15 and over
  fell by 18%;
but they also show that
• between 1981 and 1998, the years of potential life lost due to suicide
  increased by 5%.
How do we interpret these apparently conflicting data? The answer is that the major drop in suicide rates has occurred among the older age groups (45 years and over) and suicide rates in younger men have actually increased over the same time period. Suicide in a younger person leads to greater loss of potential life, so although the overall suicide rates are falling this fall masks an increasing loss of life among young men.

  These data underline how different measures of health capture different things and can give very different pictures of the health of a population. A politician hoping to demonstrate improvements in mental health could legitimately claim that suicide rates were falling, while an advocate for more funding for mental health could equally legitimately cite the increase in years of life lost.

(Gunnell and Middleton, 2003.)

economics: namely *happiness-adjusted life years* (Veenhoven, 2002). It remains to be seen whether these will be widely adopted in the health field.

  The use of measures like DALYs and YPLL can give a different sense of priorities for disease control from conventional rates (Figure 2.5 and Box 2.8). Injury,

Table 2.9 A summary of measures of disease occurrence.

Measure	Definition	Formula	Units
Prevalence (*P*)	The *proportion* of the population with disease at a specific point in time.	$$\frac{\text{No. of people with disease at a given point in time}}{\text{Total number of people in the population}}$$	Per cent or proportion (e.g., 0.01) (or per 1,000, 10,000, 100,000, etc.)
Cumulative incidence (CI)	The *proportion* of people who develop disease during a specified period. Synonyms: *attack rate, experimental* and *control event rate* (in the treated and control groups in a clinical trial)	$$\frac{\text{No. who develop disease in a specified period}}{\text{No. at risk of the disease at the start of the period}}$$	Per cent or proportion (or per 1,000, 10,000, 100,000, etc.)
Incidence rate (IR)	The *rate* at which disease is occurring, measured from individual data in a study. Synonym: *incidence density*.	$$\frac{\text{No. who develop disease in a specified period}}{\text{No. of }\textit{person-years}\text{ at risk of getting the disease}}$$	Per 100,000 person-years (or per 1,000, 10,000 person-years, etc.)
	The *rate* at which disease is occurring, measured from population data, may be *crude, specific* (e.g. age-specific) or *standardised* (direct standardisation).	$$\frac{\text{No. of people who develop disease in one year}}{\text{Average no. in the population in the same year}}$$	Per 100,000/year (or per 1,000/year, 10,000/year, etc.)
Standardised incidence or mortality ratio (SIR or SMR)	Compares incidence or mortality with a standard population using *indirect* standardisation.	$$\frac{\text{Observed no. of cases (deaths)}}{\text{No. expected for a standard population}}$$	A ratio, sometimes a percentage
Proportional mortality ratio (PMR)	Compares the *proportion* of deaths with a standard population (can be used when information is available only for deaths).	$$\frac{\text{Proportion of deaths from a specific cause}}{\text{Proportion expected for a standard population}}$$	A ratio, sometimes a percentage
Case–fatality ratio (CFR)	The proportion of people who die from a disease in a specified (usually short) time period (actually a measure of *cumulative incidence*).	$$\frac{\text{No. who die from a disease in a specified period}}{\text{Total no. with the disease}}$$	Per cent (or per 1,000, 10,000, 100,000, etc.)

for example, kills proportionally more young people than other conditions and so makes a major contribution to years of life lost due to premature death and to disability, yet far greater financial resources tend to be given to research into high-profile conditions such as breast cancer and AIDS.

Summary

You should now be able to interpret any measures of disease that you come across (the key features of the main measures are summarised in Table 2.9). It is still important to be very careful when comparing measures of disease across different groups of people because many other factors can complicate this. We will discuss some of these issues in the following chapters.

Questions

1. A thousand healthy women were followed for 10 years and 23 developed high blood pressure. What was the *cumulative incidence* of high blood pressure in this group?
2. A group of elderly men was followed for a total of 2,000 person-years and 36 of the men had a stroke during the duration of the study. What was the *incidence rate* of stroke in this group?
3. In a community with a population of 15,000 people, 9 developed diabetes during a 1-year period. What was the *incidence rate* of diabetes in the community?
4. Two thousand women aged 55 years were given a health check and 100 were found to have high blood pressure. Ten years later all 2,000 women attended a second check and another 300 women had developed high blood pressure.
   (a) What was the prevalence of high blood pressure in the women (i) at age 55 and (ii) at age 65?
   (b) How many women were 'at risk' of developing high blood pressure at the start of the 10-year period?
   (c) What was the incidence of high blood pressure in these women? Is this a measure of cumulative incidence or an incidence rate?
Assume that, on average, each of the 300 women who developed high blood pressure did so half-way through the 10 year follow-up period.
   (d) Calculate the total number of person-years at risk (of developing high blood pressure) during the 10 years.
   (e) What was the *incidence rate* of high blood pressure in these women?

REFERENCES

Agarwal, M. M. and Punnose, J. (2002). Gestational diabetes: implications of variation in diagnostic criteria. *International Journal of Gynecology and Obstetrics*, **78**: 45–46.

Anderson, R. and Rosenberg, H. (1998). Age standardization of death rates: implementation of the Year 2000 standard. *National Vital Statistics Reports*, vol. 47 no. 3. Hyattsville, Maryland: National Center for Health Statistics.

CDC National Center for Infectious Diseases. (2002). *Viral Hepatitis – U.S. Disease Burden Data, 1980–2001*. (http://www.cdc.gov/ncidod/diseases/hepatitis/resource/)

Chan, K.-L., Dumesnil, J. G., Cujec, B. *et al.* for the Investigators of the Multicenter Aspirin Study in Infective Endocarditis. (2003). A randomized trial of aspirin on the risk of embolic events in patients with infective endocarditis. *Journal of the American College of Cardiologists*, **42**: 775–780.

Gross, C. P., Anderson, G. F. and Powe, N. R. (1999). The relation between funding by the National Institutes of Health and the burden of disease. *New England Journal of Medicine*, **340**: 1881–1887.

Gunnell, D. and Middleton, N. (2003). National suicide rates as an indicator of the effect of suicide on premature mortality. *Lancet*, **362**: 961–962.

Last, J. M. (Ed.) (2001). *A Dictionary of Epidemiology*, 4th edn. Oxford: Oxford University Press.

NCHS (National Center for Health Statistics). (2003). *Health, United States, 2003*. Hyattsville, Maryland: National Center for Health Statistics.

Robinson, C. F., Petersen, M. and Palu, S. (1999). Mortality patterns among electrical workers employed in the U.S. construction industry, 1982–1987. *American Journal of Industrial Medicine*, **36**: 630–637.

UNAIDS. (2002a). *Joint United Nations Programme on HIV/AIDS. Report on the Global HIV/AIDS Epidemic 2002*. Geneva: UNAIDS. (www.unaids.org)

  (2002b). *Joint United Nations Programme on HIV/AIDS. AIDS Epidemic Update: December 2002*. Geneva: UNAIDS. (www.unaids.org)

Veenhoven, R. (2002). Commentary: the units of utility. *International Journal of Epidemiology*, **31**: 1144–1146.

WHO (World Health Organization). (2003). *The World Health Report 2003: Shaping the Future*. Geneva: World Health Organization.

3

Who, what, where and when?
Finding and using public health data

Before beginning a Hunt, it is wise to ask someone what you are looking for before you begin looking for it.

From *Pooh's Little Book of Instructions, Inspired by A. A. Milne*
(Powers, 1995)

We have discussed the ways in which we can measure the frequency of disease and some of the uses to which this information can be put, but how do we acquire the data that enable us to do this? If, for example, you were concerned about youth suicide rates in your community and wanted to compare the local rate with the state or national rates, where would you go for this information? You might have to collect it yourself or, with a bit of luck, you might be able to make use of data that have already been collected, often by a government health or statistical agency. We will consider the first option, that of collecting our own data, at more length in Chapter 6, but this process is rarely quick or cheap and it is often possible to make use of existing data that are routinely collected. Here we will introduce some of the major sources of data via selected national and international examples. The aim is to give you an idea of where to turn if you need to find specific types of health data, and also to look at some of their advantages and disadvantages.

The process of tracking down information has changed dramatically in recent years. The construction of the World Wide Web now allows instant access to mountains of data that previously mouldered in dusty reports of limited circulation. While there remains a vast array of paper-based resources, many are now mirrored by web-based electronic information. As an example, Figure 3.1 shows the wide range of information available through the World Health Organization (WHO) Statistical Information System (WHOSIS). (Note: the web addresses given throughout this chapter and elsewhere in the book are current as of early 2004 and, although most have been stable for some time, web addresses do change.)

A second change is the advance in computing technology which allows dramatic and informative visualisation of health data. For example, Figure 3.2, taken from the website of the National Center for Injury Prevention and Control (www.cdc.gov/ncipc; CDC, 2001) shows the variation in suicide rates across the USA. The new computing flexibility and lesser reliance on hard-copy publications

WHO Statistics

World Health
Organization

WHO Statistical Information System (WHOSIS)

Evidence and Information for Health Policy

The WHO Statistical Information System is the guide to health and health-related epidemiological and statistical information available from the World Health Organization. Most WHO technical programmes make statistical information available, and they will be linked from here. You also have the possibility to search by keywords within the WHOSIS or throughout the entire WHO site.

- *Look for these dots indicating downloads and links*
- *Search throughout WHO*
- *Search within WHOSIS*
- *Frequently Asked Questions*

Summary of contents (in alphabetical order)...

Burden of Disease Project | Burden of Disease statistics | Contacting the WHOSIS | Evidence for Health Policy | External sources for health-related statistical information | Genomics and World Health | Global Alcohol Database | Health Systems Performance | Health Personnel | HIV/AIDS | Immunization statistics | International Classifications and Terminology | Links to National Health-Related Websites | Maternal mortality | Micronutrient Deficiency Information System (MDIS) | Minimum Date Set on Ageing | Population statistics | Regional and Member States

Contents:

- **Severe Acute Respiratory Syndrome (SARS)**

  A web page has been created to provide the public and professionals information about Severe Acute Respiratory Syndrome (SARS). The site will be updated daily to ensure that the most current information is available.

- **Burden of Disease statistics**

  Statistical measures relating to the burden of disease, and the Burden of Disease project. Includes: Healthy Life Expectancy (HALE); Life Expectancy; Discussion Papers and methodology.

- **WHO Mortality Database**

  Data on registered deaths by age group, sex, year and cause of death for individual Member States.

- **Statistical annexes of the World Health Report**

  The Statistical Annexes of the World Health Report (in English, French and Spanish). Basic health indicators, deaths, burden of disease, healthy life expectancy, national health accounts, etc. downloadable as PDF or Excel files.

- **Statistics by disease or condition**

  Links to statistical information available throughout WHO'S technical programmes, Organized by disease, condition or topic.

- **Health Personnel**

  WHO estimates of numbers of doctors, dentists and nurses, by Member State.

- **External sources for health-related statistical information**

  External sources for health and health-related statistical and epidemiological information.

- **Population statistics**

Fig. 3.1 The WHO Statistical Information System (www3.who.int/whosis/menu, December 2003).

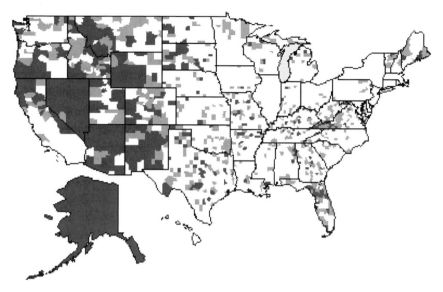

Fig. 3.2 Variation in suicide rates across the USA, 1989–1998, age-standardised to the 1940 US population: black, $\geq 17.5/10^5$ per year (top 10%); grey, 14.9–17.4/10^5 per year; white, $< 14.9/10^5$ per year. (CDC, 2001, accessed through www.cdc.gov/ncipc/on 21 April 2004.)

also make it easier to obtain customised data sets from health authorities, although there will often be a price attached. As an example of what is possible, *CDC Wonder* from the US Centers for Disease Control and Prevention (http://wonder.cdc.gov/) allows access to many data portals, and enables construction of a range of data sets of your own choice. (This was the source of the data on US mortality trends shown in Figures 1.7 and 1.8.). Don't get carried away by the technology just yet, though – if you don't know what you are looking at you can misinterpret the results wildly.

Which data?

Before embarking on a data hunt we first need to decide exactly *what* it is we want to know and this can pose a challenge. If we did want to know about youth suicide, are we interested in the suicide mortality rate, the number of hospitalisations for attempted suicide, or the proportion of teenagers who have considered killing themselves? Mortality data are probably readily available from a number of sources, but the accuracy of the underlying certification of this cause of death is known to be rather problematic. Hospital admission data are also often quite accessible, but might not capture suicide attempts that are dealt with in the emergency room and not admitted. Furthermore, separating individuals from events can be tricky – are a lot of youths making a single suicide attempt each or are there a smaller number who have made multiple attempts? The policy implications are quite different. In contrast, finding out about the prevalence (or cumulative incidence) of suicidal ideation will most probably need a special survey: it is important but you cannot easily 'look it up'.

Table 3.1 Some common health data collection or reporting systems and their primary data elements.

Data collection or reporting system	Primary information sources and information
Vital statistics (mortality)	Death certificates: death, cause, date and demographics[a]
Disease registries (e.g., cancer morbidity, mortality and survival; injuries)	Pathology reports, laboratories, hospital and medical records: diagnosis, date and demographics
Notifiable diseases (e.g., AIDS, SARS, TB, other infectious diseases, cancer)	Laboratories, practitioners and hospitals: diagnosis, date and demographics
Administrative systems (morbidity)	Hospital discharge sheets: diagnosis, date and demographics
Health surveys (morbidity, risk factors, needs, service use, etc.)	Surveys (often of population samples): usually self-reported states, sometimes examinations
Special surveillance systems	Varied: 'sentinel' primary care practices or disease registers (UK GP data base), MONICA (international CHD)
Rapid community assessments (health, nutrition)	Special surveys (sometimes of targeted groups)

[a]Basic demographic information such as age, sex and last known address.

Raw health data

Data can be accessed at two levels: the summary data – often rates in their various forms which you met in Chapter 2 – and the raw counts of health events from which the rates are calculated. Since it is the latter that determine the quality and usefulness of the former, we will deal with them first, noting some of their advantages and disadvantages as we go. Table 3.1 summarises some of the most common collection and reporting systems and the sources from which they take their information.

Mortality

As we noted in Chapter 2, many routine statistics are based on mortality data because they are generally easier to obtain and more reliable than morbidity data – but that does not mean that they are perfect . . .

Death certificates

Death certificates are a widely used primary source of information, and the basis for most reported mortality rates. They often contain additional basic demographic information about an individual, including name, date of birth, ethnicity and gender, as well as the date and cause(s) of death. Figure 3.3 shows an example of a typical form.

It is a common legal requirement that a medical practitioner complete a death certificate for someone who dies. The completion of a death certificate therefore

Medical Certificate of the Cause of Death

To the Registrar-General

I hereby certify that [   ]

(name in full)

aged [   ] years, date of birth __/__/__ who usually resided at

[   ] Postcode [   ] was attended and last

seen by me on __/__/__ (or by* Dr. [   ] on __/__/__

*if not attended by certifying medical practitioner within 3 months prior to death, insert name of medical practitioner who last attended deceased and date)

and I am informed that he/she died on __/__/__ at [   ]

(town, place etc of death)

Cause of Death (print clearly and do not abbreviate)

Duration of last illness

Disease or condition directly leading to death
(This means the disease, injury or complication which caused death – NOT ONLY, for example, the mode of dying such as 'heart failure', 'asphyxia', etc)

1a [   ] [   ]

due to, or as a consequence of

1b [   ] [   ]

due to, or as a consequence of

Antecedent causes - *morbid conditions, if any giving rise to the above cause, stating the underlying condition last*

1c [   ] [   ]

due to, or as a consequence of

1d [   ] [   ]

Other significant conditions
Contributing to the death, but not related to the diseases or condition causing it

2 [   ] [   ]

Date and type of operation in the last 4 weeks __/__/__ [   ]

Was a Coroner consulted before issuing this certificate?

No, death not subject to the provisions of the Coroners Act [   ]

Yes, issue of this certificate agreed to by [   ] , Coroner

Signature of Medical Practitioner [   ] Date __/__/__

Initials and Surname (BLOCK Letters) [   ]

Professional Qualifications [   ]

Fig. 3.3 A typical death certificate.

establishes the *fact* that someone has died with virtual certainty. Unfortunately, death certificates are less accurate when the *cause* of death is of interest, rather than the simple fact that death has occurred. This can be a consequence either of misdiagnosis (e.g., if a doctor does not know a person's full medical history) or of mis-specification on the form. The sample certificate shows the challenge of getting the sequence and content right. Look at the instructions on completing the 'cause of death' section: it will often not be easy, and those dying at older ages tend to have a number of coexisting diseases. How should the practitioner sequence the diagnoses of an overweight woman who has had diabetes for 20 years and high blood pressure for 10 years and who dies of pneumonia 1 year after suffering a stroke? Such a scenario is not uncommon, so we can be left with considerable uncertainty about the actual cause of death even on inspection of the original form. Indeed, in research studies where people are followed up for mortality, considerable extra effort often needs to be made in collecting clinical and pathology records in order to ensure accuracy in assigning cause of death. This can never be the case for routine vital statistics collections (it is far too expensive), so reports of mortality rates based on death certificates need to be used circumspectly. Generally only a single cause is extracted from the death certificate for each person who has died, that which is thought to be *underlying* any subsequent conditions. Multiple cause of death coding has recently been introduced in some countries but, while this may alleviate the problem of coding multiple conditions, it introduces another – the question of how to report and use the extra information.

What explanations can you think of for the sudden change in diabetes mortality in the USA over time shown in Figure 3.4? Which do you think is most likely?

We saw in Chapter 1 (Figures 1.7 and 1.8) that US death rates for a number of causes have been declining over time, but none as dramatically as seen here in Figure 3.4, where the mortality rate for diabetes appeared to halve between 1948 and 1949 before plateauing at the new level. This *could* be due to a spectacular new treatment (but insulin is still the mainstay, as it was in the 1940s), or to fewer cases of diabetes occurring (but no good means of preventing diabetes has been identified). So we are forced to consider artefacts in the data as a possible explanation. Here the dramatic shift in diabetes mortality was due to a coding change in the International Classification of Diseases (ICD), such that, when diabetes and coronary heart disease occurred together, diabetes was no longer listed as the underlying cause.

Not surprisingly, some diseases are recorded more accurately on death certificates than others. One that is rapidly fatal is likely to be clear cut, whereas with a long-term disease there is more chance of another illness occurring and being recorded on the death certificate instead. For example, many people like the woman above would not have diabetes recorded anywhere on their death certificates.

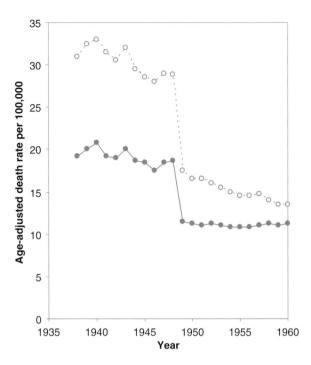

Fig. 3.4 Age-adjusted mortality rates for diabetes by gender in the USA, 1938–1960, Whites only. Figure 3-2, p. 51, from *Methods in Observational Epidemiology*, 2nd Edition, by Jennifer L. Kelsey, W. Douglas Thompson and Alfred S. Evans, copyright 1996 by Oxford University Press, Inc. Used by permission of Oxford University Press, Inc.

Similarly, diseases that are easily diagnosed tend to be more accurately recorded than those that require more complex diagnostic procedures: in the absence of an autopsy (autopsies are now uncommon), death from a motor vehicle accident would clearly be easier to recognise than one from pancreatic cancer. In an Australian study it was found that the overall accuracy of death certificates was only 77% compared with autopsy records, although cancers were accurately reported in 90% of cases (Maclaine *et al.*, 1992). A similarly high concordance for cancers was found in a UK study linking death certificates and hospital records, but chronic diseases such as diabetes and hypertension were listed as an underlying cause only about half of the time (Goldacre, 1993).

Diseases with a stigma attached may also be under-reported because of a reluctance to record the information. This might be either because of the potential stigma attached to the patient, as in the case of a death from suicide or HIV/AIDS, or because of the possibility that blame might be attached to the physician. The UK research found that conditions generally regarded as 'avoidable' causes of death were frequently omitted from the death certificate; for, example fractured neck of femur (broken hip) in the elderly was recorded in only one-quarter of cases.

Developed countries are now increasingly establishing national registers of deaths, recording both the date and the cause of death as well as key sociodemographic descriptors such as age, sex and last known address. Some of the earliest national death registries were in Scandinavia, for example Statistics Sweden (www.scb.se) provides life expectancy data back to 1750! The UK National Health Service Central Register was started in 1939 to facilitate the issue of ration books during World War II (www.gro-scotland.gov.uk), while the National Death Index in the USA (www.cdc.gov/nchs) contains information on deaths from 1979 and its Australian counterpart (www.aihw.gov.au/cancer/ndi) has information from 1980. These registries can provide information about numbers of deaths by cause, age, sex, etc., and some also have facilities to allow researchers to obtain death information for specific individuals in their studies.

Morbidity

Morbidity data provide a much greater challenge than mortality data. The scope of information is enormous and little is captured in a systematic way. As a result it is rarely simple to obtain complete information at a local level, and the problems escalate dramatically when trying to make comparisons between regions or countries. Having said that, attempts are made to record some aspects of morbidity in a routine way and these sources can provide valuable information.

Disease registries

Various disease registries exist (or have existed) to meet local health or research needs, but they cover only a small minority of conditions. For example, when it was noted that mortality from coronary heart disease (CHD) had started to fall in some countries in the late 1960s, it was not obvious what was driving this. Cardiologists of course claimed that better treatment in the newly introduced coronary care units meant that fewer patients were dying (lower case fatality). It was also possible that the number of new cases (incidence) was falling due to recent changes in smoking and dietary patterns, but no directly relevant data were available to clarify the public health debate. The WHO responded in the early 1980s by encouraging the establishment of a series of registers around the world to capture international trends in CHD incidence (the MONICA programme). These provided a wealth of data on CHD incidence, risk factors and mortality (Tunstall-Pedoe *et al.*, 1999), leading to the conclusion that both falling incidence and better clinical outcomes had contributed to the drop in death rates. Their job done, however, most have now ceased active monitoring.

Cancer is the only disease group for which good morbidity data are widely and routinely available. Some countries, most notably in Scandinavia, have cancer registries that cover the whole country and have been operating for many decades. In others such 'population-based' registries are newer and less well-established or, as in the USA, cover only part of the population. Coverage is generally increasing, however, and a wealth of data on incidence, mortality and survival is available at regional, national and international levels. In some jurisdictions cancer is a legally notifiable disease, whereas in others (e.g., the UK) comprehensive case ascertainment has come about gradually due to a combination of enthusiastic local registries and increasing awareness of the value of good morbidity data for planning and evaluating services. Cancer is an ideal candidate for such monitoring due to its relatively clear-cut diagnosis, which is usually based on a single simple record (a pathology report of histology). Rapid advances in technology now allow much of this information to be transferred electronically from the pathologist to the registry.

Many health authorities also keep registers of notifiable infectious diseases, although a prime purpose is for real-time surveillance to allow rapid response to emerging epidemics. Data for these registers usually come from medical practitioners and pathology laboratories, often under legal compunction. Despite this, and in contrast to cancers, most such diseases are poorly reported. Exceptions are those conditions which are perceived to be more severe, presenting either an acute challenge to a health system (SARS, AIDS) or a long-standing threat, such as tuberculosis. We will cover the issue of surveillance in more detail in Chapter 4.

Hospital records

Hospital records can provide useful information on major morbidity, although many hospitals are only just starting to computerise their records and it may be necessary to go through individual files by hand to collect the required information (which is clearly not suitable for 'routine' collection). The available data are usually based on discharge diagnoses as recorded and coded on the patient's record, and should be fairly reliable, although varying degrees of misdiagnosis, mis-recording and mis-coding are inevitable. It is also important to consider whether data obtained from a hospital will be representative of the general population or whether any conclusions will be restricted to the specific individuals from whom the data were obtained. This depends to a large extent both on the disease of interest and on the hospital. For diseases such as heart attacks and many cancers that almost always require hospitalisation, hospital records may provide good information on the levels of disease in the community. For conditions commonly treated outside hospital, however, the hospital-based population will not be typical: rather, it will be biased towards those with more severe disease, or towards those groups of society more likely to be hospitalised. A further limitation occurs where there is no unique patient identifier because aggregate admissions will be greater than the number of people admitted to hospital (because some will go to hospital more than once). Choosing the right numerator for a morbidity rate then becomes a challenge. Finally, most hospital data systems have no information at all regarding the vast majority of community morbidity which is treated by family practitioners or in the home.

Fig. 3.5 The prevalence of diagnosed diabetes (self-reported) in the USA, 2003, by age group and sex (dark bars, males; light bars, females). (*Source:* early release data from 2003 National Health Interview Survey, www.cdc.gov/nchs/nhis.htm, accessed 9 April 2004.)

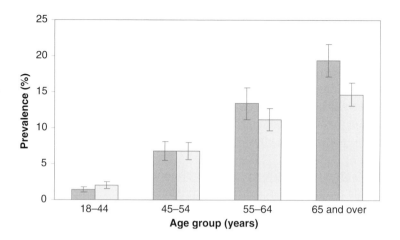

Health surveys

Spot checks on the health of a nation or region are crucial to expanding our understanding of health burdens, needs and services beyond the hospital sector. In recent decades they have become a feature of broad-based community diagnosis and health planning, using a wide range of sampling and data-capture designs. These include telephone and face-to-face interviews, and sometimes very detailed physical examinations, as in the US National Health and Nutrition Examination Surveys (NHANES I, 1973). This series was initiated in 1971, with over 30,000 people carefully selected to reflect the multi-faceted population, and it has given rich descriptions of many prevalent conditions. Such undertakings are, however, very expensive and value has sensibly been added to NHANES by using the data as baseline information for follow-up studies to identify risk factors for subsequent morbidity (requiring further personal contact) and mortality (via centrally held death records in the US National Death Index). Figure 3.5 shows some contemporary data, which will be important for future healthcare planning, drawn from a parallel series of US Health Interview Surveys.

How is the prevalence of diabetes related to age and sex?

What additional data are needed for a comprehensive planning response?

We see that, in 2003, the proportion of diabetics in US men and women rose markedly with age, affecting almost 20% of men and 15% of women over the age of 64 years. This is already a very heavy case load to manage: diabetes is a metabolic disease with many consequences, including heart and kidney damage, and adequate numbers of doctors, nutritionists and podiatrists must be provided and their care integrated. For a better view of the future we need to know time trends both in diabetes and for its risk factors. This information indicates that a major challenge is coming: the US population is ageing and also becoming more obese (a major risk factor for diabetes), so on both counts the number of cases will continue to rise.

The legend of Figure 3.5 indicates a central quality issue for many such surveys: their common reliance on self-reporting. Where reasonably accurate knowledge of disease prevalence is sought a variety of strategies can be employed to improve accuracy. In the above example respondents were asked to report only *doctor-diagnosed* diabetes. For conditions such as cancer or stroke, they may be asked whether they went to hospital or a subset, as in NHANES, may be examined to validate self-reporting for an array of conditions. For some factors, such as medication use, frequency of troublesome symptoms and visits to the doctor, choice of the time span for recall can be critical: use of shorter periods (e.g., 2–4 weeks) increases reliability but will miss less frequent events.

Rapid assessments are, as the name suggests, health surveys conducted when low-cost answers are required in a hurry, for example to justify development programmes in needy populations where baseline health data may be sparse. Although their validity has been questioned, the all-too-common combination of limited resources, rapidly changing situations and the need for 'some' information has ensured that they have persisted. At the time of writing, such data are not always accessible to those outside public health units, but we mention them here because the trend is towards increasing openness, accountability and availability of data in the future.

Confidentiality

We cannot end any section on health data without touching on the issue of confidentiality. Much of the available health data is recorded anonymously so that it is impossible to identify specific individuals, and these data can be made freely (or at least readily) available. To gain access to data on individuals it will almost certainly be necessary to sign a confidentiality agreement, have permission from a Human Research Ethics Committee and/or obtain consent from individual patients and sometimes their physicians as well before you can be given access to the material you want. Rapidly changing and expanding privacy legislation in many countries is adding to the challenges. While properly highlighting ethical use of data, the increasing emphasis on the principle of autonomy has created tensions between the need to protect personal information on the one hand and the desire for public good, which may require some access to individual data, on the other.

Summary health data

As you saw in Chapter 2, the raw health data are not particularly informative on their own. Their value comes when they are combined with population data to calculate measures of incidence and prevalence that can then be compared with pre-defined standards or rates in populations in other countries, for different time periods, etc. Traditionally, and this is still the norm, the most used (and useful) measures of health (or, more usually, ill-health) are those collected and reported at national and regional levels for internal planning and evaluation, and these statistics predominate.

As you will see below, there are many such sources of data on mortality, morbidity and other factors relevant to health and, inevitably, these are of varying reliability, quality and completeness. This is true not only across different countries (note that our emphasis here is on the better-developed data systems), but also within any country, since all public data sets will have some problems, and some of them will have many. Any comparisons should be made only with a good understanding of the accuracy and completeness of the raw data underlying the summary rates.

Gaining access to the data

This section cannot be comprehensive but it should give you a sense of the sorts of material that are available. We have given specific directions to some of the major electronic sources of data from Australia, Canada, New Zealand, the UK and the USA, but most other countries provide similar information and an internet search would lead to them. One thing to remember, however, is that the data will almost certainly have been collected for a reason other than your question of interest and therefore might not be in the ideal form for your purpose. For example, the definition of who is a 'case' might not fit your criteria exactly; the data could have been collected for age groups that do not correspond to those you want to know about, and so on. It is always important to balance these disadvantages against the major advantage of using existing data – someone else has already done the hard work.

International sources

At an international level, two incredibly rich sources of information are the WHO and the World Bank.
- The WHO publishes the *Weekly Epidemiological Record* and the annual *World Health Report* (amongst other things) and electronic copies of both are available free of charge through the WHO website (http://www.who.int). The WHO Regional Offices (Europe, Africa, etc.) also have their own sites, which are accessible through the main WHO site. They provide access to local data and an array of regional statistics, health reports and information, for example an assessment of the *Health Situation in the South-East Asia Region, 1998–2000* (available through the SE Asia Office at http://w3.whosea.org) and the European 'Health for All' Database (www.euro.who.int/HFADB).
- The World Bank site (http://www.worldbank.org) provides access to a wide range of health and economic indicators for countries and regions around the

Box 3.1 E-data – selected health departments and national statistics agencies

Australian Bureau of Statistics (http://www.abs.gov.au)

Australian Institute of Health & Welfare (AIHW) (http://www.aihw.gov.au)

New Zealand Ministry of Health, Health Information Service
 (http://www. nzhis.govt.nz)

Statistics Canada (http://www.statcan.ca)

UK Office of National Statistics (ONS) (http://www.statistics.gov.uk)

US Centers for Disease Control and Prevention (CDC) (http://www.cdc.gov)

US National Center for Health Statistics (NCHS) (http://www. cdc.gov/nchs)

US National Institutes of Health (NIH) (http://www.nih.gov)

 Contains links to the 28 separate institutes, centres and offices that make up the NIH, covering areas from child health to ageing; alcoholism to drug abuse; and allergy through deafness and eye diseases to cancer, diabetes and circulatory diseases.

US Census Bureau (http://www.census.gov)

 This site includes a comprehensive listing of other statistical agencies around the world.

world. It includes summary health data along with social, development and environmental statistics.

National data sources

Of particular value for the generalist can be publications that aim to capture the 'healthiness' of a nation or region. These often address contemporary issues via a combination of helpful and readily interpretable data, provide informed comment on implications for disease control, and may include evaluations of the positive and negative features of the health system which contribute to the nation's current 'diagnosis'. Some excellent examples that are accessible on-line (see Box 3.1 for web addresses) include

- *Australia's Health*; a biennial publication from the Australian Institute of Health and Welfare (AIHW);
- *Health, United States*; from the US National Center for Health Statistics (NCHS); and
- *UK Health Statistics Quarterly*; from the Office for National Statistics (ONS) and available through their 'virtual bookshelf'.

Other good sources of national data are the agencies in many countries that publish core health statistics, as well as demographic and other population data.

Box 3.2 E-data – disease-specific sites

Cancer

European Network of Cancer Registries (http://www.encr.com.fr/)

International Agency for Research on Cancer (IARC) (http://www.iarc.fr)

US National Cancer Institute (NCI) (http://www.nci.nih.gov/)

US Surveillance, Epidemiology and End Results (SEER) Program of
  the NCI (http://seer.cancer.gov/)

Cardiovascular disease

Global Cardiovascular Infobase available through the WHO Collaborating Centre
  for Surveillance of Cardiovascular Diseases (http://www.cvdinfobase.ca/)

Infectious diseases

Weekly Epidemiological Record (WER) from the WHO
  (http://www.who.int/wer/en/)

Morbidity and Mortality Weekly Reports (MMWR) from the US CDC
  (http://www.cdc.gov/mmwr/)

Disease-based resources

In addition to the sources listed above and in Box 3.1 there are many sites, both national and international, dedicated to specific diseases or conditions. Some of the best known are listed in Box 3.2.

Some academic and other idiosyncratic sites

Other sites that can provide a helpful starting point for a search include the following:

- The *University of California (San Francisco)* maintains a site that provides access to a wide range of epidemiology and public health-related sites (http://www. epibiostat.ucsf.edu/epidem/epidem.html).
- *Martindale's Public Health Center* has a wide-ranging and eclectic site with many data links (http://www.martindalecenter.com). (Unfortunately this site no longer includes surf and snow reports!).
- The *American Public Health Association* also has a site with multiple data and other 'public health links' (http://www.apha.org/).
- *SUMSearch* is an internet search tool designed to automate searching for medical evidence (http://sumsearch.uthscsa.edu/).

As the above references imply, today the starting point for a search for health information is the World Wide Web. You have seen the incredible array of data directly accessible through sites such as the WHO website (Figure 3.1). Additionally many of the sites listed here provide links to a broader set of data-providers worldwide, some of whom will offer a similar set of cross-links, and so on. Many of the figures in this book come directly from readily available electronic sources such as these.

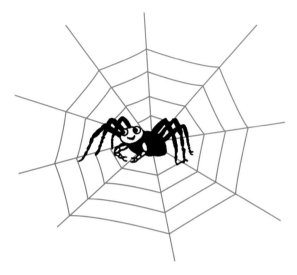

REFERENCES

CDC (Centers for Disease Control and Prevention). (2001). Injury mortality maps of the United States, 1989–1998. Atlanta, GA: CDC.

Goldacre, M. J. (1993). Cause-specific mortality: understanding uncertain tips of the disease iceberg. *Journal of Epidemiology and Community Health*, **47**: 491–496.

Kelsey, J. L., Thompson, W. D. and Evans, A. S. (1986). *Methods in Observational Epidemiology*. Oxford, Oxford University Press.

Maclaine, G. D., Macarthur, E. B. and Heathcote, C. R. (1992). A comparison of death certificates and autopsies in the Australian Capital Territory. *Medical Journal of Australia*, **156**: 462–463, 466–468.

NHANES I. (1973). Plan and operation of the health and nutrition examination survey: United States 1971–1973. *Vital Health Statistics*, **1**: 1–77.

Powers, J. 1995. *Pooh's Little Book of Instructions*. © 1995 the Trustees of the Pooh properties. Inspired by the text of A. A. Milne and illustrations of E. H. Shepard from *Winnie the Pooh and The House at Pooh Corner*. London: Egmont Books Limited.

Tunstall-Pedoe, H., Kuulasmaa, K., Mahonen, M., *et al.* for the WHO MONICA. (1999). Contribution of trends in survival and coronary event rates to changes in coronary heart disease mortality: 10-year results from 37 WHO MONICA populations. *Lancet*, **353**: 1547–1557.

4

Watching not waiting: surveillance and epidemiological intelligence

Box 4.1 Identification of the 2002–2003 SARS epidemic

November 2002: two GOARN (Global Alert and Response Network) partners, the WHO Global Influenza Surveillance Network and the US Global Emerging Infections Surveillance and Response System, noted media reports of influenza in China.

December 2002: an influenza B epidemic was virologically confirmed by Chinese authorities. In retrospect those early media reports were probably also the first indication of SARS, which also erupted at that time as seemingly unrelated clusters of atypical pneumonia in the south of China (atypical pneumonia is common in that region each winter).

20 February, 2003: Hong Kong confirmed two human cases of much-feared avian influenza (H5N1). This was soon after the Chinese government had reported that the atypical pneumonia had been unusually lethal in many cases.

21 February, 2003: just as the WHO prepared for an influenza pandemic, a Chinese doctor was admitted to a local Hong Kong hospital; staff adopted strict precautions against bird influenza but he had already infected several people at the hotel he occupied the night before. They spread the virus to other hospitals, the Hong Kong community, Canada, Vietnam and Singapore.

12 March, 2003: GOARN had gathered enough data from those countries and Hong Kong for the WHO to issue its first global alert.

15 March, 2003: the disease was given the name severe acute respiratory syndrome (SARS). GOARN then linked laboratory scientists, clinicians and epidemiologists all over the world.

July 2003: the causative agent, incubation period, infectious period and usual modes of transmission had been determined, good diagnostic tests and surveillance and control programmes had been devised and implemented, and human transmission ceased.

(From Heyman and Rodier, 2003.)

Without information on our ever-changing health problems, public health is paralysed. In this chapter we discuss the design and use of the special information systems that allow health officials to detect new risks and diseases, track old problems, and generate data needed for health planning and allocating resources. This is the population health surveillance system. It is complex in practice but simple in its aims – to generate timely and useful information on the occurrence of health events. It covers infections, chronic diseases and injuries, as well as many of the exposures known to cause ill-health. It is inter-connected within and among regions and has grown much more accessible since the advent of the Internet. Surveillance is the eyes (and ears) of public health and is its most important sensory organ.

The word surveillance, meaning 'the constant watching of subversives', came into use during the time of the Napoleonic wars. The modern epidemiological meaning is consistent with the idea of constant watching, but usually of diseases rather than suspects. However, surveillance of people does still occur for public health purposes; for example, close contacts of infectious persons who have been isolated (or quarantined) to interrupt community transmission are observed until the end of the incubation period for that infection. Similarly, those emerging from a zone with an ongoing epidemic may be monitored; for example, the temperature (thermal screening) and respiratory symptom checks (by questionnaire) of travellers moving in and out of Hong Kong during the SARS epidemic in 2003. During that epidemic even high-rise apartment buildings were placed under watch in Hong Kong if two or more cases of SARS occurred.

Dynamic surveillance data on population risks, morbidity and mortality are the key indicators for epidemiological intelligence on community health. When surveillance data vary from the expected they may provide a justification for investing in basic or strategic research to respond to the anomalies. Surveillance is used to detect outbreaks of new or old diseases and, over recent years, has increasingly been recognised as a crucial component of national and global defences against catastrophic epidemics. Globally, regionally and locally, it also provides evidence and data for health planning and evaluation. Surveillance detects and quantifies the occurrence of important or potentially important health risks or outcomes, revealing their distribution, incidence and prevalence. For many infections (such as HIV/AIDS, TB, malaria, meningitis and dengue) local and regional transmission rates are of central interest in deciding whether to activate and justify control programmes or to monitor their effects. For other infections (such as new strains of influenza) the surveillance data lead to rapid global responses.

A definition of surveillance that incorporates the essentials is the following.

Surveillance is the continuous monitoring of the occurrence and distribution of diseases and other conditions of ill-health, and their determinants, for their effective control and prevention. It includes the collection, analysis and interpretation of relevant data and the distribution of information to all who need to know.

The essential features of a surveillance system are practical, clear case definitions for each disease; workable, uniform and continuous data collection methods; and rapidity of collection, analysis, interpretation and dissemination of data. Ultimately, the purpose of surveillance is disease control and prevention. Practical intermediate goals include identifying and monitoring outbreaks, limiting transmission of infectious agents, prompt treatment of illness, evaluation of disease control programmes and planning health services.

The scope of surveillance

Traditionally the term surveillance has been applied to monitoring acute infectious diseases, but its scope has widened substantially. Today, surveillance also covers morbidity and mortality for many non-infectious diseases (e.g., congenital malformations, injuries and cancer); hospital discharges; use of vaccines and prescription drugs and their adverse reactions; and even environmental hazards in the workplace and the general environment (air, water, soil). In addition, health information systems are beginning to extend surveillance to risk factors themselves, an interest reinforced by *The World Health Report* in 2002 which highlighted the need to reduce risks in order to lower the avoidable burden of disease. The WHO identified the ten leading risk factors accounting for over one-third of all deaths worldwide: being underweight; unsafe sex; high blood pressure; tobacco consumption; alcohol consumption; unsafe water, sanitation and hygiene; iron deficiency; indoor smoke from solid fuels; high cholesterol level and obesity (WHO, 2002). It is not possible to tackle these risks without good surveillance to monitor their trends and distributions. Some of these are monitored by specialised units while others are rolled into general health service information collections.

At the same time as a risk-oriented re-focussing has occurred in public health, there has been growing awareness (or rediscovery) of the role of poverty and other fundamental social determinants of health. The last decade of active research on social epidemiology has brought the concern with health inequities into the consideration of many health ministries. Surveillance and geo-social mapping of these socioeconomic trends is in its infancy but is growing quickly. This development involves partnerships between the health and social service sectors, as well as with national statistics offices and treasuries, information technologists and statisticians.

The most developed surveillance systems are to be found in the USA. There the Centers for Disease Control and Prevention (CDC) provide an excellent example of integrated disease surveillance. Their website (http://www.cdc.gov/scientific.htm) lists many surveillance activities, related scientific data (e.g., injury maps and information on hazardous materials), health statistics (including the National Center for Health Statistics database) and up-to-date laboratory information on

Box 4.2 CDC (USA) Surveillance Programmes

121 Cities Mortality Reporting System
Assisted Reproductive Technology Success Rates
Behavioral Risk Factor Surveillance System
Birth Defects Surveillance
Cancer Registries Programme
HIV/AIDS Surveillance Report
National Notifiable Diseases Surveillance System (NNDSS)
National Oral Health Surveillance System
Pediatric Nutrition Surveillance System (PedNSS)
Pregnancy Nutrition Surveillance System (PNSS)
Pregnancy Risk Assessment Monitoring System
Sexually Transmitted Diseases
Surveillance Resources (infectious diseases)
Tuberculosis Surveillance Reports
Workplace Safety and Health Surveillance
Youth Risk Behavior Surveillance System

(From http://www.cdc.gov/scientific.htm#survey.)

disease organisms. Sixteen surveillance programme categories were listed in March 2004 (Box 4.2).

The CDC integrates surveillance with its Public Health Information Network (PHIN) and uses on-line methods to enhance the system. The latest initiative is called the National Electronic Disease Surveillance System (NEDSS) (http://www.cdc.gov/nedss/) and it promotes integrated systems at federal, state and local levels. This will monitor the health of the nation, detect outbreaks rapidly, simplify electronic transfer of information from clinical to public health systems, make it easier to provide information, and boost the timeliness and quality of information.

The WHO is also a leading global agency for disease surveillance. It compiles global data and is the central resource for monitoring infectious diseases and detecting and reporting outbreaks. The WHO is especially important for helping resource-poor areas respond to epidemics. Since 1997 it has operated the Global Alert and Response Network (GOARN). This network includes 120 partners throughout the world and identifies and responds to over 50 national outbreaks per year in developing countries. It includes tracking of media reports in its surveillance strategies and has found that it is helpful to monitor and plot rumours of outbreaks as well as respond to reports from member countries or its network. The utility of GOARN for multi-country epidemics was revealed by the SARS emergency in 2003 (see Box 4.1 at the start of the chapter).

Notifiable diseases

What issues do you think should be considered before a disease is included on a notifiable list as a disease to be watched?

In the first instance, this is a matter of assigning a level of public health importance to a disease. When doing this, the first issue to be considered is the incidence of the disease (if it is of long duration, its prevalence might be more appropriate). How many people are affected and how many more are likely to be? How severe is the illness? What is its expected mortality? Infectivity? Other pertinent factors include the degree of preventability of the disease, the potential effects on productivity and medical costs, media exposure and political and economic costs. The recent global focus on the explosive SARS epidemic was driven by a powerful combination of its high case–fatality ratio, mysterious origins and cause, apparent rapidity of long-distance spread and the severe consequences for the travel industry.

Clearly, any schedule of notifiable diseases should be reviewed regularly. Are there new problems we need a handle on? Have laboratory advances meant that we need to review this or that case definition? Also, in a system that relies heavily on the co-operation of busy clinicians, is everything being done to maximise co-operation? This includes keeping the list of notifiable diseases as short as possible (in practice it seems to be a lot harder for a disease to 'leave' a list than to join it); using simple reporting forms or procedures (electronic forms are increasingly common); and giving timely feedback to show how the data collected are used to enhance health care.

Sometimes surveillance information is available within the health system but there is a slow response (or no response) or further dissemination is actually suppressed. Response failures have been shown to lead to much avoidable national morbidity and mortality for infections such as plague, cholera, Ebola haemorrhagic fever, West Nile virus and SARS. It is even worse when the infection spreads to multiple countries, or around the world. Early responses to outbreaks of lethal transmissible infections, or to diseases caused by new exposures to environmental toxins, may save many lives.

Types of surveillance

Surveillance systems essentially fall into three broad types, all of which may co-exist in any one geographical area or health system: active, passive and sentinel systems.

Active surveillance

This is based on specific collection of data from healthcare providers or institutions, both as a need arises and in the longer term. It is used, for example, during outbreaks of food-borne pathogens or measles when healthcare providers are contacted and asked to provide details of any cases they have seen. Laboratory data defining strains of prevalent organisms are used for forward planning (e.g., choosing the right influenza vaccine for the next winter epidemic); and knowledge of patterns of resistance to antibiotics can influence local choices of treatment for bacterial diseases. A further example is the requirement that hospitals provide data on all discharges. Expansion to non-infectious diseases has come with legal requirements to report incidence of cancers in many countries, establishing high-quality networks that permit research as well as monitoring (see Chapter 3).

Active surveillance may also include household surveys to detect ongoing transmission of infections. For example, this can be done serologically for malaria in at-risk areas if incidence rates are low and reports by health workers are unreliable. It may also be done for TB or schistosomiasis, by using skin tests to detect past infection, or for polio, by searching for floppy paralysis. In the latter example the detection of non-polio floppy paralysis at a minimum rate indicates that the surveillance system is working. Active surveillance may extend to environmental assessment for ongoing, reappearing or even new disease risks, including the presence or abundance of relevant vectors of infection such as specific species of mosquitoes or snails.

Active surveillance can produce more complete data of better quality than that provided by other systems. However, it is resource-intensive to maintain, especially to produce timely output of information. In those jurisdictions that permit it, and when the technology makes it feasible, active surveillance can be done using *record linkage* to link records from different sources to extract information that would otherwise be sought by passive surveillance systems. Examples include the use of clinical and treatment records to detect iatrogenesis (illness as a result of treatment by a physician), especially adverse reactions to drugs. This can be taken further by anticipating such events even before they occur (e.g., when potentially adversely interacting drugs are prescribed but before they are dispensed), so linking surveillance with prevention in a most direct manner.

Passive surveillance

As the name implies, a passive surveillance system depends on the discretion or whim of the healthcare provider, even where notification is required by law. Although a passive system is likely to be inexpensive, it will be less complete than an active system because not all events will be reported. An exception to this might be the reporting of a condition with a high level of media coverage at a particular time (e.g., SARS, dengue haemorrhagic fever, Ebola, haemolytic–uraemic syndrome and anthrax).

Media-driven alerts can also assist passive surveillance of non-infectious diseases. An example is the spectacular epidemic of eosinophilia–myalgia syndrome

Box 4.3 Polio eradication – surveillance and progress in India

By 2001, polio had largely been limited to two states in India, with only 268 new cases that year, but in 2002 there was a major resurgence with 1,600 new cases. In 2003, a network of 248 medical officers trained in surveillance assisted Indian health authorities with surveillance for acute flaccid paralysis (AFP), the critical clinical marker of polio. The WHO criteria for assessing the quality of polio surveillance require that

- *non-polio* AFP should be detected at a rate of ≥1 per 100,000 in the population aged <15 years (to ensure that 'background' AFP cases are being detected at a level showing good coverage) and
- adequate stool specimens should be collected from ≥80% of people with AFP for polio diagnosis.

India had been meeting these criteria since 2000, but in 2003 the non-polio AFP rate was <1/100,000 in seven small states and stool specimens were inadequate in 11 states (covering 35% of India's population). During 2002, the proportion of infants aged less than 1 year who received three or more routine doses of oral poliovirus vaccine was only 21% in some states. Vaccination increased again in 2003 and only 225 wild poliovirus cases were reported that year, the lowest level yet (Anonymous, 2004).

Post-marketing surveillance of the safety of the drug cimetidine

Almost 10,000 patients who took cimetidine (mostly for peptic ulcer) between 1977 and 1980 were followed for 15 years to observe their long-term health outcomes. The findings were reassuring, providing no evidence of any long-term adverse effects of cimetidine (at least not ones that could be detected by monitoring mortality rates). The data have also been used to examine the possible positive relationships between ingestion of aluminium and Alzheimer's disease, and *H. pylori* infection and ischaemic heart disease, but no significant relationships were found (Beresford *et al.*, 1998).

(a rare autoimmune disease) in the USA. Over 1,500 cases and more than 25 deaths were detected in 1989 and 1990. This painful and mysterious non-infectious condition was investigated epidemiologically by contacting many cases detected by the passive surveillance system. The cause was found to be the chemical composition of a single source of L-tryptophan, a common over-the-counter dietary supplement for which the method of manufacture had been altered just before the epidemic began (Jimenez and Varga, 1991).

Surveillance of the majority of notifiable diseases in many countries relies heavily on a passive system, whereby the diagnosing doctor initiates a report to the monitoring authority (although often only a minority of cases is actually reported). In addition, laboratories notify the authority when they come across an individual with any one of a specific set of diseases for which notification is required by law (including cancer as well as infectious diseases). These laboratory reports are likely to be much more complete than the primary-care-initiated reports.

Absolute figures from passive surveillance may underestimate the true illness burden. It is likely, however, that patterns and changes over time, across regions and among differing groups of people (age, sex, ethnicity) will still be informative. It is also possible to perform active surveillance in representative sub-sets of a passive-surveillance population and thus derive multipliers to convert the passive rates into more accurate estimates. Of course this is cheaper than a population-wide active surveillance system but it will miss small outbreaks and other sub-regional variation if those areas were not included in the active-surveillance samples.

Sentinel surveillance

Sentinel surveillance relies on the reporting of cases of specific diseases or risk factors that may indicate that a particular preventive or therapeutic activity is not working as planned. Examples of sentinel health events would include a case of poliomyelitis, which might indicate that there has been a breakdown in the vaccine cold chain (such that a batch of vaccine has not been stored correctly) or that vaccination coverage has fallen to a low level; or a case of mesothelioma linked to a past history of exposure to asbestos. In some countries (Australia and the UK to name two), there is also a network of sentinel primary care practices that report a number of diseases on a regular basis. Their list of diseases reported varies from year to year but typically includes things like influenza-like illnesses, culture-confirmed influenza, chickenpox and shingles. Sentinel surveillance of the staff in large hospitals that treat cases arising from an epidemic in the community can also be useful. For example, annual influenza trends among staff in large Hong Kong hospitals amplify early trends in the community and could be used as an early warning system, provided that the staff are not vaccinated against influenza (and many are not). Similarly, presentations of community-acquired pneumonia to such hospitals can be monitored to discern trends of respiratory illness in the community, detect unusual pathogens and track incidence rates for year-to-year comparisons and early detection of epidemics.

Surveillance in practice

Box 4.4 gives an example of the historical development and scope of a sophisticated use of several complementary data sources to plan, evaluate and update an evolving vaccination strategy for measles, mumps and rubella (MMR) in the UK.

Box 4.4 Surveillance of MMR (measles–mumps–rubella) in England and Wales

Methods of monitoring vaccine coverage

(i) Estimate *vaccine coverage* in 2- and 5-year olds (since 1960s for 2-year olds); done quarterly, using sentinel antigens with rapid feedback to immunisation services.

(ii) Introduce *statutory notification* of clinical measles (1940), mumps (1988) and rubella (1988).

(iii) Widespread *laboratory confirmation* of clinical reports (since 1994) – a critical addition because with the low prevalence <20% of clinical diagnoses were actually confirmed as cases (also genotyping for diagnosis and outbreak tracing).

(iv) *Antibody prevalence monitoring* of MMR (1986) in residues of general specimens submitted to public health laboratories; plus *sentinel laboratory monitoring* of rubella susceptibility in antenatal women (1984).

(v) Supplementation by other data sources: death certificates, hospital admissions, primary care surveillance of mumps (sentinel practices), and congenital abnormality surveillance for rubella.

Vaccine policy

Guided by modelling based on the above data and vaccine availability, delivery strategies moved through a number of stages:

1968: measles vaccine introduced (80% coverage by 1988);

1970: rubella vaccine introduced for schoolgirls and susceptible women (>95% protection of young adult women by 1988);

1988: combined MMR vaccination of infants commenced (plus initial catch-up for 2–4-year olds and selective vaccination of older females susceptible to rubella);

1994: one-off measles–rubella campaign in 5–16-year olds to head off possible measles epidemic and 'top up' rubella coverage;

1996: two-dose MMR strategy implemented (second dose before school entry).

(Vyse *et al.*, 2002.)

The original article (Vyse *et al.*, 2002) shows elegantly how each element has contributed to the increasingly subtle analyses required as vaccine coverage has improved, local disease rates have declined (causing more misdiagnosis), imported disease has increased and vaccine resistance has emerged in some population subgroups. Figure 4.1 shows the very positive overall disease trends, but the continuing challenge is to maintain and extend control of these diseases. The WHO is committed to eliminating measles as a global problem, but this will be difficult.

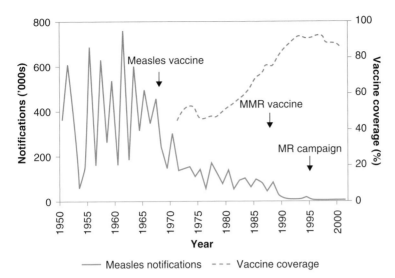

Fig. 4.1 Evolution of surveillance for measles, mumps and rubella in England and Wales: providing the platform for evidence-based vaccination policy. (From Vyse *et al.*, Evolution of surveillance of measles, mumps and rubella in England and Wales, *Epidemiologic Reviews*, 2002; 24: 125–136, by permission of Oxford University Press.)

Describe the overall pattern of measles occurrence. Comment on the likely role played by vaccination in its control.

We see a regular see-saw of epidemic peaks (with hundreds of thousands of extra cases) and troughs from 1950 through to the commencement of measles vaccination in 1968, although their amplitude was lessening somewhat. Thereafter there is an initial sharp drop in the number of notified cases (even though vaccine coverage expanded slowly at first), followed by a general pattern of steady decline interrupted by occasional peaks. The switch to MMR vaccination and extra coverage pushed notifications down sharply again towards zero (this would show better on a logarithmic scale); and the 1994 campaign does look as if it might have killed off a possible small epidemic. This is a very successful public health intervention that has required a lot of thought and hard work to implement.

Disease surveillance in Queensland, Australia – a regional example

As a fairly standard example of a practical overall surveillance scheme at a regional level, we describe below the Queensland (Australia) notifiable-diseases system. Queensland is a geographically large state (seven times the area of the UK) but has a population of only 3.7 million. Queensland Health currently conducts surveillance for over 50 diseases, primarily using passive surveillance based on combinations of clinical and laboratory notifications. Data are collated centrally and then disseminated for local action. Regular improvements to the underlying information technology aim to enhance the system's sensitivity, timeliness, uniformity and acceptability. Giving good feedback to clinicians and increasing their involvement in the process are also expected to add substantially to the system's quality. Some case studies give examples of the varied ways in which surveillance data are used, which are often a function of the nature, severity and frequency of the disease concerned.

> ***Hepatitis C.*** Most notifications are of chronic (i.e., prevalent) infections (acute clinical presentations are rare), so reported numbers give no idea of incidence. There is no active public health response to a notification, and the data are used for health planning only.

> ***Poliomyelitis.*** This is now a very rare disease (as in most developed countries). Apart from local needs, this viral illness is monitored as an element of the WHO programme to eradicate polio. There is enhanced surveillance seeking all cases of acute flaccid paralysis (clinical diagnosis) with very strict guidelines on laboratory samples and testing. There is a direct public health response to every case notified.

> ***Ross River virus.*** Queensland has large annual outbreaks of this often debilitating mosquito-spread viral illness. Actual notifications received are only a small proportion of cases, and there is a lag time in notification reflecting both the long incubation period of the disease and the time needed for confirmatory laboratory testing. The data are used for health planning, including responses at the community level (mosquito control), and in public awareness campaigns.

Within any regional health jurisdiction, useful contributions to health surveillance activities can come from many other types of information. This could include, for example, reports on climatic conditions, which would be of interest with respect to patterns of respiratory disease, mosquito-borne infections or even heat- or cold-induced thermal stress. Information on animal health is always an important component of regional public health surveillance. Contemporary examples include avian influenza, Q fever and leptospirosis – all subject to surveillance in animal populations. Historical examples in developed countries since World War II include surveillance for brucellosis, tuberculosis in dairy herds (to control human TB in the 1950s) and then tuberculosis in beef cattle (to protect abattoir workers). Today, meat inspection remains a very important component of all infectious-disease surveillance systems intended to protect human populations from zoonoses – infections that cross from animals to humans. Information from environmental health staff on potential infection vectors, and detailed data from special surveys and field investigations (including epidemics), also remain indispensable elements of modern surveillance.

International risk-factor surveillance

The above historical and typical regional examples of surveillance in practice are complemented by a look at recent developments in global surveillance under the leadership of the WHO. In 2003 the Non-Communicable Diseases and

Mental Health team at the WHO launched the first 'SuRF' report on Surveillance of Risk Factors related to non-communicable disease (http://www.who.int/ncd_surveillance/infobase/). This report assembles existing data on the prevalence of major risk factors related to non-communicable diseases for WHO member states for the first time. The information comes from the WHO Global NCD (non-communicable disease) Infobase. The eight risk factors reported make the major contribution to mortality and morbidity from chronic diseases, can be changed by primary interventions, and can be easily measured in populations. These factors are tobacco and alcohol use, patterns of physical inactivity, low fruit/vegetable intake, obesity, raised blood pressure, raised blood cholesterol level and diabetes. Future SuRF reports will contain harmonised estimates to enable comparisons between countries. Health planners will be able to track trends over time and across the globe and this will help identify the best focus for any preventive programmes aimed squarely at established or emerging chronic disease.

Evaluation of surveillance

Surveillance systems have (or should have) stated goals and objectives. These are the logical starting points for evaluations and the following attributes should be the focus.

1. *Is the system detecting what it is supposed to detect?*
   The surveillance system data need to be compared with data produced by another detection mechanism set up especially for the evaluation.
2. *Is the system producing data in time for appropriate responses?*
3. *Can the system cope with anomalies and changes?*
   The disease, or our knowledge of it (or both), may be changing quickly. A surveillance system should be able to adapt to such changes and should not rigidly adhere to outdated definitions or criteria. A good system needs to have a mechanism to enable such flexibility.
4. *Is the system as simple and cheap as possible?*
5. *Are the public health responses timely and appropriate?*
   Any system that does not lead to appropriate responses is flawed. Evidence that the responses are appropriate should be sought.

Summary

Surveillance is an important tool for public health and routine surveillance data are available in regular reports produced by national and international sources all over the world (we discussed some of these in the previous chapter). Any system that provides for the rapid collection, analysis and interpretation of data in order to prevent disease is highly valuable, but here is a word of caution from one of the world's pre-eminent epidemiologists, Sir Richard Doll. In an article on 'Surveillance and monitoring' (1974), he warned that 'It is almost as easy to be drowned in useless information as it is to be starved of essential elements.'

REFERENCES

Anonymous. (2004). Progress toward poliomyelitis eradication – India, 2003. *Morbidity Mortality Weekly Report*, **53**: 238–241.

Beresford, J., Colin-Jones, D. G., Flind, A. C. *et al.* (1998). Postmarketing surveillance of the safety of cimetidine: 15-year mortality report. *Pharmacoepidemiology and Drug Safety*, **7**: 319–322.

Doll, R. (1974). Surveillance and monitoring. *International Journal of Epidemiology*, **3**: 305–313.

Heyman, D. L. and Rodier, G. (2003). Global surveillance, national surveillance, and SARS. *Emerging Infectious Diseases*, **10**: 173–175. Available from www.cdc.gov/ncidod/EID/vol10no2/03-1038.htm

Jimenez, S. A. and Varga, J. (1991). The eosinophilia–myalgia syndrome and eosinophilic fasciitis. *Current Opinion in Rheumatology*, **3**: 986–994.

Vyse, A. J., Gay, N. J., White, M. E. *et al.* (2002). Evolution of surveillance of measles, mumps and rubella in England and Wales: providing the platform for evidence-based vaccination policy. *Epidemiologic Reviews*, **24**: 125–136.

WHO (World Health Organization). (2002). *The World Health Report 2002. Reducing Risks, Promoting Healthy Life*. Geneva: World Health Organization.

Why? Linking exposure and disease

Box 5.1 Who does all the housework?

His view: Australian men do **three times more** housework today than they
  did 40 years ago . . .
Her view: Australian men spend 5 minutes a day on laundry now compared
  to 1.6 minutes 40 years ago – an **extra 3½ minutes a day** . . .

(Maushart, 2003.)

One of the main uses of epidemiology is to identify the causes of disease and
this is of fundamental importance in all areas of public health – if we can work
out what is causing ill-health then we can work to prevent it. In Chapter 2 we
looked at the ways in which we can measure the occurrence of disease and
touched on some ways in which we can compare different populations. In this
chapter we will look more closely at the ways in which we look for associations
between 'exposures', or potential causes of disease, and the disease itself. An
understanding of these measures will help you to interpret epidemiological
reports regarding the causes of ill-health and the effects of particular exposures
or interventions on the burden of illness in a community. (Note that, while we
will discuss the measures in the context of an 'exposure' and 'disease', they can be
used to assess the association between any measure of health status and any
potential 'cause'.)

Measuring the occurrence of a disease in a population can tell us about the
health of that population but it does not directly shed much light on the underlying causes of the disease. To identify the aspects of people or their environment
(exposures) that might lead to the onset of disease, we need to *compare* disease
occurrence in groups with and without the exposures of interest. By measuring
the association between an exposure and disease we can start to make judgements as to whether the exposure might actually cause the disease (we will discuss causality in more detail in Chapter 10). If we believe that it is causing
disease, we can then identify the importance of that exposure in terms of its

overall effect on the health of a community. In this chapter we will look at the ways in which we calculate, use and interpret these measures.

Looking for associations

We all know that smoking is a cause of lung cancer but might it also increase the risk of stroke? To answer this question we could compare the incidence of stroke in a group of women who smoke with that in a group of non-smokers.

   Table 5.1 displays data from a cohort study in which the investigators followed a large group of women for several years (person-years of observation). They classified the women as never smokers, ex-smokers and current smokers, recorded how many women had a stroke during the follow-up period and calculated the *incidence rate* of stroke in each group.

How many **times more likely** was
(i)   a current smoker to have a stroke than a never smoker and
(ii) an ex-smoker to have a stroke than a never smoker?

Compared with non-smokers, how many **extra** strokes were there per 100,000 person-years in
(i)   ex-smokers and
(ii) current smokers?

There are two main ways in which we can compare smokers and non-smokers. First, ex-smokers were *1.6 times* (27.9 ÷ 17.7) and current smokers were *2.8 times* (49.6 ÷ 17.7) as likely to have a stroke as never smokers during the follow-up period. An alternative way to look at the data would be to say that, all other things being equal, if the smokers had never smoked we would have expected them to have

Table 5.1 Stroke incidence rates by smoking category in female nurses.

Smoking category	No. of cases of stroke	Person-years of observation	Incidence rate per 100,000 person-years
Never smoked	70	395,594	17.7
Ex-smoker	65	232,712	27.9
Current smoker	139	280,141	49.6
Total	274	908,447	30.2

(Colditz *et al.*, 1988.)

the same rate of stroke as the never smokers, i.e. 17.7/100,000 person-years. This means that, compared with never smokers, there were an *extra 10.2 strokes per 100,000 person-years* (27.9 − 17.7) in ex-smokers and an *extra 31.9 strokes per 100,000 person-years* (49.6 − 17.7) in current smokers.

What we calculated above were, first, the **rate ratio** and, second, the **rate difference** for the association between smoking and stroke. These measures give us two different ways of quantifying the relation between an exposure and a disease. The **rate ratio** tells us how many times higher the rate of disease is in one group than in another group. This gives an indication of the *strength* of the association and can help us to decide whether smoking could be a cause of stroke. The **rate difference** tells us how many extra strokes occurred among smokers. If we believe that smoking is a cause of stroke then this extra disease can be attributed to the fact that the women had smoked and, theoretically, it would not have occurred if they had never smoked. This information gives some sense of the potential value of a preventive intervention, in this case a programme aimed at stopping women from taking up smoking. (Of course, if such an intervention were successful it would reduce the incidence of many diseases, not just stroke.)

From www.CartoonStock.com

"What do you mean I never help out around the house - Right now I'm cleaning out the fridge!"

It is important to remember that ratio and difference measures give us very different perspectives on a given situation. Look back to Box 5.1 at the start of the chapter. Men would probably prefer to look at the **ratio** or **relative** measure: they do three times more housework now than 40 years ago. In contrast, women would focus on the **difference** or **absolute** measure: men may do three times more laundry now than 40 years ago but they still do an average of only 5 minutes (3.5 minutes extra) per day.

The measures that we use to compare populations in this way are often described as 'measures of association' because they describe the association between an exposure and a health outcome. They are calculated by comparing the frequencies of disease in two groups of people – one group of people who have been exposed to something (the potential cause) and a second 'unexposed' group.

Ratio measures (relative risk)

The cholera was therefore **fourteen times as fatal** at this period amongst persons having the impure water of the Southwark and Vauxhall Company, as amongst those having the purer water from Thames Ditton (Snow, 1855)

People who ate cold chicken at the youth camp were **almost four times more likely** to become ill than people who did not eat cold chicken (from Table 1.2)

Ratio or relative measures tell us how many times more likely it is that someone who is exposed to something will develop a certain disease or experience a particular health outcome than (or *relative* to) someone who is not exposed. *They do not tell us anything about the actual amount of disease occurring in either group.* They provide information about the *strength* of the association between the exposure and the outcome and, as you will see in Chapter 10, a strong association is more suggestive that the exposure is actually causing the outcome. For example, the rate ratio for stroke and current smoking was 2.8. This is a fairly strong association and would add weight to an argument that smoking was actually causing strokes, although it is not as compelling as the much stronger relation between smoking and lung cancer, for which the rate ratio for current smoking is somewhere between 10 and 15.

As the example shows, ratio measures are very easy to calculate – you simply divide the frequency of disease (or of any health outcome) in the group that is exposed to the factor of interest by the frequency in the group that is not exposed to it. This can be done using either of the measures of disease incidence that you met in Chapter 2. If you divide two incidence rates you end up with a **rate ratio** (as for the stroke example above); if you divide two measures of cumulative incidence or risk then it is a **risk ratio**. It is also possible to divide two measures of prevalence to calculate a **prevalence ratio**. (Note that you must always divide two measures of the same type – you cannot usefully divide an incidence rate by a measure of cumulative incidence.)

Rate ratios

As you saw above, a **rate ratio** is calculated by simply dividing the incidence rate of disease in a group of people exposed to the factor of interest (often denoted by a subscript 'e') by the incidence rate in a group of people who are not exposed to the same factor (denoted by a subscript 'o'):

$$\text{Rate ratio} = \frac{\text{Incidence rate in exposed}}{\text{Incidence rate in unexposed}} = \frac{IR_e}{IR_o} \qquad (5.1)$$

This factor could be a potential cause of disease, it could be a characteristic of a person, such as their age or where they live, or it could be something that influences behaviour. Equally, it could be a preventive measure or, in the clinical context, a drug or other treatment that we hope will reduce the incidence of disease.

Risk ratios

Similarly, the **risk ratio** (also called the **relative risk**) is calculated by dividing the cumulative incidence or risk of disease in an exposed group by the cumulative incidence in an unexposed group:

$$\text{Risk ratio} = \frac{\text{Cumulative incidence in exposed}}{\text{Cumulative incidence in unexposed}} = \frac{CI_e}{CI_o} \qquad (5.2)$$

For example, in Chapter 2 we considered a randomised trial to evaluate whether taking aspirin would reduce the risk of blood clots in people with infective endocarditis.

Look back at Table 2.3 and calculate the risk ratio for the association between aspirin and blood clots.

In this trial, the risk ratio was 28.3% ÷ 20.0% = 1.4; those who took aspirin were 1.4 times as likely to develop blood clots as those who did not take aspirin. A risk ratio of 1.0 would mean that there was no difference between the groups, so those taking aspirin were 40% *more likely* to develop blood clots than those not taking aspirin (in the context of clinical epidemiology this may be described as the *relative risk increase* or *RRI*). Clearly this intervention did not work the way the investigators had hoped it would.

This approach can be used much more widely than in the search for the causes of disease. As an example, a trial carried out in three general practices in the UK set out to find out whether telephoning patients to offer them an appointment

Table 5.2 The results of a study evaluating the effects of calling patients on influenza immunisation rates.

	Outcome		
Exposure	Immunised	Not immunised	Percentage immunised (%)
Received a call	328	332	50
No call	288	370	44
Total	616	702	47

(Hull *et al.*, 2002.)

for immunisation against influenza would increase immunisation uptake rates (Hull *et al.*, 2002). In this study, attending for immunisation was the outcome of interest and receiving a telephone call was the exposure. A total of 1,318 patients aged 65 to 74 years were randomly assigned to two groups. Patients in one group (n = 660) received a telephone call from the receptionist at their general practice inviting them to make an appointment for immunisation (the intervention or exposed group). Patients in the other group (n = 658) were not called (the control or unexposed group). The investigators then waited to see who turned up for immunisation. They found that 328 of the patients who received a phone call attended, as did 288 of those who did not receive a call.

The easiest way to look at these data is in the form of a '2 × 2 table'. These tables are usually set out so that the two columns show the numbers of people with and without the outcome of interest while the rows show the numbers in the exposed and unexposed groups (Table 5.2).

What was the cumulative incidence of immunisation or, in other words, what percentage of patients attended for immunisation in each of the two groups?

How many times more likely were patients to attend if they had received a personal call to make an appointment than if they had not been telephoned?

In the intervention group 50% of patients were immunised, compared with 44% of those in the control group (despite the intervention the immunisation rates were still below the government target of 60%). This means that patients who received an invitation were 1.14 times (50% ÷ 44%) more likely to attend for immunisation. This measure is still a relative risk because it has the same structure – the cumulative incidence (or risk) of a particular health outcome in one group is divided by the cumulative incidence in a second group. In this case the word 'risk' seems less appropriate but the term relative risk is still regularly used.

Prevalence ratios

It is also possible to use measures of prevalence instead of incidence to compare the burden of disease in two groups and in this situation you end up with a **prevalence ratio**:

$$\text{Prevalence ratio} = \frac{\text{Prevalence in exposed}}{\text{Prevalence in unexposed}} = \frac{P_e}{P_o} \qquad (5.3)$$

As we discussed in Chapter 2, measures of prevalence are harder to interpret than measures of incidence and for this reason prevalence ratios are used much less frequently than rate and risk ratios.

A note about relative risks

We noted above that the term *relative risk* is synonymous with *risk ratio*. In practice, it is also commonly used to describe a *rate ratio*, since both the rate ratio and the risk ratio compare the amount of disease in one group *relative* to that in another. If a disease is rare (cumulative incidence or risk less than about 10%), then the rate ratio and risk ratio will be almost identical; if it is not so rare then the risk ratio will be closer to 1.0 than the rate ratio. The three terms are also commonly and conveniently abbreviated as RR. When we use the term relative risk it will refer to both the rate ratio and the risk ratio.

Standardised incidence and mortality ratios

We discussed these measures in Chapter 2 because of the links between direct and indirect standardisation, but they also deserve a mention here since they compare the rate of disease (or death) in two populations and so, in effect, are also measures of relative risk.

Difference measures (attributable risk)

As we noted above, the relative risk tells us nothing about the actual amount of disease that is occurring. If the cumulative incidences or risks of disease in exposed and unexposed groups were 0.5% and 0.1%, respectively, the relative risk would be 5.0. Similarly, if the risks were 50% and 10% the relative risk would also be 5.0. The major difference between these two situations is obvious: the actual amount of disease that is occurring is vastly different – in fact in the second example it is 100 times greater. This vital public health information cannot be obtained from the relative risk.

The approach to measuring the excess amount of disease occurring among those exposed to a potential risk factor is just as intuitive and as simple to calculate

Box 5.2　Relative risks in clinical epidemiology

Although relative risks are also used in the context of clinical trials, several other related measures are also used.

In 1998, Botti *et al.* reported a trial of the use of pressure bandages for patients undergoing coronary angiography. Some of their results are shown in Table 5.3.

Table 5.3 Use of pressure bandages in patients undergoing coronary angiography.

Pressure bandages	Total	Number with bleeding	Cumulative incidence or event rate
Yes	519	18	EER^a = 3.5%
No	556	37	CER^b = 6.7%
Total	1,075	55	5.1%

[a] EER = experimental event rate or cumulative incidence in the treatment group.
[b] CER = control event rate or cumulative incidence in the comparison group.
(Botti *et al.*, 1998.)

The ***relative risk*** of bleeding among those given pressure bandages compared with those without is 3.5 ÷ 6.7 = 0.52. This tells us that those given pressure bandages were about half as likely to develop bleeding as those who were not given bandages. The results of treatment trials are sometimes also reported as a ***relative risk reduction* (RRR)**. This is the amount by which the treatment has reduced the relative risk and it is calculated by subtracting the relative risk from 1.0. It may then be expressed as a percentage by multiplying by 100:

$$\text{Relative risk reduction (RRR)} = 1.0 - RR \tag{5.4}$$

So the RRR = 1.0 − 0.52 = 0.48 or 48%.

Alternatively, it can be calculated directly from the cumulative incidence or ***event rates*** among the experimental (EER) and control (CER) groups:

$$\text{Relative risk reduction (RRR)} = (CER - EER) \div CER \tag{5.5}$$

In this case the RRR = (6.7 − 3.5) ÷ 6.7 = 0.48.

In other words, use of the pressure bandages has reduced the risk of bleeding among patients undergoing coronary angiography by 48%. Obviously, the greater the RRR the better the intervention.

For studies with a positive association (RR > 1.0) the results are turned around to give what is logically called the ***relative risk increase (RRI)***. In the

(continued)

Box 5.2 (*continued*)

aspirin study discussed previously, aspirin increased the risk of bleeding by 40% (RR = 1.4).

Note that you will see associations described in this way in all fields of epidemiology, e.g., 'The risk of disease was 20% lower among those who exercised more'. It is a simple, informative mode of description that just happens to have been given a separate name in the area of clinical epidemiology.

as the relative risk. As you saw in the smoking and stroke example at the start of the chapter, we can calculate the *extra* amount of disease that is occurring in the exposed group by simply subtracting the incidence in the unexposed group (IR_o, CI_o or *background risk*) from the incidence in the exposed group (IR_e, CI_e). This can again be done using either of the measures of disease incidence (incidence rate or cumulative incidence) that you met in Chapter 2. If you are subtracting two incidence rates (as in the stroke example) you end up with a **rate difference**, whereas if you are subtracting two measures of cumulative incidence or risk (as in the immunisation example) you have a **risk difference**. Both of these measures can also be described as the **attributable risk** (in the same way that *relative risk* is used to describe both rate ratios and risk ratios). (Note, however, that it is appropriate to use this term only if it is reasonable to assume that the excess disease can be *attributed* to the exposure, i.e., the exposure is causing the disease.)

Rate differences

Consider the smoking and stroke example again (Table 5.1). Compared with never smokers, there were an extra 10.2 strokes (27.9 − 17.7) per 100,000 person-years in ex-smokers and an extra 31.9 strokes (49.6 − 17.7) per 100,000 person-years in current smokers. These effects are illustrated in Figure 5.1. The left-hand bar (a) shows the incidence rate of stroke in non-smokers. This is often called the background or *reference rate* because it reflects the natural occurrence of the disease in an unexposed population. We expect this to operate on all members of the population regardless of their smoking status, and this is shown for the ex- and current smokers. This lets us visualise directly the extra burden of stroke added by past and present smoking habits. Thus the second bar shows the extra incidence of stroke in ex-smokers (b) that is presumably due to the fact that the women had smoked in the past. Similarly, the third bar shows the far greater added rate of stroke in current smokers (c) that is attributable to their smoking. This extra disease is simply the difference between the rate in the exposed group (smokers) and the rate in the unexposed group (non-smokers). The total

Fig. 5.1 Attributable risks: the
results of a study of smoking
and stroke. (Drawn from Colditz
et al., 1988.)

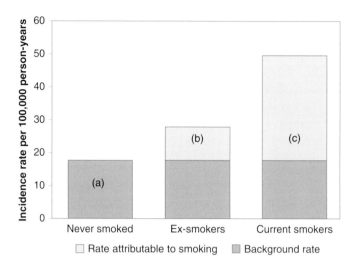

rate of disease in exposed individuals is therefore the sum of the background rate
(due to other causes) and the additional rate due to the exposure in question.

If the groups differ only in their smoking habit *and if we believe that smoking
is actually causing strokes to occur* then we can say that the extra disease in the
smokers is attributable to their smoking – if they had not smoked then it would
not have occurred. This *rate difference* is also called the *attributable risk* (AR)
because it measures the actual amount of disease that can be attributed to a particular exposure:

Rate difference or attributable risk
  = Incidence rate in exposed – Incidence rate in unexposed
  = $IR_e - IR_o$ (5.6)

Risk differences

Look back to the example of immunisation against influenza in Table 5.2.

What percentage of patients in the intervention group would have been
expected to attend for immunisation even if they hadn't received a phone call
(background 'risk')?

What extra percentage of patients presumably attended only because they had
received a call (i.e., how many attendances could be attributed to the phone call)?

We would have expected 44% of patients in the intervention group to go for
immunisation even if the practice receptionists had not called to offer them an
appointment. We can therefore say that an extra 6% of patients (50% − 44%) in
the intervention group presumably went for immunisation only because they
had received a call, i.e., their immunisation can be attributed to this. Here we

have calculated a risk difference (as opposed to a rate difference) since we are subtracting cumulative incidences (or risks):

Risk difference or attributable risk

= Cumulative incidence in exposed − Cumulative incidence in unexposed

$$= CI_e - CI_o \qquad (5.7)$$

Attributable fractions (AFs)

A further way to consider attributable risk that can also be informative is as the *proportion* or *percentage* of disease in the exposed group that would not have occurred in the absence of the exposure. This measure is often called the **attributable fraction** or **attributable proportion**, although you will also come across it described as the **attributable risk per cent**. To calculate the attributable fraction you simply divide the attributable risk by the incidence in the exposed group:

$$\text{Attributable fraction (AF)} = \frac{\text{Attributable risk}}{\text{Incidence in exposed}}$$

$$= \frac{\text{Incidence in exposed} - \text{Incidence in unexposed}}{\text{Incidence in exposed}}$$

Again this can be done using either the incidence rate or the cumulative incidence:

$$\text{Attributable fraction (AF)} = \frac{AR}{IR_e} \quad \text{or} \quad \frac{AR}{CI_e} \qquad (5.8)$$

$$= \frac{IR_e - IR_o}{IR_e} \quad \text{or} \quad \frac{CI_e - CI_o}{CI_e} \qquad (5.9)$$

Consider the smoking and stroke example again. The rate of stroke among current smokers was $49.6/10^5$ person-years and the rate difference or attributable risk was $31.9/10^5$ person-years. The attributable fraction is therefore 0.64 or 64%, i.e., of all the strokes occurring *among current smokers*, about two thirds could be attributed to the fact that the women smoked:

$$\text{Attributable fraction (AF)} = \frac{49.6 - 17.7}{49.6} = 0.64 = 64\%$$

Interpretation of the attributable risk

The attributable risk tells us how much extra disease is actually occurring in the *exposed* group as a result of the exposure. By implication, we can then say that, *if the association is causal*, this is the amount of disease that we could prevent in a comparable group of people in the future *if* we could prevent them from being

Box 5.3 Attributable risks in clinical epidemiology

In the field of clinical epidemiology, what we have called the *attributable risk* is often called the **absolute risk reduction** (**ARR**) or **absolute risk increase** (**ARI**) depending on whether the event rate is reduced or increased in the treatment group. (N.B. The ARR and ARI are identical to the attributable risks used elsewhere in epidemiology and are calculated in exactly the same way – the only difference is in the names.)

For example, in the trial of the use of pressure bandages for patients undergoing coronary angiography (Table 5.3) the absolute risk reduction (ARR) of bleeding would be

$$\text{ARR} = \text{CER} - \text{EER} = 6.7 - 3.5 = 3.2\% \tag{5.10}$$

In other words, the use of pressure bandages has prevented bleeding in 3.2% of patients.

Another quite useful way of looking at these data is in terms of the **number needed to treat** (**NNT**). The NNT is the number of patients who would have to be given the experimental therapy in order to prevent one adverse event (death, complication) from occurring. It is calculated by simply dividing 1.0 by the ARR:

$$\text{NNT} = 1 \div \text{ARR} \tag{5.11}$$

In the study of pressure bandages the ARR was 3.2% or 0.032, so

$$\text{NNT} = 1 \div 0.032 = 31.3$$

This means that about 30 patients undergoing coronary angiography would need to be given pressure bandages in order to prevent one case of bleeding. (Note that, unlike in most other situations, the NNT should be *rounded up* to the nearest whole number because you cannot treat part of a person.) This gives a good intuitive feel for the treatment benefit, and can aid communication with patients.

exposed. This measure is, therefore, of direct use to health planning and policy setting.

In practice, of course, it is often impossible to remove or prevent an exposure altogether. Someone who smokes cannot go back to being a never-smoker but they can become an ex-smoker. This means that current smokers who stop smoking will not realise the full benefit predicted by the standard attributable risk (which would compare smokers with the unexposed group, in this case never smokers). Rather, the best we can achieve with a 100% effective 'stop smoking'

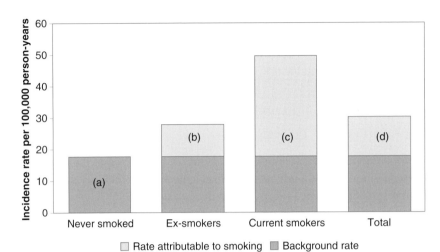

Fig. 5.2 Attributable and population attributable risks: the results of a study of smoking and stroke. (Drawn from Colditz *et al.*, 1988.)

campaign is to reduce the rate of stroke among smokers to the level seen among ex-smokers, a rate difference given by

$$IR_{current} - IR_{ex} = 49.6 - 27.9 = 21.7 \text{ strokes}/100{,}000 \text{ person-years}$$

Population attributable risks (PARs)

The attributable risk tells us about the amount of extra disease occurring in the exposed group because of the exposure. An alternative way to look at this is to consider *how much disease in the whole community* can be attributed to the exposure. To do this we need to compare the incidence of disease in the whole population or community (some of whom will be exposed and some unexposed) with the amount of disease in an unexposed group (the amount that we would expect if no one had been exposed). In the smoking and stroke example in Table 5.1 we know that the overall incidence rate of stroke among the women was $30.2/10^5$ person-years.

What would this rate have been if no one had smoked?

How much of the incidence of stroke in the total population is due to the fact that some women smoke or are ex-smokers?

What fraction of the overall rate of stroke in the total population is due to smoking?

If none of the women had smoked the overall rate of stroke in the population would be the same as the rate in never smokers ($17.7/10^5$ person-years). This means that, in the whole population, there are an extra 12.5 cases ($30.2 - 17.7$) per 100,000 person-years that can be attributed to the fact that *some* of the women in the population smoke or are ex-smokers. This is the **population attributable risk** (PAR) and is depicted (d) in the fourth bar in Figure 5.2.

There are two ways to calculate the PAR. One way, analogous to the calculation of attributable risk (formulae (5.6) and (5.7)), is to subtract the incidence in the unexposed group (IR_o, CI_o) from the incidence in the *whole population* (IR_T, CI_T). As for the attributable risk, this can be done using either incidence rates or cumulative incidence:

PAR = Incidence rate in population – Incidence rate in unexposed

$$= IR_T - IR_o \quad \text{or} \quad CI_T - CI_o \tag{5.12}$$

The population attributable risk depends on the prevalence of the exposure in the population and an alternative way to calculate it is to multiply the attributable risk by the prevalence of exposure in the population (P_e):

$$PAR = AR \times P_e \tag{5.13}$$

(Note that, while this is straightforward when there are only two levels of exposure, it is more tricky when there are more than two levels, as in the stroke and smoking example. In this situation it is much easier to use Equation (5.12).)

Population attributable fractions (PAFs)

As with the attributable risk and attributable fraction, we can also calculate the **population attributable fraction** (or **population attributable risk per cent**) which indicates the proportion of all the strokes that occurred in the population that could potentially have been avoided if no-one had smoked. The formula to calculate the population attributable fraction is analogous to that used for the attributable fraction but with the incidence in the total population used instead of the incidence in the exposed group:

Population attributable fraction

$$= \frac{\text{Population attributable risk}}{\text{Incidence in total population}} \times 100$$

$$= \frac{\text{Incidence in total population} - \text{Incidence in unexposed}}{\text{Incidence in total population}} \times 100$$

Again this can be done using either incidence rates or cumulative incidence:

$$\text{Population attributable fraction} = \frac{PAR}{IR_T} \quad \text{or} \quad \frac{PAR}{CI_T} \tag{5.14}$$

$$= \frac{IR_T - IR_o}{IR_T} \quad \text{or} \quad \frac{CI_T - CI_o}{CI_T} \tag{5.15}$$

So, in the stroke example, approximately 41% ($12.5 \div 30.2 = 0.41$) of strokes in the whole population could be attributed to smoking and, in theory, would not have occurred *if no-one had ever smoked.*

Interpretation of the population attributable risk

The population attributable risk (PAR) is exactly analogous to the attributable risk (AR) but, while the attributable risk tells us how much disease in the *exposed* group can be attributed to the exposure, the population attributable risk tells us how much disease in the *whole population* can be attributed to the exposure. The population attributable risk and population attributable fraction are functions both of the *incidence of disease* due to an exposure and of the *prevalence of the exposure*. An exposure may be associated with a very high attributable risk of a disease such that those exposed have a very high chance of developing it, but if the exposure is rare then this high risk will only affect a small proportion of the population. It will therefore have little impact in a whole community (a low population attributable risk). The population attributable risk is the best way to measure the burden of disease in a whole community that can be attributed to a particular exposure.

As we have noted above for the AR, in practice there is no intervention that we could implement to change a woman who is a current smoker into a never smoker; the most we could do would be to persuade her to stop smoking. If we could do this we could estimate the incidence rate of strokes in the whole group as 23.4 per 100,000 person-years (based on the new mix of never smokers and ex-smokers[1]). This means that, if we could have persuaded all current smokers to give up smoking, we could potentially have prevented 6.8 strokes per 100,000 person-years (PAR = 30.2 − 23.4) or 22.5% of all strokes in the population (PAF = 6.8 ÷ 30.2).

When thinking about the possibilities for intervention and prevention of disease we should bear in mind that changing someone's smoking habit will reduce not just their risk of stroke but also their risk of many other diseases, so the public health benefits of a 'stop smoking' campaign are not limited to stroke reduction. While the overall benefits of stopping smoking are clear cut, it is less obvious where an intervention reduces risk of one disease but increases that of another. For example, moderate alcohol consumption can reduce the risk of heart disease but it can also increase the risk of breast cancer. These benefits and risks have to be weighed up and no-one would recommend that women should drink more alcohol to prevent heart disease.

A word of caution regarding attributable risks

There are possibly more terms used to describe attributable risks than any other measure in epidemiology. People use different names for the same thing and, what is even more confusing, the same name for different things. This emphasises

---

[1] If all the current smokers became ex-smokers at the start of the study their rate of stroke would have been $27.9/10^5$ person-years and about 78 strokes would have occurred in the 280,141 person-years of follow-up. This gives a total of 213 strokes (70 + 65 + 78) in 908,447 person years or a rate of $23.4/10^5$ person-years in the whole population. *Note that this assumes that the full benefit is seen immediately after stopping.*

Box 5.4 Use of population attributable risks

At the global level, population attributable risks and population attributable fractions are used to calculate the impacts of various exposures on world health. For example, it has been estimated that in the year 2000 almost five million premature deaths around the world were attributable to smoking (Ezzati and Lopez, 2003). Similarly, the World Health Report 2002 (WHO, 2002) presents estimates of the amount of ill-health, measured this time in DALYs, that can be attributed to various risk factors (Table 5.4). Note the variation in the relative importance of some causes (e.g., nutritional deficiency) depending on the affluence of the population. Note also that, for a particular disease, the DALYs attributable to various causes can add up to more than 100%. This is because several factors commonly act together to cause disease. This means that getting rid of any one of them might reduce the incidence of disease quite considerably but, once this cause has been removed, getting rid of a second cause may provide relatively little additional benefit.

Table 5.4 The percentages of DALYs due to ischaemic heart disease and diarrhoeal diseases in males which can be attributed to various risk factors, shown separately for developing countries with high and low mortality and developed countries.

	Percentage of DALYs in men attributable to various risk factors		
	Developing countries with high mortality (%)	Developing countries with low mortality (%)	Developed countries (%)
Ischaemic heart disease			
High blood pressure	45	45	59
High cholesterol level	50	48	53
Low fruit and vegetable intake	32	31	29
Inactivity	21	22	23
Drinking alcohol	7	5	2
Diarrhoeal diseases in childhood			
Being underweight	49	24	13
Vitamin A deficiency	19	10	0
Zinc deficiency	11	3	2
Drinking unsafe water	88	88	80

(*World Health Report*, WHO, 2002.)

the importance of never taking things at face value – always take time to check what are being presented. Here the key distinction is whether people are talking about only the exposed group (what we call the attributable risk or, in clinical epidemiology, the absolute risk reduction) or the whole population (what we call the population attributable risk). It is also important to distinguish between absolute differences (what we have called attributable risks) and percentage differences (attributable fractions).

Relative risk versus attributable risk

In the British Doctors Study (discussed in Chapter 1) mortality rates were calculated for deaths both from lung cancer and from coronary heart disease (CHD). These rates, together with the relative risks, attributable risks and attributable fractions, are shown in Table 5.5.

Is the association with smoking stronger for lung cancer or CHD?

If everyone stopped smoking, would we prevent more cases of lung cancer or CHD?

In these data there is a very strong *relative* association between smoking and lung cancer (RR = 14), but only a modest link between cigarettes and CHD (RR = 1.6). On its own, this offers powerful support to a belief in smoking as a cause of lung cancer, but leaves quite a few doubts as to whether it has a causal role in the development of CHD (see also Chapter 10). Given that smoking does cause CHD as well as lung cancer (and there is plenty of other evidence to support this), the *attributable fraction* supports the view that smoking is a more important cause of lung cancer than it is of CHD: among smokers 93% of lung cancers but only 38% of CHD can be attributed to smoking. In contrast, the *attributable risks* show that the *public health impact* of smoking is twice as great

Table 5.5 Lung cancer and CHD mortality rates in the British Doctors Study.

Disease	Smoking status	Mortality rate per 10^5 person-years	Relative risk	Attributable risk per 10^5 person-years	Attributable fraction (%)
Lung cancer	Yes	140	14.0	130	93
	No	10			
Coronary heart disease	Yes	669	1.6	256	38
	No	413			

(Doll and Peto, 1976.)

for CHD mortality as for lung cancer deaths: there are almost 260 additional deaths from CHD in smokers for every 100,000 person-years compared with only 130 from lung cancer.

The background rate of CHD (the rate in non-smokers) is very high, so a large difference in rate does not look so impressive when we calculate the RR. In contrast, the background rate of lung cancer is very low, so a much smaller increase in rate leads to a very high RR. This example shows very clearly the striking difference in what these measures describe and the different implications of a large relative risk (or attributable faction) versus a large attributable risk.

To recapitulate, the *relative risk* is particularly useful to evaluate the strength of an association between exposure and disease, and can be best used to help identify causes of a disease. The *attributable fraction* can be used to pinpoint the most important causes of a particular disease and thus to identify potential targets for prevention. The *attributable risk* and *population attributable risk* are the best measures of the burden of disease due to the exposure (either in the exposed group, AR, or in the whole population, PAR) and each can be used to assess the magnitude of a public health problem associated with exposure. With respect to smoking, this is clearly a stronger cause of lung cancer than it is of coronary heart disease but, from the public health perspective, it causes many more deaths from heart disease than it does from lung cancer.

Case–control studies

All of the above measures relate to situations in which we can measure the incidence of disease. This information usually comes from a follow-up or **cohort study** in which we identify groups of exposed and unexposed individuals who do not have the disease of interest and then follow them over time to see how many develop the disease. Now, imagine that we were interested in a rare disease. If we did a cohort study we would have to identify a very large group of people and follow them for a very long time before many people developed the disease. In this situation an alternative study design called a **case–control study** is often used. (We will discuss different types of study in Chapter 6.) Instead of identifying people on the basis of their exposure status and waiting to see who develops disease, we select people with (cases) and without (controls) the disease we are interested in and then ask them about their previous exposures. In a case–control study we generally aim to identify as many of the people in a community with the disease as possible, but usually select only a sample of all possible people without disease as controls. This often means that we can no longer calculate disease incidence, so we need different methods to calculate measures of association in a case–control study.

In the early 1990s a case–control study of ovarian cancer was conducted in Australia. It included the majority of women newly diagnosed with ovarian

Table 5.6 A case–control study of oral contraceptive (OC) use and ovarian cancer.

	Cases	Controls	Total
Used OC pill	416	555	971
Did not use OC pill	408	305	713
Total	824	860	1,684

(Purdie *et al.*, 1995.)

cancer in three Australian states (Queensland, New South Wales and Victoria) between 1991 and 1993, a total of 824 cases. The controls were a sample of 860 women who did not have ovarian cancer and were chosen at random from the same states. The investigators found that 416 of the cases and 555 of the controls had previously used the oral contraceptive (OC) pill (Purdie *et al.*, 1995), as shown in Table 5.6.

What percentage of the OC users have ovarian cancer? Does this reflect the likely incidence of ovarian cancer in OC users?

In this case–control study 43% (416 ÷ 971) of the OC users have ovarian cancer. It is tempting to interpret this as meaning that the incidence of ovarian cancer among oral contraceptive users was 43% but, even if you don't know anything about ovarian cancer, this should ring some warning bells! It is clearly ridiculous to imagine that almost half of women who use the OC pill would develop the rare disease of ovarian cancer. The numerator (the number of women with cancer) is fine because most of the women with cancer were included, but the denominator (the total population) is very wrong because only a tiny proportion of all the women without ovarian cancer have been included. This means that, in a case–control study, we often cannot calculate the usual measures of disease incidence and so cannot calculate relative risks in the same way.

Relative risk in case–control studies

In a case–control study we calculate another measure of association known as the **odds ratio** (OR). This involves calculating the '*odds*' that a case had used OCs in exactly the same way as odds are calculated in horse racing. Among the cases, 416 women had used the OC pill and 408 had not, so the 'odds' of a case having used the pill are '416 to 408' or 416 ÷ 408 = 1.02.

What are the odds that a control had used the OC pill?

Among the controls, 555 women had used the pill and 305 had not. The odds that a control had used the pill are therefore 555 ÷ 305 = 1.82. We can then calculate

Table 5.7 Calculation of the odds ratio in a case–control study.

	Cases	Controls	Total
Exposed	a	b	$a + b$
Unexposed	c	d	$c + d$
Total	$a + c$	$b + d$	$a + b + c + d$

the **odds ratio** by dividing the odds that a case had used the pill (i.e., was exposed) by the odds that a control had used the pill. In this example:

Odds ratio (OR) $= 1.02 \div 1.82 = 0.56$

An alternative and simple way to calculate the odds ratio that is often used in practice is as follows. Your data must be arranged in a standard way as shown in Table 5.7 (note that this is the same as the way in which the data are shown in Table 5.6).

The odds that a case used the OC pill $= a \div c$

The odds that a control used the OC pill $= b \div d$

Therefore the ratio of these odds $= (a \div c) \div (b \div d)$

or

$$\text{Odds ratio} = \frac{a \times d}{b \times c} \tag{5.16}$$

So, for the ovarian cancer data, the OR associated with OC use is

$$\text{Odds ratio} = \frac{416 \times 305}{555 \times 408} = 0.56$$

In many situations, the odds ratio will be approximately equal to the relative risk that we calculated earlier from cohort studies and it can be interpreted in the same way. This is the case in the following situations.

- The disease is rare – and for the purposes of epidemiology most diseases are rare. (See Box 5.5 for a mathematical derivation of why this is true.)
- The controls for the study were recruited using what is called *density sampling.* This means that the controls must have been identified during the period when the cases were occurring, *not* at the end of the study. In practice this does not make a lot of difference if the disease is rare, but if the disease is common it means that it is possible for someone to be recruited as a control early in the study and then to be recruited again as a case if they later develop the disease of interest. Although ovarian cancer is rare by any standards, one woman participated in the case–control study described above as a cancer-free control but was diagnosed with ovarian cancer a year later. She then participated in the study a second time as a case. This is not only valid but essential for true density sampling.

Box 5.5 Why the odds ratio approximates the relative risk for a rare disease

Table 5.8 shows the results of a hypothetical cohort study.

Table 5.8 Results of a hypothetical cohort study.

	Cases	Non-cases	Total	CI (%)
Exposed	75 (a)	9,925 (b)	10,000 ($a + b$)	0.75
Unexposed	25 (c)	9,975 (d)	10,000 ($c + d$)	0.25
Total	100	19,900	20,000	

$$\text{Relative risk} = \frac{CI_e}{CI_o} = \frac{a}{a+b} \div \frac{c}{c+d} = 0.75\% \div 0.25\% = 3.0$$

However, if the disease is rare then

a (=75) is very small in comparison to b (=9,925), so $a + b \approx b$

and

c (=25) is very small in comparison to d (=9,975) so $c + d \approx d$

This means that the

$$\text{Relative risk} = \frac{a}{a+b} \div \frac{c}{c+d} \approx \frac{a}{b} \div \frac{c}{d} = \frac{a \times d}{b \times c} = \text{Odds ratio}$$

If we were to do a case–control study in this population we might include all 100 cases and then select the same number of controls. Half of the population is exposed and half is unexposed, so if we chose 100 controls at random we would expect about 50 to be exposed and 50 to be unexposed, as shown in Table 5.9.

Table 5.9 Results of a hypothetical case–control study.

	Cases	Controls
Exposed	75	50
Unexposed	25	50

So the

$$\text{Odds ratio} = \frac{75 \times 50}{25 \times 50} = 3.0$$

Box 5.6 Rate ratios, risk ratios and odds ratios

Each of the three measures of association is a valid measure in its own right but the relationship among them varies in different situations.

If a disease is rare it can be shown that all three measures are approximately equal and all can be interpreted as a relative risk:

Rate ratio ≈ Risk Ratio ≈ Odds ratio

If a disease is not rare then the relationship between the odds ratio and the risk and rate ratios depends on how the controls were selected for the study (see Rodrigues and Kirkwood, 1990).

- If they were selected at the *start* of the case-recruitment period and so included anyone who was disease-free at that point in time (regardless of whether they went on to develop disease) then

  Odds ratio ≈ Risk ratio

  so an OR of 3.0 can be interpreted as meaning that the risk of disease in those who were exposed was three times greater than that among those who were not exposed.

- If they were selected at the *same* time as cases were being recruited (i.e., density sampling), as is usually the case in practice, then

  Odds ratio ≈ Rate ratio

  so an OR of 3.0 can be interpreted as meaning that the rate of disease in those who were exposed was three times greater than that among those who were not exposed.

- If they were selected to include only people who were still disease-free at the end of the study then the odds ratio will still provide information about the strength of the association but, if the disease is not rare, it might not be a good estimate of the relative risk. That is, if an OR = 3.0 it tells us that the association is strong but it does *not* necessarily mean that those who were exposed were three times more likely to develop disease than those who were not exposed.

Attributable risk in case–control studies

Because we cannot usually calculate the actual incidence of disease in exposed and unexposed subjects in a case–control study, we cannot calculate the attributable risk of disease associated with the exposure. We can, however, calculate the *attributable fraction* using the following formula:

$$\text{Attributable fraction (AF)} = \frac{\text{OR} - 1}{\text{OR}} \times 100 \tag{5.17}$$

We can also calculate the **population attributable fraction**, as follows:

$$\text{Population attributable fraction (PAF)} = \frac{P_e(\text{OR} - 1)}{P_e(\text{OR} - 1) + 1} \times 100 \qquad (5.18)$$

where P_e is the prevalence of exposure in the population, estimated by measuring the prevalence in the *control* group.

Or, alternatively,

$$\text{Population attributable fraction} = \text{AF} \times P_{e(cases)} \qquad (5.19)$$

where $P_{e(cases)}$ is the prevalence of exposure among the *cases*.

These measures are the only way of assessing the potential public health importance of an exposure from a case–control study. (Note that these formulae can also be used for follow-up studies by substituting the RR for the OR.)

Another example comes from a study of the effectiveness of bicycle helmets for preventing head injury in children (Thomas *et al.*, 1994). The cases were 98 children who presented to the local children's hospital with bicycle-related head injuries and the controls were 266 children treated for other bicycle-related injuries. In total 207 children, 67 of the cases and 140 controls, were not wearing a helmet at the time of the accident. (Note that we will consider '*not wearing a helmet*' as the exposure in this example.)

What is the OR for the association between not wearing a helmet and head injury?

What percentage of head injuries occurring among the children not wearing a helmet could be attributed to the fact that they were not wearing a helmet (AF)?

What proportion of the control children were not wearing a helmet (P_e)?

What percentage of all bicycle-related head injuries in children could be attributed to not wearing a helmet (PAF)?

Table 5.10 shows the results of the study laid out in a standard 2 × 2 table. The odds ratio for the association between not wearing a bicycle helmet and head injury is

$$\text{OR} = \frac{a \times d}{b \times c} = \frac{67 \times 126}{140 \times 31} = 1.95$$

Table 5.10 A case–control study of bicycle helmets and head injury

	Cases	Controls	Total
No helmet (exposed)	67	140	207
Wearing a helmet (unexposed)	31	126	157
Total	98	266	364

(Thomas *et al.*, 1994.)

Box 5.7 An example – obesity and type-2 diabetes

The following example summarises the various measures of association. It is based on *incidence rates* of type-2 diabetes but the formulae also apply to *cumulative incidence* or risk data – simply substitute CI for IR. In a case–control study it is not usually possible to calculate the AR or PAR but we can use the odds ratio (formula (5.16)) in place of the RR to calculate the AF and PAF.

Imagine that 30% of the population in a particular community is overweight, 82.5% of diabetics are overweight and the rate of type-2 diabetes is

- $330/10^5$ person-years in the obese (IR_e),
- $30/10^5$ person-years in the non-obese (IR_o) and
- $120/10^5$ person-years in the whole population (IR_T).

Then we can calculate the following.

(1) The **rate ratio** or **relative risk** (RR) using Equation (5.1):

$$RR = \frac{IR_e}{IR_o} = \frac{330}{30} = 11.0$$

The **relative risk** tells us that the rate of type-2 diabetes is 11 times higher among people who are obese than among non-obese people.

(2) The **rate difference** or **attributable risk** (AR) using Equation (5.6):

$$AR = IR_e - IR_o = 330 - 30 = 300 \text{ per } 10^5 \text{ person-years}$$

The **attributable risk** tells us that, if obesity is a cause of type-2 diabetes, then, *among obese people*, 300 cases per 10^5 person-years can be attributed to their obesity.

(3) The **attributable fraction** (AF) using Equation (5.9):

$$AF = \frac{IR_e - IR_o}{IR_e} \times 100 = \frac{330 - 30}{330} \times 100 = 91\%$$

or Equation (5.17) (using the RR instead of the OR):

$$AF = \frac{RR - 1}{RR} \times 100 = \frac{11 - 1}{11} \times 100 = 91\%$$

The **attributable fraction** tells us that more than 90% of type-2 diabetes in obese people would not occur if they were not overweight.

(4) The **population attributable risk** (PAR) using Equation (5.12):

$$PAR = IR_T - IR_o = 120 - 30 = 90/10^5 \text{ person-years}$$

or using Equation (5.13):

$$PAR = AR \times P_e = 300 \times 0.3 = 90/10^5 \text{ person-years}$$

where P_e = prevalence of exposure in the population = 30% or 0.3.

(continued)

Box 5.7 (*continued*)

The **population attributable risk** tells us that, in the **whole population**, 90 cases of type-2 diabetes per 10^5 person-years can be attributed to obesity

(5) The **population attributable fraction** (PAF) using Equation (5.14):

$$\text{PAF} = \frac{\text{PAR}}{\text{IR}_T} \times 100 = (90 \div 120) \times 100 = 75\%$$

or Equation (5.18) (using the RR instead of OR):

$$\text{PAF} = \frac{P_e(\text{RR} - 1)}{P_e(\text{RR} - 1) + 1} \times 100 = \frac{0.3 \times (11 - 1)}{[0.3 \times (11 - 1)] + 1} \times 100 = \frac{3}{4} \times 100 = 75\%$$

or Equation (5.19):

$$\text{PAF} = \text{AF} \times P_{e(\text{cases})} = 91\% \times 0.825 = 75\%$$

The **population attributable fraction** tells us that 75% of all cases of type-2 diabetes would not occur if no one was grossly overweight.

This indicates that children who do not wear helmets are more likely to sustain a head injury in a bicycle accident than children who do wear helmets.

The attributable fraction tells us the proportion of head injuries among those not wearing a helmet that could be attributed to the fact that they were not wearing a helmet:

$$\text{AF} = \frac{\text{OR} - 1}{\text{OR}} \times 100 = \frac{1.95 - 1}{1.95} \times 100 = 49\%$$

This tells us that 49% of head injuries *among children not wearing helmets* could be attributed to the fact they were not helmeted and were therefore potentially preventable if they had been wearing a helmet.

Out of the 266 controls, 140 or 53% were not wearing a helmet. We can use this information to calculate the population attributable fraction to estimate the proportion of all head injuries that could be attributed to the fact that some children were not wearing a helmet:

$$\text{PAF} = \frac{P_e(\text{OR} - 1)}{P_e(\text{OR} - 1) + 1} \times 100 = \frac{0.53 \times 0.95}{(0.53 \times 0.95) + 1} \times 100 = \frac{0.5035}{1.5035} \times 100 = 33\%$$

The results suggest that, in the study population, almost one-third of all child head injuries incurred while cycling could be prevented if all children wore bicycle helmets. (Note that it is important not to round off the numbers during calculations like this because this may make the answer inaccurate. Rounding should be used only for communication of the final answer.)

Questions

1. In an industry employing 10,000 people, 2,500 were employed in areas where they were exposed to ionising radiation, while the remaining 7,500 were not exposed. At the beginning of the study, all employees were free of disease. The entire population of 10,000 was followed for 10 years to determine whether exposure to radiation increased the risk of developing a particular disease. For this disease, the findings were as given in Table 5.11.
   (a) Calculate the cumulative incidence of the disease in
       (i) the exposed workers,
       (ii) the unexposed workers and
       (iii) all workers combined.
   (b) Calculate the relative risk of this disease in those exposed to radiation. What does this tell us?
   (c) How much disease in the exposed workers could be due to their exposure (attributable risk)?
   (d) Calculate the population attributable fraction. What does this tell us?
2. The Family Planning Association in Oxford, England studied 17,000 women who had been enrolled in a cohort study between 1968 and 1974 to look at the association between oral contraceptive (OC) use and venous thromboembolism (Vessey *et al.*, 1989). For current users of OCs, person-time was counted from the time a woman began using OCs. For never or past users, it was counted from the time a woman enrolled in the study. Woman-years were counted until venous thromboembolism occurred, the woman was lost-to-follow-up, or the end of the study.
   (a) The incidence rate of venous thromboembolism was 53 per 100,000 woman-years among current OC users and 6 per 100,000 woman-years among never or past users. Calculate the relative risk of venous thromboembolism for current users compared with never or past users.

Table 5.11 The results of a hypothetical study of the effects of ionising radiation.

	Developed disease	Did not develop disease	Total
Exposed to radiation	30	2,470	2,500
Not exposed	60	7,440	7,500
Total	90	9,910	10,000

(b) The incidence rate of thromboembolism was 62 per 100,000 among users of OCs containing higher dosages of oestrogen and 39 per 100,000 among users of lower-dose OCs. Calculate the relative risk of venous thromboembolism for

  (i) low-dose users compared with never or past users and

  (ii) high-dose users compared with never or past users.

(c) What can you conclude about the risk of thromboembolism for users of OCs containing different doses of oestrogen?

3. Doll and Hill first evaluated the proposition that smoking was a risk factor for lung cancer in a case–control study (Doll and Hill, 1950). They found that, of 649 men with lung cancer (cases), 647 had smoked at some time, compared with 622 of the 649 men without lung cancer (controls).

(a) Draw up a clearly labelled and appropriate 2×2 table to show these data.

(b) How many times more likely was a smoker to develop lung cancer than a non-smoker?

(c) Calculate the proportion of lung cancers attributable to smoking among (i) *smokers* and (ii) the *whole population*.

(d) What are these measures called and how does their interpretation differ?

4. The association between decreased duration of sleep and incidence of coronary heart disease (CHD) was studied among women enrolled in the Nurses' Health Study (Ayas *et al.*, 2003). Among women who reported sleeping 7 or 8 hours per night there were 541 incident cases of CHD during 451,393 person-years of follow-up. Among those who slept for 6 hours per night there were 267 cases in 175,629 person-years, and among those sleeping 5 or fewer hours per night there were 67 cases during 30,115 person-years of follow-up.

(a) Calculate the incidence rate of CHD among

  (i) women who reported sleeping 7–8 hours per night,

  (ii) women who reported sleeping for 6 hours per night,

  (iii) women who slept 5 or less hours per night and

  (iv) all women.

(b) How strong is the association between sleep duration and the incidence of CHD?

(c) What percentage of CHD cases could theoretically be prevented if all women slept for 7–8 hours per night?

REFERENCES

Ayas, N. T., White, D. P., Manson, J. E. *et al.* (2003). A prospective study of sleep duration and coronary heart disease in women. *Archives of Internal Medicine,* **163**: 205–209.

Botti, M., Williamson, B., Steen, K., McTaggart, J. and Reid, E. (1998). The effect of pressure bandaging on complications and comfort in patients undergoing coronary angiography: a multicentre randomized trial. *Heart and Lung,* **27**: 360–373.

Colditz, G. A., Bonita, R., Stampfer, M. J. *et al.* (1988). Cigarette smoking and risk of stroke in middle-aged women. *New England Journal of Medicine*, **318**: 937–941.

Doll, R. and Hill, A. B. (1950). Smoking and carcinoma of the lung. *British Medical Journal*, **2**: 739–748.

Doll, R. and Peto, R. (1976). Mortality in relation to smoking: 20 years' observations on male British doctors. *British Medical Journal*, **2**: 1525–1536.

Ezzati, M. and Lopez, A. D. (2003). Estimates of global mortality attributable to smoking in 2000. *Lancet*, **362**: 847–852.

Hull, S., Hagdrup, N., Hart, B., Griffiths, C. and Hennessy, E. (2002). Boosting uptake of influenza immunisation in a randomised controlled trial of telephone appointing in general practice. *British Journal of General Practice*, **52**: 712–716.

Maushart, S. (2003). Domesticator: rise of the machines. *The Weekend Australian Magazine*, August 16–17.

Purdie, D., Green, A., Bain, C. *et al.* (1995). Reproductive and other factors and risk of epithelial ovarian cancer: an Australian case–control study. *International Journal of Cancer*, **62**: 678–684.

Rodrigues, L. and Kirkwood, E. R. (1990). Case–control designs in the study of common diseases: updates on the demise of the rare disease assumption and the choice of sampling scheme for controls. *International Journal of Epidemiology*, **19**: 205–213.

Snow, J. (1855). *On the Mode of Communication of Cholera*, 2nd edn. London: Churchill. (http://www.ph.ucla.edu/epi/snow/snowbook.html)

Thomas, S., Acton, C., Nixon, J. *et al.* (1994). Effectiveness of bicycle helmets in preventing head injury in children: case–control study. *British Medical Journal*, **308**: 173–176.

Vessey, M. P., Villard-Mackintosh, L., McPherson, K. and Yeates, D. (1989). Mortality among oral contraceptive users: 20 year follow up of women in a cohort study. *British Medical Journal*, **299**: 1487–1491.

WHO (World Health Organization). (2002). *The World Health Report 2002: Reducing Risks, Promoting Healthy Life*. Geneva: WHO. (www.who.int/whr/2002)

Solid foundations: research designs for public health

Box 6.1 Oranges and lemons

In 1747, James Lind conducted an experiment to test six different cures for scurvy. While at sea, he identified twelve patients with scurvy whose 'cases were as similar as I could find them' and prescribed a different treatment to each pair of patients. After a few days he found that the two patients fortunate enough to have been prescribed oranges and lemons were almost fully recovered whilst no improvement was seen in the other ten, who had been subjected to various regimens including sea-water, gruel, cider and various elixirs. From this, Lind inferred that inclusion of citrus fruit in the diet of sailors would not only cure, but also prevent scurvy. Limes or lime juice thus became a part of the diet on ships, earning British sailors their nickname of 'limeys' (Lind, 1753).

In this chapter we will introduce the main epidemiological research designs. We will discuss the descriptive studies that provide the 'bread-and-butter' information of public health and the analytic studies that are our main tools for identifying the causes of disease and evaluating health interventions. Together they provide information needed at all stages of health planning, from the identification of problems to the funding of public health solutions and evaluation of whether they really work in practice.

It is worth bearing in mind that the approaches that we will discuss are also applied in situations in which we are not directly interested in disease per se, but rather in upstream influences, i.e., personal, community or environmental risk factors known to affect disease rates. For instance, we might want to identify factors that influence children to take up smoking, in which case smoking or perhaps the amount of smoking is the outcome of interest. Or we might be interested in the reasons why some parents have their children vaccinated and others do not, with the child's vaccination status as the relevant outcome.

Likewise, the range of exposures or study factors that might influence health – for good or bad – is incredibly broad. The 'exposure' we are interested in could well be an environmental factor such as an infectious agent, radiation or some chemical, but it could equally well be a behavioural factor like smoking or drinking habits, or an intrinsic characteristic (phenotype) of the individual such as sex, age, skin colour or an underlying genetic factor (after all, we are all 'exposed' to our own genes). Traditionally, most of these are personal exposures that affect us at the individual level, but epidemiology is expanding to encompass the additional influences of the social environment, and *lifecourse epidemiology* attempts to integrate exposures over long periods of time. While all these questions place different demands on the specifics of data collection, all can be addressed via the same suite of research designs, although different designs will be more or less appropriate in different situations.

When we discuss study designs in this chapter we will do so mainly in the context of 'exposure' and 'disease', but you should be aware of the broader application of the ideas.

Types of study

You will come across several schemes used to classify studies and you may also find that the same studies have different names in different fields (for example the social or behavioural sciences), but, generally, the variations are minor and semantic. The key to any classification scheme is that it should give insight into the likely utility and validity of a well-conducted study of a given type. We present here a fairly widely accepted approach on two overlapping axes.

Observational versus experimental studies

Epidemiology is rarely an experimental science. Most of the time an epidemiologist will just go out (after a lot of thoughtful planning) and measure the rate of occurrence of a disease or other health outcome, or will compare patterns of exposure and disease to identify particular exposures or risk factors associated with that disease. This is purely an *observational* role: the researcher does not intervene in any way. He or she leaves nature to take its course, and records what happens, or what happened in the past. These are commonly described as **observational studies**.

These contrast with formal **experimental** or **intervention studies**. Here an investigator actively attempts to change something to see what effect this has on disease occurrence. These designs include *clinical trials*, in which an investigator wants to compare two (or more) forms of treatment for patients with a disease, as well as *preventive trials*, in which we aim to intervene to reduce individuals' risk of developing disease in the first place. These experimental epidemiological studies are analogous to experiments in other sciences because the investigator controls who is exposed and who is not, who is allocated to a new treatment regimen and who receives the old treatment, and who is enrolled in a 'stop smoking' campaign and who is not.

Descriptive versus analytic studies

Observational studies can be further classified as **descriptive** or **analytic**. This subdivision attempts to distinguish between research that *describes* the occurrence of disease and/or exposures – **descriptive studies** – and that which goes further to incorporate analysis of associations *between* exposure and disease – **analytic studies**. There is, however, a grey area between the two and epidemiologists may disagree about which group a particular study falls into. A large part of this ambiguity reflects the fact that creative use of data can allow both purposes to be achieved within a single design. Hence, whether a particular study is classified as descriptive or analytic is not too important. What is important is an understanding of the types of questions that can be answered by different types of study and the particular advantages and disadvantages, theoretical and practical, of each.

Descriptive studies are most commonly used to look for patterns of disease and to measure the occurrence of disease or risk factors for disease (exposures) in a population. They are concerned with the 'person, place and time' aspect of epidemiology and are used to answer the questions 'Who?', 'What?', 'Where?' and 'When?'. Although they might lead to suggestions as to why something has occurred, they do not usually produce the sort of data that would give an answer to the question 'Why?' because they often do not involve an explicit comparison or control group. The national health surveys conducted in many countries (see Chapter 3) are good examples of descriptive studies since they aim to document the prevalences of various health conditions and health-related behaviours in the population at a given point in time. Most reports of routine population data, including changing rates of disease over time (time trends) and variations in rates of disease in different geographical areas and in various groups of people within a single geographical area, also come under this heading. Note that, while in the first place these routine data are collected for a single population at a specific time, their utility goes beyond local planning for health services to the extent that they can lead to comparison, both internal (e.g., time trends in a single region) and external (e.g., comparisons with other nations).

Analytic studies, on the other hand, involve planned comparisons between people with and without disease, or between people with and without exposures thought to cause disease. They try to answer the questions 'Why (do some people develop disease)?' and 'How strong is the association between exposure and outcome?'. This group of studies includes both the follow-up or **cohort studies**, as they are commonly known, and **case–control studies** that you have already met.

Some other types of study fall into the grey zone between these two extremes. **Ecological** (or **correlation**) **studies** involve statistical comparisons of group data on exposure and disease from whole populations and you will find them classed as either descriptive or analytic by different authors. **Cross-sectional studies** that measure the prevalence of disease or risk factors for disease among a sample of individuals in a population are often called prevalence surveys and fit best under the heading of descriptive studies, but they can also be used to study the association between exposure and disease among the individuals in the population, in which case they are clearly analytic.

We will now look at how descriptive epidemiology can contribute to an understanding of health and disease and will then consider the more complex analytic and experimental studies. This is the general sequence in which research tends to be performed in practice since it corresponds, more or less, both to a general increase in complexity and cost of the study and also to an increase in the quality of the evidence that each study can provide. Descriptive studies or reports are essential to identify health problems in the first place and to provide the first ideas about causality (to generate hypotheses), but more formal analytic studies are then required in order to test these hypotheses.

Descriptive studies

Descriptive epidemiology can be anything from a description of disease in a single person (a case report) to the description of patterns and trends seen among routine data collected at a population level, or a survey especially designed to collect information from individuals to describe the prevalence of some attribute in that population. It describes the occurrence of disease in relation to *person*, for instance, by age group, sex, race, occupation or lifestyle; in relation to *place*, such as for different countries, different regions of the same country or urban and rural areas of a single region; and in relation to *time*, either calendar time or life events, for example, birth, puberty, menopause, graduation, marriage or divorce.

Case reports and case series

All scientific studies begin by naming and describing the phenomenon of interest. In epidemiology the process often begins with a **case report** or **case series**. These are detailed descriptions, usually by a doctor or group of doctors, of one or more cases of a disease that are unusual for some reason. This might be because the disease has not been seen before, not been noted before or not been named before, or because it is rarely seen in that form. Occasionally the cases may have occurred in individuals who would not normally be expected to develop that disease or they may have arisen in an area where it had not previously been reported or was thought to have been controlled. The cases might be reported in conjunction with a previous exposure to something that, it is speculated, may have caused the disease.

The selective nature of these reports and the limited amount of information they contain mean that they provide little evidence of causality and cannot say much about patterns of disease occurrence. However, they can help identify potential health problems and thus stimulate interest in an area, leading on to more detailed studies, and some have been seminal in advancing knowledge (Box 6.2).

Routine data

As you have seen, an enormous volume of routine data is generated in a wide variety of forms. Figure 6.1 shows another example: trends in lung cancer mortality over time in Hungary, the UK and the USA.

What does this graph tell us about lung cancer? Why might rates have risen in Hungary but fallen in the UK and USA? Do we need any other information before we can draw any conclusions from this information?

Figure 6.1 suggests that lung cancer mortality rates in the UK have fallen dramatically since the early 1970s, whereas in the USA they are gradually falling after

Fig. 6.1 Age-standardised death rates from lung cancer among men aged 40–69 years in Hungary (▲), the USA (○) and the UK (●). (*Data source:* WHO Statistical Information System, accessed via http://www-depdb.iarc.fr/who/menu.htm, December 2003.)

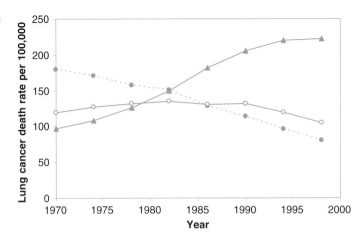

Box 6.2 Case reports and case series that were instrumental in the early identification of health problems

- The classic description of a series of infants born with congenital cataracts, some with additional cardiac abnormalities, in Australia in 1941. This led Dr N. M. Gregg in Sydney to postulate a causal link between a severe epidemic of rubella (German measles) that had occurred six to nine months before the children were born and the subsequent abnormalities (Gregg, 1941). It is now well known that if a woman develops rubella during pregnancy it may affect her unborn baby.

- A case report published in the UK in 1961 described the development of a pulmonary embolism in a 40-year-old pre-menopausal woman, five weeks after she had started using an oral contraceptive (OC) to treat endometriosis (Jordan, 1961). Because pulmonary embolism is rare in women of that age, the author suggested that it might have been caused by the OC, particularly since it was a novel exposure at that time. A report of one case could not provide conclusive evidence that it was the OC rather than some other characteristic of the patient that led to the embolism – but it did pave the way for more detailed studies. These have consistently shown that there is an association between the use of OCs and the risk of this condition.

- A report of a series of five cases of *Pneumocystis carinii* pneumonia that occurred in young, previously healthy, homosexual men in three Los Angeles hospitals in a six-month period during 1980–81 (CDC, 1981). Until then, this disease had been seen almost exclusively in the elderly, the severely malnourished and those on anti-cancer chemotherapy whose immune systems were suppressed. This cluster of cases in young men suggested that the men were suffering from a previously unknown disease, possibly related to sexual behaviour. We now know this as HIV/AIDS.

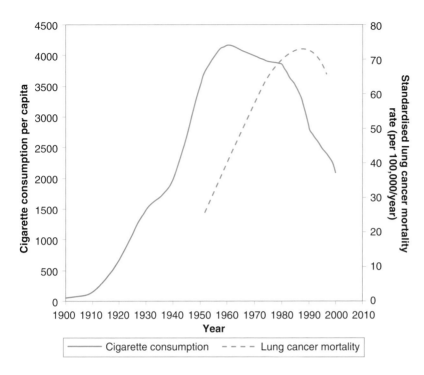

Fig. 6.2 Cigarette consumption (——) and lung cancer mortality rates (----) in males, age standardised to the 1970 US population. (Cigarette consumption data from www.infoplease.com, accessed February 2004; lung cancer mortality rates from Devesa *et al.*, 1999.)

having peaked in the 1980s. In contrast, the rates in Hungary rose markedly in the 1980s and are just starting to level out. However, before we accept that this is a real effect, we must consider a variety of alternative explanations. Is lung cancer diagnosed in the same way in each country? Have either the method of diagnosis or the criteria for diagnosis changed over time and have they changed differently in the three countries? Does lung cancer mortality mirror the incidence of lung cancer (i.e., is lung cancer really more common in Hungary?), or are the mortality rates higher in Hungary simply because treatment is less effective and the case–fatality ratio higher? Are lung cancer mortality rates in the UK and USA falling because the incidence is falling or because treatment has improved? If this is a real effect, does the fall in rates in the western countries reflect the reduction in cigarette smoking?

Data of this type leave us with many questions but few definitive answers. However, if we can relate them to changes in other factors that might influence mortality they can add support to a hypothesis. For example, by plotting a graph of per-capita cigarette consumption over time and comparing this with lung cancer mortality rates (Figure 6.2), we find that the rise in lung cancer mortality in the USA parallels increasing cigarette sales, but it occurred 20–30 years later. This represents the two to three decades that it takes smoking to cause lung cancer and kill someone. The fact that lung cancer rates started to fall again 20–30 years after the decline in smoking adds further weight to the hypothesis that smoking causes lung cancer: if this fall had not occurred then the hypothesis would have failed a critical test – removal of the cause should reduce the incidence of disease. So, although these data do not prove that smoking causes lung cancer, they add weight to the belief that it could. If we found that an increase in cigarette consumption in Hungary occurred much later than the increases seen in the UK and US this would strengthen the belief even further.

Prevalence surveys

Surveys are conducted to measure the prevalence of a wide variety of aspects of health, including diseases that are not captured by other routine statistics; conditions such as obesity; health-related behaviours such as smoking, sun-exposure and diet; and use of health services. To a large extent these are purely descriptive and their aim is primarily to determine the prevalence of these factors in the community, often to aid health planning. In many cases, however, the breadth of information collected allows much more in-depth analysis of the relationships between health behaviours and conditions and we will discuss this aspect under analytic studies.

Migrant studies

Another creative use of descriptive data comes from what are often called *migrant studies*. One of the challenges in even starting to interpret differences in disease rates between countries is separating the effects of nature and nurture. Do Japanese women have very low rates of breast cancer compared with White American women because they are Japanese (i.e., because of a different genetic predisposition) or because they live differently (i.e., have different environmental exposures, such as diet)? For some populations we are fortunate to have what could be called 'natural experiments' when large numbers of people have migrated from a country with a low risk of a particular disease to a high-risk country, or vice versa, which can help to answer these questions. For example, large numbers of Japanese have migrated to Hawaii and California, and their overall rates of some diseases (e.g., breast cancer and coronary heart disease) have changed dramatically within one or two generations, moving away from the low rates in Japan towards the higher rates of the USA. The converse is true for rates of stroke and stomach cancer, which are lower in Japanese people residing in the USA than in those who live in Japan. If these diseases were largely genetic in origin then the rates could not have changed so quickly when the migrants moved to the USA. This strongly implicates the importance of the environment in increasing or decreasing the migrants' risk of disease and has led to enthusiasm for the idea that diet plays an important causal role in these diseases. However, the only specific causal hypothesis that is directly tested by such data is that large-scale international variation in these diseases is not primarily genetic in origin.

Analytic studies

We will now consider the main types of analytic research that you are likely to come across in the health literature. The primary purpose of these studies is to evaluate the association between an exposure or characteristic and the development of a particular disease. In order to make causal inferences about this association we need to eliminate **bias** as a possible explanation. All research should be designed to minimise bias, but some types of study are more prone to it than others. We will discuss the problem of bias in greater depth as we look at each design in turn (and will pick it up again in Chapter 7).

Ecological or correlation studies

Figure 6.3 shows the relation or correlation between the prevalence of infection with *Helicobacter pylori* (a bacterium that infects the stomach) and stomach cancer mortality rates in 46 Chinese counties (Forman *et al.*, 1990). In this study, the prevalence of infection was measured as the percentage of the population in the county with antibodies to the bacterium and the cumulative gastric cancer mortality rate is the rate per 1,000 men and women (summed from birth to age 64). Each spot on the graph represents one of the 46 counties. There is not a perfect

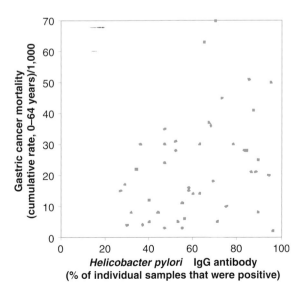

Fig. 6.3 An ecological study comparing the prevalence of serum antibodies to *H. pylori* (a gastric infection) and gastric cancer mortality rates in 46 rural Chinese counties. (From Forman *et al.*, Geographical association of *Helicobacter pylori* antibody prevalence and gastric cancer mortality in rural China. *Int. J. Cancer*, 1990; 46: 608–611, reprinted by permission of Wiley-Liss, Inc., a subsidiary of John Wiley & Sons, Inc.)

association, but the graph indicates that counties with a higher prevalence of *H. pylori* infection also tend to have higher stomach cancer rates and, perhaps more importantly, counties with a low prevalence of *H. pylori* have low stomach cancer rates. This hints that *H. pylori* might play a role in the development of stomach cancer; however, the fact that some counties have a high *H. pylori* prevalence but a low stomach cancer rate suggests that infection alone is not enough to cause cancer. Other factors must also play a role.

This example illustrates the key characteristic of ecological studies – they compare the prevalence of exposure and occurrence of disease in *populations* or groups of people, not individuals. The points on the graph represent the population prevalence of infection (in this case, taken from special surveys of individuals in each county) and the rate of disease in the population. The focus is on whether counties or populations with a high prevalence of infection also had a high cancer rate. A problem with this type of study is that an observed association between variables at the *group* level might not represent the association at the *individual* level: in this example, we have no way of knowing whether the people who developed cancer were actually infected with *H. pylori*. Ascribing characteristics to members of a group that they might not possess as individuals is called an **ecological fallacy**.

In general, ecological studies are attractive because they are easy to do if the routine data are readily available, but they can be difficult to interpret. The populations being compared may well differ in ways other than their exposure to the factor of interest and it is possible that something else that is related to the exposure is actually responsible for the observed differences in morbidity or mortality (i.e., an apparent relation could be due to confounding – see Chapter 8). For these reasons, ecological studies rarely give a strong test of a causal hypothesis but, more often, they help to generate or develop hypotheses.

Cross-sectional studies

A group of researchers in South Africa set out to determine the extent of abuse against women in three of the nine provinces in South Africa. Randomly selected women between the ages of 18 and 49 years were interviewed in their homes and the participation rate was 90%. The investigators found that 9.5% of the 1,279 women reported abuse from a current or former husband or boyfriend in the previous year and almost 25% of women had been abused at some time during their lives. Multiple factors were associated with the abuse, including violence in the women's childhood, limited education and alcohol abuse by the women themselves (Jewkes *et al.*, 2002).

This study combined descriptive and analytic components. It both defined the scope of the problem (descriptive) and identified a number of possible causal risk factors (analytic). It also captured the prevalences of those factors.

Box 6.3 Ecological studies that have been instrumental in suggesting associations between exposures and disease

- In a classic study, Armstrong and Doll (1975) reported the correlation between 27 cancers and a wide range of dietary and other variables in 23 countries. Diet was strongly correlated with several types of cancer, particularly consumption of meat with cancer of the colon. Countries with low per-capita daily consumption of meat had the lowest rates of colon cancer. The findings from this study suggested that dietary factors play a role in the development of cancer and led to a burgeoning of research in this area.
- In 1979, the authors of another study reported a strong inverse association between average per-capita consumption of wine and mortality from ischaemic heart disease (high wine consumption was associated with low IHD mortality) (St Leger *et al.*, 1979). Since then more than 60 ecological, case–control and cohort studies have been conducted and most have shown that *moderate consumption* of wine and other alcohol has a protective effect against heart disease.

All these data, descriptive and analytic, can be valuable for planning health and social system responses.

The key feature of the study is that the women were not recruited because they had (or had not) been abused or because of their particular histories. Rather, they were invited to participate because they were assumed to be typical of all South African women. This then is a cross-sectional study, i.e., the study group is chosen to be a cross-section of a population. The idea is to select people in such a way that they are representative of the whole population so that information collected from the study sample can be generalised directly to the whole population. Surveys such as this may be conducted to gather information about any aspects of health and lifestyle. As in the example, people should be recruited without knowledge of either their exposure status (presence or absence of the exposures of interest) or their disease status (presence or absence of the diseases of interest) in order to avoid **selection bias** (we will discuss this further in Chapter 7). Exposure and out-come are then both assessed at the same point in time. The data can be analysed using similar methods to those for case–control studies, enabling the calculation of odds ratios to describe the association between exposure and disease. Alternatively, comparisons between the prevalences of disease in exposed and unexposed participants can be made using prevalence ratios (see Chapter 5).

Figure 6.4 shows the major features of a cross-sectional study. In the example above, information on abuse (outcome) and previous abuse, education, alcohol use, etc. (the exposures) was obtained simultaneously. For this reason, in this

Fig. 6.4 The design of a
cross–sectional study.

type of study it can be difficult to identify which came first – the exposure or the outcome (disease). Cross-sectional studies can, however, be particularly useful for examining exposures that do not change over time (for example, personal characteristics like sex and blood group) or that occurred many years previously.

Studies of this type evaluate prevalent cases of disease – those that are already present in the population at the time of the survey. As we discussed in Chapter 2, prevalence is a function both of the incidence and of the duration of a disease. People who have a disease for longer are more likely to be ill at the time of a cross-sectional study than those who are sick for a shorter time. An association between exposure and prevalence of disease can thus reflect not only a link between exposure and the occurrence of new disease, but also a link between exposure and factors that affect survival or persistence of a diseased state. Thus, it is not always easy to interpret cross-sectional data in causal terms with respect to disease aetiology.

Is there any problem here with the time-directionality of the link between level of education and abuse?

Are the South African women studied likely to be typical of all South African women? What are the implications for interpreting the findings?

In this study it is unlikely that there is a problem with the time-directionality of this exposure–outcome link. The level of education attained by the women prior to their relationships is not likely to change much over time and so can be assumed to have preceded the abuse. In relation to the generalisability of the findings, the results from the study were based on a random sample of women from three of nine provinces in South Africa. The participation rate was high, but the three provinces were chosen for pragmatic reasons and may be quite different from the other provinces. Thus it might not be reasonable to generalise the results to *all* South African women, but they will be directly applicable to women from the areas studied.

Cross-sectional surveys such as the national health surveys conducted in many countries are often carried out at regular intervals. They recruit a *different* sample of people for each survey and then study changes in the population prevalence of disease, disability or potential risk factors for disease. In this regard they differ from cohort studies, which follow the *same* group of people over a period of time.

Box 6.4 Diagnostic studies

A study to evaluate the accuracy of a diagnostic test can be thought of as a special type of cross-sectional study in which the data are collected from diagnostic test results or physical examination rather than from interviews or questionnaires. Typically, individuals with symptoms of disease are selected randomly or consecutively from a clinic or hospital to undergo the test of interest (the **index test**). Then independently (and blinded to the results of the index test) the same individuals undergo the best test available to diagnose the disease (the *reference test* or '**gold standard**'). The results of the two tests are then compared and the accuracy of the index test (its **sensitivity** and **specificity**) can be determined (we will discuss the mechanisms of this in Chapter 14). As in all cross-sectional studies, it is important that the people selected are representative of the target population – in this case patients in whom the test would be used in real life.

Case–control studies

In a case–control study we choose individuals with the disease or outcome of interest (cases) and a comparison group without the disease (controls), and then measure their past exposure to certain risk factors. (Some authors prefer to call the comparison group the 'reference' group and will describe the study as a *case–reference* or *case–referent* study.) The odds of exposures of interest for the cases and controls are then compared (see Chapter 5). For instance, if we wanted to know whether smoking was associated with lung cancer we would compare the odds of smoking among lung cancer cases with that among controls without lung cancer, exactly as Doll and Hill did back in 1950 (see Chapter 1). Figure 6.5 shows the design features of a typical case–control study.

A classic case–control study was conducted in Germany in 1961 (Mellin and Katzenstein, 1962). The mothers of children born with unusual limb malformations (cases) were compared with mothers of normal children (controls) with respect to their exposures in pregnancy. Forty-one of the 46 case mothers (89%), but none of 300 control mothers, had taken thalidomide early in their pregnancy. This strongly suggested that thalidomide use early in pregnancy could be responsible for the birth defects. (It should be noted that this study was stimulated by data from an earlier case series.)

In the Australian ovarian cancer case–control study described in Chapter 5, more than 800 women who developed ovarian cancer were interviewed, together with a similar number of cancer-free control women. Table 6.1 shows some more results from this study (Purdie *et al.*, 1995).

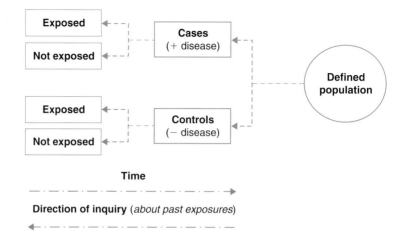

Table 6.1 Results from an Australian case–control study of ovarian cancer and use of oral contraceptive (OC) pills.

Exposure (use of OC pills)	Cases (n)	Control (n)	Odds ratio (crude)	95% Confidence interval
Never	408	305	1.0	(Reference group)
<5 years	213	230	0.7	0.5–0.9
5–9 years	110	143	0.6	0.4–0.8
≥10 years	66	167	0.3	0.2–0.4

(Purdie *et al.*, 1995.)

What does Table 6.1 tell us about the relation between oral contraceptive (OC) use and development of ovarian cancer?

Table 6.1 presents the raw data (the actual numbers of women in each group) and the crude odds ratios for the association between the duration of use of the OC pill and the risk of ovarian cancer in Australian women. The odds ratio falls with increasing duration of use of the OC pill (a *dose–response* relationship), suggesting that longer duration of use is associated with a lower risk of ovarian cancer. The 95% confidence limits for all three categories of exposure are narrow and the upper limits are all below 1.0, indicating that the reduction in risk is statistically significant. (We will discuss crude odds ratios, confidence intervals and statistical significance further in Chapters 7 and 8.)

A wide range of other possible causes have also been examined within this one study and this is one of the major appeals of the case–control design. Participants can be asked about many different exposures, allowing multiple factors to be evaluated within the same study.

Ideally case–control studies include only incident or new cases of disease as they arise. However, some studies, especially those of very rare diseases, will also include prevalent cases. This makes them rather like cross-sectional studies, with the possible problem of determining a clear time sequence for the exposure–disease relation. (That is, a factor may appear to be related to disease risk simply because it enhances the duration of disease.) This issue can also arise in an incidence-based study using biological measures, because sub-clinical disease present before diagnosis may have influenced metabolism and, for instance, led to low plasma vitamin levels or loss of weight, rather than low vitamin levels or loss of weight having led to disease.

Case–control studies offer a number of advantages over follow-up studies. They are generally quicker and more economical to perform (but still not a trivial undertaking) and are good for evaluating rare outcomes. (If you wanted to investigate the causes of a rare cancer using a follow-up study design, you would have to recruit an enormous number of people and follow them for a long time before enough cancers occurred to allow a useful analysis.) Case–control studies are also good for evaluating many different exposures, all of which can be asked about at the one interview as we noted above. Their use is largely restricted to causal investigations, although they have been used in other areas, for example to identify factors that predict whether individuals attend for vaccination.

The central problem in the design of a case–control study is selection of the control group. Controls should represent the population from which the cases have come such that their exposure prevalence is very similar to that of the whole population. In practice this means that appropriately selected controls should have been identified as cases if they had developed the condition of interest. If the cases form a population-based series (e.g., if all cases from a defined geographical region are included), then the appropriate control group should be representative of that population. **Population controls** can be selected in a number of ways, including from population registers or comprehensive electoral rolls and, in recent times, by sampling residential telephone numbers at random (random-digit dialling). In the ovarian cancer study described above, the controls were selected from the electoral roll because enrolment to vote is compulsory in Australia, but this strategy would not work in other countries where voting is not mandatory. (Note, to ensure comparability between cases and controls, in terms of source population, any case not on the electoral roll was excluded from the study.) In the UK, selection of controls from the patient lists of the general practitioners (GPs) who referred the cases would be a viable alternative because most of the population is registered with a GP.

Where the case group does not originate from a clearly defined geographical population, a traditional approach employed to identify controls from the likely

Box 6.5 When hospital controls may be the best way to go

Tertiary referral clinics may attract patients from an unpredictably wide variety of geographical and social origins. If cases are identified through these clinics it can then be a major challenge to find a group of disease-free controls that represent the same geographical and social backgrounds as the cases. For example, a colonoscopy is needed to diagnose adenoma (polyps) of the large bowel so a colonoscopy clinic is an ideal place to identify cases for a study. If controls are selected at random from the local population there is no guarantee that they would have been picked up as cases if they had adenoma – they might have gone to a different facility. Similarly, we would miss all of those people from outside the local population who would, nonetheless, have travelled to that clinic for treatment. An alternative then is to select controls from among other patients attending the clinic who have a colonoscopy but do *not* have bowel polyps. This solution ensures that the controls will represent the geographical and social distribution of the cases, but it is important to be aware that it might also introduce other biases. For example, if there are characteristics, such as a family history of bowel cancer, that make someone more likely to be referred for colonoscopy then these characteristics will be over-represented in the control group. This example serves to emphasise that epidemiological studies will rarely be perfect – the important thing is to do the best that is possible in a given situation and then to consider the likely effects of any bias (we will discuss this further in Chapter 7).

source population utilises the local neighbourhood of the case as a sampling frame. This is time-consuming and expensive, but effective; and a modern variant is based on matching telephone numbers with random selection of the last few digits.

Whilst population or neighbourhood controls are ideal, practical reasons mean that **hospital controls** are still used, although not as frequently as in the past. This is usually accomplished by selecting controls from patients admitted to the same hospitals as the cases, but for conditions other than the one being studied. Although this is a much more efficient and economical process than selecting population controls, it is associated with an obvious major drawback. The controls are themselves ill and thus different from most healthy people in the source population from which the cases come. Indeed, their distribution of risk factors (especially personal habits such as smoking, excessive alcohol consumption, etc.) may well resemble that of the cases rather more than that of the source population, resulting in biased estimates of effect. However, thoughtful use of such designs can provide good public health information, e.g., for post-marketing drug surveillance (pharmacoepidemiology). There are also situations in which it

Box 6.6 Case–control studies

- Phenacetin was introduced as an analgesic in 1887 and used extensively until it was suggested that it might be associated with kidney disease. A case–control study involving 554 adults with newly diagnosed kidney disease and 516 matched control subjects selected randomly from the same geographical area was conducted in the USA to investigate this (Sandler *et al.*, 1989). After allowing for the effects of other types of analgesic, the risk of kidney disease was five-fold higher among daily users of phenacetin (OR = 5.1; 95% confidence interval (CI) 1.8–14.9) and it was also three-fold higher (OR = 3.2; 95% CI 1.1–9.8) among daily users of paracetamol (acetaminophen, a metabolite of phenacetin) than it was among infrequent users of these drugs. There was little association between aspirin use and renal disease (OR = 1.3; 95% CI 0.7–2.5). Results from this study and others confirmed the risks of phenacetin, which was withdrawn from the market.

- In a case–control study conducted in Tasmania, Australia, the parents of 58 children who had died from SIDS (sudden infant death syndrome) and of 120 control children were interviewed about the sleeping practices of their children. Children who were placed face-down had a four-fold higher risk of SIDS than children placed in other positions. This risk was increased even further if the child slept in a heated room, was tightly wrapped or had recently been ill (Ponsonby *et al.*, 1993). The results of this study and others have led to campaigns aimed at persuading parents to place babies on their backs to sleep in order to reduce rates of SIDS.

may be impossible to identify an appropriate population-based series of controls such that each control would fit the criterion that they would have been included as a case *if* they had the disease of interest.

An important issue related to the selection of both cases and controls is that they must be chosen *independently of their exposure status*. In a case–control study of oral contraceptive pill use and deep vein thrombosis, for example, whether or not a woman is using the pill should not affect her chances of being recruited as either a case or control. Knowledge of the exposure status of individuals could lead to bias in participant recruitment called **selection bias**. Another type of bias that can occur within case–control studies arises when the information collected from the cases and controls is not comparable. This can occur if an interviewer elicits or interprets exposure information differently when the disease status of the individual is known (**interviewer bias**) or because people with disease recall their exposures or experiences more precisely than or otherwise differently from those without disease (**recall bias**). We will revisit bias and other forms of inaccuracy in data collection and discuss the potential impact of these types of error on the results of a study in Chapter 7.

There are several modern variants of the case–control study design, the most common being *nested case–control, case–cohort* and *case–crossover* designs. We will consider the first two under cohort studies as they are essentially different ways of analysing cohort data but will look briefly at the third type here.

Case–crossover studies

The **case–crossover** design is especially suited to identifying the effects of brief exposures on the risk of an acute-onset disease. Instead of recruiting a separate group of controls, each case is also their own control and their exposure in a defined period prior to the onset of disease is compared with their normal exposure frequency. This innovative design eliminates many of the problems inherent in studies that compare different groups of people and comes closest to the theoretical (but unattainable) ideal, which would be to study an exposed population and then wind back the clock and study exactly the same population again when they had not been exposed.

In the seminal case–crossover study, Maclure (1991) examined the influence of a variety of possible precipitating factors, including sexual activity, on the occurrence of myocardial infarction (MI, or heart attack). He classified cases as exposed if they had been sexually active in the two hours before their MI and then compared this with their usual frequency of sexual activity over a one-year period. He hypothesised that, if sexual activity were a risk factor for MI, then more cases would have been sexually active shortly before their MI than would be expected from their usual frequency. After interviewing 300 cases he estimated that sexual activity increased an individual's risk of MI more than two-fold (RR = 2.6; 95% confidence interval 0.9–7.1).

Cohort studies

Cohort studies are also known as 'follow-up' (or sometimes prospective) studies because they follow people over time to see what happens to them. The cohort[1] might be a group of initially healthy people whom we follow to observe the occurrence of disease among them or a group of patients whom we follow to study their disease outcomes, i.e., their prognosis. A classic example of a cohort study is the Framingham Heart Study (Dawber, 1980). It was started in 1948 at a time when heart disease had become the USA's number one killer, and the principal aim was to learn which biological and environmental factors were contributing to the rapid rise in cardiovascular death and disability. The epidemiological approach was quite novel at the time and it was designed to identify how and

---

[1] In Ancient Rome, a cohort was one of ten divisions of a Roman military legion. It comprised young men of similar age from one region. In service its members were often injured or killed and they were not replaced. The cohort was then disbanded when the term of enlistment was over – a good model for the epidemiological version.

Table 6.2 Contributions made by the Framingham Heart Study.

Year	Significant contribution
1956	Findings on progression (natural history) of rheumatic heart disease reported.
1959	Factors found that increase the likelihood of heart disease. Some heart attacks discovered to be 'silent' (causing no pain).
1960	Cigarette smoking found to increase the risk of heart disease.
1961	Cholesterol level, blood pressure and electrocardiogram abnormalities found to increase the risk of heart disease.
1967	Physical activity found to reduce, and obesity to increase, the risk of heart disease.
1970	High blood pressure found to increase the risk of stroke.
1974	Overview of diabetes. Its complications and association with development of cardiovascular disease described.
1976	Menopause found to increase the risk of heart disease.
1977	Effects of triglycerides and LDL ('bad') and HDL ('good') cholesterol described.
1987	Oestrogen replacement therapy found to reduce risk of hip fractures in post-menopausal women.
1988	High levels of HDL cholesterol found to reduce risk of death. Cigarette smoking found to increase risk of stroke.
1990	Homocysteine (an amino acid) found to be possible risk factor for heart disease.
1993	Major report predicts survival after diagnosis of heart failure.
1998	New 'risk prediction' formulae to calculate a patient's risk of CHD in the next 10 years.

(*Source:* www.framingham.com/heart, accessed 15 March 2004.)

why those who developed heart disease differed from those who escaped it. The town of Framingham, Massachusetts was selected by the US Public Health Service as the study site, and 5,209 healthy residents between 30 and 60 years of age, both men and women, were enrolled. Framingham was appealing because it had a stable population and a single medical facility, suggesting that it would be relatively easy to carry out the follow-up. The study was expanded in 1971 when 5,124 children (and their spouses) of the original cohort were recruited for a second study, the Offspring Study.

Before Framingham, the notion that scientists could identify, and individuals could modify, '*risk factors*' (a term coined by the authors of the study) tied to heart disease, stroke and other diseases was not part of standard medical practice. With over 50 years of data collected from residents of Framingham (and the publication of more than 1,000 scientific papers), the Framingham researchers have identified major risk factors associated with heart disease, stroke and other

Fig. 6.6 The design of a cohort study (adapted from Beaglehole *et al.* (1993) with permission).

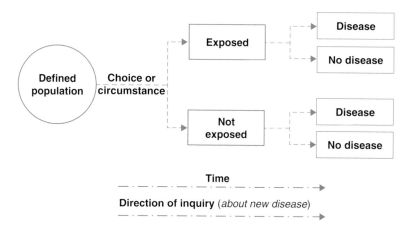

diseases and created a revolution in preventive medicine. Most of the risk factors that were identified are so commonly accepted today, both by health professionals and by the lay public, that it is difficult to imagine a time when we did not know about them. Table 6.2 provides a timeline of just some of the many contributions the study has made to our knowledge of cardiovascular disease.

The Framingham Study is quite small by modern standards: the Nurses' Health Study initiated in 1976 and run from Boston, USA, included 120,000 women (Stampfer *et al.*, 1988) and the Million Women Study was initiated in the UK in 1996 (The Million Women Study Collaborative Group, 1999). The Framingham study therefore needed particularly long follow-up to accumulate enough endpoints to give robust results. A crucial trade-off is that the smaller size and the setting permitted regular detailed physical examination and other 'hands-on' investigations such as the recording of electrocardiograms, giving a rich array of high-quality exposure data that cannot be gathered on a very large scale. The Nurses' Health and Million Women studies rely primarily, but not exclusively, on questionnaires.

In a cohort study we compare the rates of occurrence of disease in groups of people with and without a particular exposure (Figure 6.6). The participants must be free of the outcome of interest at the start of the follow-up, which makes it easier to be sure that the exposure preceded the outcome. (If there is a long pre-clinical phase before a disease is diagnosed, the exposure–disease sequence can still be muddled.) Of all the observational designs, cohort studies generally provide the best information concerning the causes of disease and the most direct measurements of the risk of developing disease. The other advantage of collecting exposure information before people develop disease is that measurement of exposure is not biased by knowledge of outcome status. Bias in outcome measurement is still possible, but this can generally be avoided or minimised by the use of objective measures (e.g., death) or independent or blinded observers to assign outcomes.

Cohort studies are by nature very time-consuming and expensive. However, the benefit : cost ratio of a well-run cohort study is high, given the enhanced validity over case–control studies and the multitude of associations that can be assessed. For example, over the last decade the Nurses' Health Study has been the basis for between 30 and 50 publications every year. In principle, a long-term cohort study also has the potential to deliver the public health knowledge of most value, by showing the full array of harms and benefits associated with a given exposure. The British Doctors Study is an outstanding example of this with regard to cigarette smoking because while it, like other studies, shows that there is a potential benefit of cigarette smoking with regard to Parkinson's disease, this is overwhelmed by the many negative effects of smoking, which puts control of smoking at the top of the public health agenda.

Selection of participants is an issue at two points of a cohort study: who is *selected into* the cohort at the start of the study and who is *lost from* the cohort during

Box 6.7 Some other notable cohort studies

- The British Doctors Study cohort was established in 1951 and is still being followed, although many of the original 40,701 participants are now dead. It has been of enormous value, particularly in relation to identifying the manifold health consequences of smoking, despite the fact that, compared with studies today, only limited exposure data were collected on a very short postal questionnaire mailed to the doctors at 10-year intervals since 1951 (Doll and Hill, 1964).
- The US Nurses' Health Study started in 1976 with 121,964 female nurses aged 30–55, and 5 years of funding. Since then its focus has widened enormously from the oral contraceptive–breast cancer links for which it was first funded (Stampfer *et al.*, 1988) to cover many exposures (including diet) and a multitude of outcomes. It celebrated its 25th year of follow-up in 2001 and is still going strong. It is very expensive to run, but the scientific and public health yield has been exceptional. There is now also a Nurses' Health Study II that began in 1989 with 117,000 nurses aged 25–42 (Rockhill *et al.*, 1998).
- ALSPAC (The Avon Longitudinal Study of Parents and Children) was started in 1990 to determine ways in which an individual's genes combine with environmental pressures to influence health and development. Comprehensive data on over 10,000 children and their parents, from early pregnancy until the children are aged between 8 and 9, have now been collected. Since the study is based in one geographical area of the UK, linkage to medical and educational records is relatively simple, and hands-on assessments of children and parents using local facilities allows good quality control (Golding *et al.*, 2001).

follow-up. Who is selected into a cohort can influence the generalisability of its findings since they may apply only to the sorts of people who agreed to take part, but generally in a cohort study the more important issue is to avoid or minimise selective losses from the cohort. Regardless of the length of the follow-up period, one of the most important criteria for a high-quality cohort study is to ensure that complete *follow-up* of all participants is carried out. The more people who are 'lost to follow-up' with unknown health status, the more likely it is that the results will be biased. (We will discuss selection bias further in Chapter 7.)

Historical cohort studies

It is sometimes possible to avoid the long follow-up period common to many cohort studies by establishing a retrospective or **historical** cohort. This requires good records of past exposure for a group of people who can be traced to determine their current health. Such a study is most common in industry or the military where good personnel records exist, but they have also been used to study the development of disease in relation to characteristics at birth (e.g., weight and length at birth) because this information can often be obtained retrospectively from birth records. In the absence of close follow-up – the usual situation – they are generally limited to studying mortality or cancer outcomes, given the lack of universal records for other non-fatal endpoints. Some interesting and useful variations include the use of college alumni records in the USA to study benefits of physical activity as a young adult (Paffenbarger *et al.*, 1986) and the Boyd Orr Study based on detailed dietary records collected from over 4,000 British children in the 1930s (Frankel *et al.*, 1998).

Nested case–control studies

In many cohort studies, all participants provide a wide range of information at the time of recruitment, including answers to detailed dietary questionnaires and blood and urine samples. Because of the large numbers and cost, these resources – especially the biological samples – are often not analysed in detail at the time but are stored for future use. It is then possible to use this information efficiently by conducting a case–control study 'nested' within the cohort. This involves identifying people in the cohort who develop the disease of interest and then selecting controls from among those who were disease-free at the time the cases were diagnosed (i.e., the controls are 'matched' to the cases for follow-up). Detailed exposure information can then be retrieved for this sub-set of participants from the full cohort. This design maintains the major advantage of a cohort study in that the exposure data were originally collected before the development of disease, but on a much smaller scale.

Case–cohort studies

The case–cohort design is similar in principle to the nested case–control study with the difference that the comparison group is selected from the full cohort at

Box 6.8 Prognostic studies

A common way to investigate the prognosis of people with a particular condition is to assemble a cohort of patients with the condition at the same point in the course of their illness (e.g., at diagnosis) and follow them until they experience the outcome of interest (e.g., death). The term *inception cohort* is often used to describe a group of people who are assembled near the onset ('inception') of disease. The outcome or prognosis for an individual can be more precisely predicted when the individual characteristics of a patient are taken into account. Characteristics that may affect an outcome include demographic factors (e.g., age, gender and socioeconomic status), disease-specific factors (e.g., extent or stage of disease) and co-morbidities (other health conditions). Such characteristics are called *prognostic factors*; they do not need to *cause* the outcome, but must be associated with it strongly enough to *predict* it. Event rates tend to be high, so prognostic studies are usually much smaller than cohort studies of risk factors.

baseline, allowing it to be used for comparison with multiple different case groups. The drawback of a case–cohort study is that it requires more sophisticated data analysis than the traditional cohort and nested case–control analyses.

Record linkage

Many investigators performing cohort studies enhance their follow-up by using external sources of health data to which they link their cohort members in order to pick up new outcomes, commonly occurrence of cancer or mortality (since these data are often routinely available from central registries). The matches are made in a variety of ways, including using a common personal identification number as in many Scandinavian countries and the USA (social security number), or through probabilistic approaches based on a variety of personal identifiers (e.g., name, date of birth and address).

There is also an interesting and often informative sub-set of studies that are based on record linkage alone. They are effectively cohort studies in which both exposure and outcome information comes from electronic records. While they have been used mostly to link health services and outcomes, increasing computerisation of medical information makes more conventional aetiological research possible by this means. As an example, Swedish investigators were able to use the Swedish Inpatient Register to identify a cohort of 29,187 patients hospitalised for type-1 diabetes between 1965 and 1999. They then 'linked' these names to the Swedish Cancer, Total Population, Migration and Death Registers. This told them who had been diagnosed with cancer, the type of cancer and date of diagnosis, and also who had migrated or died from some other cause and so was no longer at risk of being diagnosed with cancer in Sweden. They calculated standardised incidence ratios for the cohort compared with the general population and found that diabetes was associated with significantly increased risks of cancer of the stomach (SIR = 2.3), cervix (SIR = 1.6) and uterus (SIR = 2.7) (Zendehdel *et al.*, 2003).

Current privacy concerns and legislation in some countries have the potential to limit this avenue of epidemiological research in particular, although the general issue of access to non-anonymised health records for public health research is being debated widely. Much effort is being expended to enable a constructive resolution of the tensions between maximising individual autonomy (by protecting against inappropriate access to personal health data) while ensuring that the public good delivered by health research is not compromised (Lawlor and Stone, 2001).

Intervention studies or experiments

If a laboratory scientist wanted to see whether something causes a particular effect he or she would set up an experiment. This would involve creating two identical test systems under identical conditions, adding the particular factor of interest to one of them and then waiting to see what happened. Any differences between the outcomes in the two systems could then be attributed to the presence of that factor. How then can we apply this scientific approach to the study of human populations?

Clearly, it would be acceptable to conduct such an experiment only if we thought that the factor under test would improve health; it would not be ethical to expose people to something thought to be harmful.

The examples in Box 6.9 give a hint of the range of interventions that can be studied experimentally. In each study the investigators 'intervened' to change something in the hope that this would improve the future health of the participants. The participants in the ISIS trials were already sick (patients who had had an MI), and the intervention was intended to improve their duration of survival – aspirin and streptokinase were shown to be very effective. In contrast, the children in the polio vaccine trial were healthy and it was hoped that the vaccine would prevent them from becoming ill. Similarly, it was hoped that vitamin A supplementation would reduce childhood mortality but, in this example, the intervention was given to whole villages rather than individual children.

These examples cover three major types of intervention study: clinical trials in patients, field or prevention trials in healthy people and community trials in which we intervene at the community level on groups of people instead of individuals. The principles of sound design and conduct are common to all. We will now look at each of these in more detail, taking the clinical randomised controlled trial (RCT) as the model and giving practical examples of each.

Box 6.9 Some large-scale intervention studies

- The ISIS (International Studies of Infarct Survival) investigators compared various treatments for myocardial infarction (heart attack), including the use of aspirin and streptokinase in ISIS-2 (ISIS-2 Collaborative Group, 1988). Since the first trial, the number of collaborators has increased enormously, so huge numbers of patients throughout the world were recruited into these studies.
- In the early 1950s, one of the largest epidemiological studies, and almost certainly the largest formal human 'experiment', was conducted in the USA. This was a field trial of polio vaccine in which over 400,000 school children were assigned to receive either the vaccine or a placebo (inactive) injection. The trial clearly demonstrated both the efficacy and the safety of the vaccine, which was then given to millions of children throughout the world (Francis *et al.*, 1955). This has led to a major drop in the incidence of polio not only in industrialised countries but also in many developing countries, which have recently been declared polio-free by the WHO.
- A randomised, controlled community trial was conducted to evaluate the effectiveness of vitamin A supplementation to prevent childhood mortality in Indonesia (Sommer *et al.*, 1986). In 229 villages, children aged 1–5 years were given two doses of vitamin A while children in the 221 control villages were not given vitamin A until after the study. Mortality among children in the control villages was 50% higher than that in the villages given vitamin A.

Randomised controlled (clinical) trials (RCTs)

The best way to evaluate a new treatment is to identify a group of patients with the same condition and then allocate them to receive the various treatments at *random*. **Random allocation** (also called **randomisation**) ensures that all of the groups are as similar as possible at the start of the study. (Note that equality of the groups at baseline is highly dependent on group size – with very small groups it is unlikely that the groups will be similar in terms of all important variables that could affect the outcome.) Random allocation is important because if one group were in some way more ill than the other at the start, this might make one treatment look better or worse, even if there were really no difference. (This problem is called confounding and we will discuss this in more detail in Chapter 8.) It is because of this aspect of RCTs – the close similarity of the groups in all respects other than the intervention – that they are generally considered to give the best evidence of all epidemiological studies. In a cohort study investigating potentially harmful risk factors, people cannot be randomly allocated to the various study

From www.CartoonStock.com

"Do a double-blind test. Give the new drug to rich patients and a placebo to the poor. No sense getting their hopes up. They couldn't afford it even if it works."

groups and, for example, a group of alcohol drinkers will certainly differ from a group of non-drinkers in more ways than just their alcohol consumption. While we can deal with some of these factors in our analysis, there may also be other important factors that we either do not know about or cannot measure well. The real strength of randomisation is that, on average, it will also balance these other unknown or unmeasured factors across the groups.

Randomised controlled trials also include a **control** or comparison group so that outcomes in the treated group can be compared with those in a group that is not treated. Generally, the patients in the control group either receive no treatment or, preferably, they are given a placebo (something that resembles the real treatment but is not active). If an acceptable standard treatment is available the control group must be given this – it would be unethical to withhold it – and this is compared with the new experimental treatment. It is these features of an ideal clinical trial that have led to them being called 'randomised controlled trials'. Figure 6.7 shows the design features of a simple randomised controlled trial. In practice it is just a special form of the standard prospective cohort study – the only difference being that participants are allocated to the exposed and unexposed groups at random.

Ideally, the trial investigators and patients should be unaware of which treatment patients are receiving, creating a 'double-blind' or 'masked' study. If only the patient is unaware of the treatment, it is a single-blind study. Blinding is important because knowledge of the treatment might affect both the patient's response – quite a few people become well after taking a placebo simply because they believe it will cure them – and an observer's measurement of outcome. In some situations (e.g., comparing medical treatment with surgery) there may be no feasible way of blinding patients and study personnel to the differences in treatments. Minimising measurement bias in this situation may be best accomplished by bringing in an independent 'blinded' observer whose only involvement is to

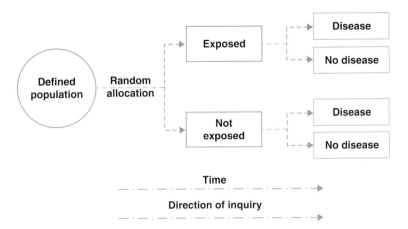

Fig. 6.7 The design of a randomised controlled trial.

assess the outcome measure. Blinding of outcome measurements obviously becomes more crucial as the measurement becomes more subjective. When the outcome measure is objective and less dependent on interpretation, as in a biochemical parameter or death, blinding is less important.

Apart from patients and trial investigators, there are many others (e.g., healthcare providers, data collectors, outcome assessors, data analysts) involved in the conduct of a trial who can introduce bias through their knowledge of treatment allocation. For this reason there is a growing tendency to abandon the terms single- and double-blind in favour of a transparent reporting of the blinding status of each group involved in the trial.

As for a cohort study, the other crucial feature of an RCT is good follow-up. It is important to know what has happened to all of the patients in the study.

Preventive trials

A preventive trial differs from an RCT in only one respect. Instead of patients, it involves people who are disease-free but thought to be at risk of developing disease. Ideally these studies should be conducted in the same way as randomised controlled trials.

Some other examples of major preventive trials include the following.

The US Physicians' Health Study (we have already met the British Doctors and the US Nurses' Health studies!) in which 22,000 physicians were randomly allocated to take aspirin, in an attempt to reduce cardiovascular morbidity and mortality, and/or capsules of β-carotene, in an attempt to reduce rates of cancer (Hennekens and Eberlein, 1985). After 12 years of follow-up, rates of cancer were very similar in the β-carotene and placebo groups, and, while aspirin was shown to lower the rates of heart attack, so few of these very healthy doctors died that the trial could not determine whether aspirin saved lives from cardiovascular disease.

Box 6.10 Randomised crossover trials

The design of randomised clinical trials can be categorised as either **parallel group** or **crossover**. Figure 6.7 shows the design of a parallel group RCT, in which patients are randomly allocated to one of the two groups, which are then followed in parallel. In a crossover design, the participants serve as their own controls (this is analogous to the case–crossover study we described earlier). For example, in a simple two-period crossover study to assess the efficacy of an intervention we would assign each participant to either the intervention or the control (I or C) for a specified period of time and then the alternative for a similar period of time. The order in which each participant receives I and C is randomly assigned. Thus, approximately half of the participants receive the intervention in the sequence I–C and the other half in the sequence C–I. This eliminates any trend from the first period to the second period from the estimate of group differences in response. One of the biggest advantages of this design is that it can produce statistically and clinically valid results with fewer participants than would be required with a parallel design. However, not all interventions are suitable for assessment in this way. If the effects of the intervention during the first period are likely to carry over into the second period then this design is clearly inappropriate, as it is for assessing long-term benefits and harms.

A variant of the crossover trial is single patient trials, often called **n-of-1 trials**. An individual patient receives the experimental and control treatments in random order on multiple occasions, with specific outcomes being monitored throughout the trial period. Ideally both the patient and the treating doctor are blinded to the treatment being received and the trial usually ends when it becomes clear that there are (or are not) important differences between the treatments. Although the results of n-of-1 trials are not generalisable to the same extent as those of typical RCTs, they do provide a good guide to individual clinical decisions.

MRFIT – the Multiple Risk Factor Intervention Trial, in which almost 13,000 American men at risk of coronary heart disease (CHD) were randomly allocated to either a special programme aimed to help them stop smoking and reduce their blood pressure and cholesterol levels, or to a control group who received their usual care. There was a (non-significant) 7% reduction in CHD in the intervention group (MRFIT Research Group, 1982). The authors speculated that this difference might have been so small because many men in the control group also changed their behaviour, for instance, by giving up smoking.

Community trials

These are preventive trials in which the intervention is implemented at the community level and are generally conducted when it would be impossible to offer (or evaluate) the intervention at the individual level. An example is the studies of water fluoridation and dental health conducted in various countries. When investigators wanted to study the effects of adding fluoride to the water supply on dental health it was clearly impossible to add fluoride to some people's water and not to others', so whole towns were allocated to receive fluoride in their water or not. The controlled trial of water fluoridation which gave the most striking results was carried out in the towns of Newburgh and Kingston in New York State. After 10 years of fluoridation, the DMF (decayed, missing or filled teeth) score for Newburgh children aged 6–16 was 50% lower than that for children in the unfluoridated town of Kingston (Ast and Schlesinger, 1956). The assumption underlying this result was that, apart from the water, there was no other major difference between the towns that could explain the effect (i.e., there was no confounding). (Note that, although this and other studies clearly showed the benefits of low levels of fluoride on dental health, continuing controversy about the possible adverse effects of fluoride on other organs in the body, particularly the bones, has meant that universal fluoridation of water supplies has not occurred.)

Because only two towns were included in this study, in practice it is little different from a non-randomised comparison. Other cluster designs involve larger numbers of groups, so that the random allocation of multiple groups to intervention or no intervention gives more of the benefits of randomisation in terms of balancing out other factors across the groups (e.g. the vitamin A study, Box 6.9).

Experimental studies like those described above are theoretically the ideal way to look for associations between exposure and disease or health outcome. They do, however, have to be designed, run and reported rigorously to realise this potential in terms of providing convincing evidence concerning causality. Unfortunately, they are often inappropriate (for ethical reasons), not feasible or unaffordable. Furthermore, since they are often conducted in highly selected groups of volunteers, it can be challenging to generalise their findings. The other non-experimental study designs are therefore still of great importance.

REFERENCES

Armstrong, B. and Doll, R. (1975). Environmental factors and cancer incidence and mortality in different countries, with special reference to dietary practices. *International Journal of Cancer*, **15**: 617–631.

Ast, D. B. and Schlesinger, E. R. (1956). The conclusion of a ten-year study of water fluoridation. *American Journal of Public Health*, **46**: 265–271.

Beaglehole, R., Bonita, R. and Kjellström, T. (1993). *Basic Epidemiology*. Geneva: World Health Organization.

CDC (Centres for Disease Control). (1981). *Pneumocystis* pneumonia – Los Angeles. *Morbidity and Mortality Weekly Review*, **30**: 250.

Dawber, T. R. (1980). *The Framingham Study. The Epidemiology of Atherosclerotic Disease.* Harvard: Harvard University Press.

Devesa, S. S., Graumann, D. J., Blot, W. J. *et al.* (1999). *Atlas of Cancer Mortality in the United States, 1950–94.* Washington: US Government Print Office.

Doll, R. and Hill, A. B. (1964). Mortality in relation to smoking: ten years' observations of British doctors. *British Medical Journal*, **1**: 1399–1410, 1460–1467.

Forman, D., Sitas, F., Newell, D. G. *et al.* (1990). Geographical association of *Helicobacter pylori* antibody prevalence and gastric cancer mortality in rural China. *International Journal of Cancer*, **46**: 608–611.

Francis Jr, T., Korns, R. F., Voight, R. B. *et al.* (1955). An evaluation of the 1954 poliomyelitis vaccine trials: summary report. *American Journal of Public Health*, **45**: 1–65.

Frankel, S., Gunnell, D. J., Peters, T. J., Maynard, M. and Davey Smith, G. (1998). Childhood energy intake and adult mortality from cancer: the Boyd Orr cohort study. *British Medical Journal*, **316**: 499–504.

Golding, J., Pembrey, M., Jones, R. and the ALSPAC Study Team. (2001). ALSPAC – the Avon Longitudinal Study of Parents and Children. I. Study methodology. *Paediatric and Perinatal Epidemiology*, **15**: 74–87.

Gregg, N. M. (1941). Congenital cataract following German measles in the mother. *Transactions of the Ophthalmological Society of Australia*, **3**: 35–46. Reprinted (1991) *Australian and New Zealand Journal of Opthalmology*, **19**: 267–276.

Hennekens, C. H. and Eberlein, K. (1985). A randomised trial of aspirin and β-carotene among U.S. physicians. *Preventive Medicine*, **14**: 165–168.

ISIS-2 Collaborative Group. (1988). Randomised trial of intravenous streptokinase, oral aspirin, both or neither among 17187 cases of suspected acute myocardial infarction: ISIS-2. *Lancet*, **2**: 349–360.

Jewkes, R., Levin, J. and Penn-Kekana, L. (2002). Risk factors for domestic violence: findings from a South African cross-sectional study. *Social Science and Medicine*, **55**: 1603–1617.

Jordan, W. M. (1961). Pulmonary embolism. *Lancet*, **2**: 1146.

Lawlor D. A. and Stone, T. (2001). Public health and data protection: an inevitable collision or potential for a meeting of minds? *International Journal of Epidemiology*, **30**: 1221–1225.

Lind, J. (1753). *A Treatise of the Scurvy. A Bicentenary Volume.* Edinburgh: Sands, Murray and Cochran.

Maclure, M. (1991). The case–crossover design: a method for studying transient effects on the risk of acute events. *American Journal of Epidemiology*, **133**: 144–153.

Mellin, G. W. and Katzenstein, M. (1962). The saga of thalidomide: neuropathy to embryopathy, with case reports of congenital anomalies. *New England Journal of Medicine*, **267**: 1184–1193, 1238–1244.

MRFIT Research Group. (1982). Multiple risk factor intervention trial. Risk factor changes and mortality results. *Journal of the American Medical Association*, **248**: 1465–1481.

Paffenbarger Jr, R. S., Hyde, R. T., Wing, A. L. and Hsieh, C. C. (1986). Physical activity, all-cause mortality, and longevity of college alumni. *New England Journal of Medicine*, **314**: 605–613.

Ponsonby, A. L., Dwyer, T., Gibbons, L. E., Cochrane, J. A. and Wang, Y-G. (1993). Factors potentiating the risk of sudden death syndrome associated with the prone position. *New England Journal of Medicine*, **329**: 377–382.

Purdie, D., Green, A., Bain, C. *et al.* (1995). Reproductive and other factors and risk of epithelial ovarian cancer: an Australian case–control study. *International Journal of Cancer*, **62**: 678–684.

Rockhill, B., Willett, W. C., Hunter, D. J. *et al.* (1998). Physical activity and breast cancer risk in a cohort of young women. *Journal of the National Cancer Institute*, **90**: 1155–1160.

Sandler, D. P., Smith, J. C., Weinberg, C. R. *et al.* (1989). Analgesic use and chronic renal disease. *New England Journal of Medicine*, **320**: 1238–1243.

Sommer, A., Tarwotjo, I., Djunaedi, E. *et al.* (1986). Impact of vitamin A supplementation on childhood mortality. A randomised controlled community trial. *The Lancet*, **327**: 1169–1173.

Stampfer, M. J., Willett, W. C., Colditz, G. A., Speizer, F. E. and Hennekens, C. H. (1988). A prospective study of past use of oral contraceptive agents and risk of cardiovascular diseases. *New England Journal of Medicine*, **319**: 1313–1317.

St Leger, A. S., Cochrane, A. L. and Moore, F. (1979). Factors associated with cardiac mortality in developed countries with particular reference to the consumption of wine. *Lancet*, **1**: 1017–1020.

The Million Women Study Collaborative Group. (1999). The Million Women Study: design and characteristics of the study population. *Breast Cancer Research*, **1**: 73–80.

Zendehdel, K., Nyrén O., Östenson, C.-G. *et al.* (2003). Cancer incidence in patients with type 1 diabetes: a population-based cohort study in Sweden. *Journal of the National Cancer Institute*, **95**: 1797–1800.

All that glitters is not gold: the problem of error

Box 7.1 Bigger isn't always better!

In the run-up to the 1936 presidential election in America, the *Literary Digest* conducted a poll of more than 2,000,000 voters and confidently predicted that the Republican candidate, Alf Landon, would win. On the day it was the Democrat candidate, Franklin D. Roosevelt, who won a landslide victory. The *Digest* had correctly predicted the winner of the previous five elections, so what went wrong in 1936?

The *Digest* sent polling papers to households listed in telephone directories and car registration records. In 1936, however, telephone and car ownership were more common among more affluent households and these were the people who were also more likely to vote Republican. The generally less affluent Democrat voters were thus under-represented in the sample of voters polled. In contrast, a young George Gallup conducted a much smaller poll of a few thousand representative voters and correctly predicted the Roosevelt win. As a result of this fiasco the *Digest* folded but Gallup polls are still conducted today.

If the results of a study reveal an interesting association between some exposure and health there is a natural tendency to assume that it is real. (Note that we are considering whether two things are *associated*. This does not imply a causal association. We will discuss causality further in Chapter 10.) However, before we can claim this we have to be able to rule out all alternative explanations for the results. There are three main 'alternative explanations' that we have to consider whenever we analyse epidemiological data or read the reports of others: could the results be due to

- chance (random error),
- bias (systematic error) or
- confounding?

We will discuss the first two, *chance* and *bias*, in this chapter and will cover the third, *confounding*, in Chapter 8.

Error

The results of any research are only as good as the data upon which they are based. In epidemiology we frequently rely on records that have been collected for some other purpose, and we have already discussed some of the problems inherent in this in Chapter 3. Even when the data have been collected specifically for research they are unlikely to be completely free of error. We can never study as many people as we would like, so how representative are the people we do study of everybody in the population? We often rely on people's memories, but how accurate are they? We also take biological measurements, such as blood pressure and weight, and these are often subject to natural variation as well as being affected by the performance of the measurement system that we use.

People live complicated lives and, unlike laboratory scientists who can control all aspects of their experiments, epidemiologists have to work with that complexity. As a result, no epidemiological study will ever be perfect. Even an apparently straightforward survey of, say, alcohol consumption in a community can be fraught with problems. Who should be included in the survey? How do you measure alcohol consumption reliably? All we can do when we conduct a study is aim to *minimise* error as far as possible, and then *assess the practical effects* of any unavoidable error. An important aspect of epidemiology is, therefore, the ability to recognise potential sources of error and, more importantly, to assess the likely effects of any error, both in your own work and in the work of others. In this chapter we will point out some of the most common sources of such error in epidemiological studies and how these can best be avoided. We also want to emphasise from the outset that some degree of error is inevitable and that this need not invalidate the results of a study.

Sources of error in epidemiological studies

In an epidemiological study we usually want to measure the proportion of people with a particular characteristic or to identify the association between an exposure and an outcome. To do this we have to recruit people into the study, measure their exposure and/or outcome status and then, if appropriate, calculate a measure of association between the exposure and outcome. We also want the results we obtain to be as close to the truth as possible. (Note that, although we will discuss error in the context of exposure and disease, as previously when we talk about exposure we mean anything from a gene to a particular behaviour, and the outcome need not be a disease but could be any health-related state.)

As you will discover, there are dozens of different names that have been given to the kinds of error that can occur in epidemiological studies. Fortunately, in practice, all types of error can be classified into one of two main areas: they relate either to the **selection** of participants for study or comparison, or to the **measurement** of exposure and/or outcome. These errors can in turn be either **random** or **systematic**. Random error or poor precision is the divergence, by chance alone, of a measurement from the true value. Systematic error occurs when measurements differ from the truth in a systematic way.

Random error

If you were to weigh yourself several times on the same set of scales, how similar would the results be? If there is little variation between the results we say that the measuring device is *precise*. If there is a lot of variation between the results then the precision is poor or, conversely, we have a lot of *random* error. Some measuring instruments will be better than others, but if we measured the same thing several times we would not expect to obtain exactly the same result every time, although we would hope that the results would be close. If, for example, we measured someone's systolic blood pressure and the reading was 140 millimetres of mercury (mm Hg), then, ideally, if we measured it again and again the results would all be close to this value – perhaps ranging from 137 to 143 mm Hg. This would indicate that the measuring device was quite *precise*, i.e., it always gives approximately the same answer when measuring the same thing. Note that this tells us nothing about the *accuracy* of the measurement, i.e., whether the person's systolic blood pressure really is 140 mm Hg.

Systematic error

Although our measuring instrument was not 100% precise and we would expect some results to be a bit too high and some a bit too low, we would hope that the *average* results would be close to the true value. In other words, we want the device to be *accurate*. Consider the measurement of blood pressure again. If we use a sphygmomanometer that has not been calibrated for a year it might consistently read 10 mm Hg too high. The person with a blood pressure of 140 mmHg would now appear to have a blood pressure of 150 mm Hg. The precision of the measurements will be unchanged but, if we were to make several measurements on each person and average them, we would find that the average value was always 10 mm Hg too high. In this situation our measurements might be precise but they are not accurate because we are systematically recording everybody's blood pressure as 10 mm Hg greater than it should be. We have, therefore, introduced *systematic* error or *bias* into our measurements.

We can summarise the effects of systematic and random error, or their inverse accuracy and precision, by analogy with target shooting (Figure 7.1). If someone is a good shot and they are using a gun with the sights properly aligned, their shots will tend to cluster closely around the bull's-eye in the centre (situation (a)). The shots are, therefore, both accurate (close to the centre) and precise (close to each other). If, however, the sights on the gun are not aligned correctly, it will not be so accurate and the shooter might always hit a spot to the right of

Fig. 7.1 Accuracy and precision (systematic and random error).

(a) Accurate and precise
Little systematic or random error

(b) Precise, not accurate
Systematic error but little random error

(c) Accurate, not precise
Random error but little systematic error

(d) Neither accurate, nor precise
Random and systematic error

the centre (situation (b)). The results are still precise because they are tightly clustered around this point, but they are no longer accurate because they are consistently falling too far to the right. We have introduced a systematic error. If a less experienced shooter were to use the first gun then their shots would be more spread out, but they would still land around the bull's-eye (situation (c)). In this situation we have good accuracy because, on average, the shots are centred around the bull's-eye, but the shots are very spread out so we have more random error and thus less precision. Finally, an inexperienced shooter with a faulty gun would both miss the centre of the target and cover a wide area (situation (d)). In this situation we have neither accuracy nor precision. We can, therefore, separate the effects of accuracy and precision, i.e., systematic and random error.

Random and systematic errors can also occur during the process of subject selection and in this context they are usually thought of as *chance* and *bias*. If we select a sample of people for a study at random, we may obtain the wrong result just by *chance*, but if there is some systematic bias in how people are recruited the results of the study may also be *biased*.

We will now discuss the main types of both selection and measurement error in more detail and will also consider the effects that they may have on the results of a study. Remember that in practice it is impossible to eliminate all error and the most important thing is therefore to consider the likely practical effects of any remaining error.

Subject selection

When we conduct a study or collect any epidemiological information, one of the first decisions we have to make is who we will include in the study. This decision is important for two reasons. If the way in which people are selected for the study, and particularly the way they are allocated to the various study groups, is biased in some way, we may end up with misleading results (as did the *Literary Digest* US presidential election poll in 1936). This is known as *selection bias* and is a problem of *internal validity* (we will discuss this in Chapter 9). The selection of our study subjects will also determine how applicable our results are to other groups of people in other places. Imagine, for example, that you were interested in the association between physical activity and health. If, for practical reasons, you conducted a study in Italian men aged 20–30, would the results also apply to older men? Non-Italians? Women? This is a question of *generalisability* or *external validity*.

Since we can rarely study a whole population, we usually have to rely on a *sample* of that population and trust that this sample will give us an answer that holds true for the general population. If we select the sample of people wisely and they are truly representative of the target population (the population that we want to study) then we will not introduce any *systematic* error into the study. However, if we were to study several different samples of people from the same population it is unlikely that we would find exactly the same answer each time, and unlikely that any of the answers would be exactly the same as the true population value. Thus, in any study there will always be an element of chance as to who is studied and who is not – this is *random* or *sampling error*. Statistical methods have been developed to assess the amount of sampling error that is likely to be present in any particular study. Nonetheless, if we do not select the study participants carefully and they are not representative of the wider population (i.e., they differ from the target population in a *systematic* way) then we will introduce *selection bias* into the study and the results we find may be misleading.

Random sampling error (chance)

Imagine that you were interested in the health effects of obesity and wanted to know the average body-mass index (BMI) of 10-year-old children in your community. If you weighed and measured just one or two children you would not obtain a very good picture of the average BMI of all children – but the more children you studied, the better your picture would be. In general, if we select a small sample of a population then our results are more likely to be different from the whole population values than if we had a larger sample. The best way to reduce sampling error is thus to increase the size of the study sample as far as is practical. (Of course, there is always a trade-off between study size and cost.)

There are ways in which we can calculate how many people we should include in a study to reduce sampling error to an acceptable level. In an analytic study these calculations involve some knowledge, first, of the likely size of the effect we expect to see and, secondly, of the prevalence of the factor of interest in the population. They also require a decision as to how precisely we wish to measure the effect, i.e., how much sampling error we are prepared to accept in our result. If we are looking for a large effect and the exposure and/or disease are quite common then we do not need a large study to show this. For example, in 1971 a tiny case–control study showed that young women who had been exposed in utero to diethylstilboestrol (DES) had an increased risk of developing a rare type of vaginal cancer (clear cell adenocarcinoma) (Herbst *et al.*, 1971). (DES is a synthetic oestrogen that was used between 1940 and 1970 to prevent spontaneous abortion and premature delivery.) In this situation, the frequency of DES use among the mothers of the cases was so high (7 out of 8) and the difference was so large (none of 32 control mothers had used DES) that the investigators needed to study only those 40 women to show that there was a clear association. Unfortunately, in modern epidemiology we are often looking for much smaller effects and our studies have to be much larger than this to detect them with certainty. We will not discuss the statistical methods for performing what are called '*sample size*' or '*power*' calculations further here; the formulae for these can be found in many standard textbooks on medical statistics.

Confidence intervals (CI)

Confidence intervals provide a useful measure of the amount of sampling error in a study. They reflect the fact that the results we obtain from a study may vary from the truth simply because of chance variation in the people who ended up in the study. They are in effect an explicit admission that the result of a study (the 'point' or 'effect' estimate) is probably not exactly right, but that the real answer is likely to lie somewhere within a given range – the confidence interval. A narrow confidence interval therefore indicates good precision or little random error and, conversely, a wide confidence interval indicates poor precision.

The most commonly used confidence intervals are 95% intervals (95% CI) and they are often described as meaning that we can be '95% confident' that the real value is within the range covered by the confidence interval. What this really means is that if we were to repeat the study many times with different samples of people, then 95% of the 95% confidence intervals would include the true value. Note that this also means that 5% of the time (or 1 in 20 times) the 95% CI will not include the true value (and we will never know which times these are). Other percentages can be used, such as 90%, which gives a narrower confidence interval but less certainty that it will contain the true value (we will be wrong about 1 time in 10); and 99%, which will give a wider interval and be more likely to contain the true value (we will only be wrong about 1 time in 100).

Imagine two studies that have evaluated the association between exposure to air pollution and asthma.

Study 1 finds a relative risk of 1.5 with a 95% confidence interval (CI) of 1.2–1.9. What does this tell us about the association between air pollution and asthma?

This is a fairly precise estimate. It tells us that people who are exposed to air pollution are about one and a half times as likely (or 50% more likely), to develop asthma than those who are not exposed, that the risk might be as high as 1.9 times and that it is probably at least 1.2 times (i.e., a 20% increase). It also tells us that the relative risk is *unlikely* to be more than 1.9 or less than 1.2 (but it still could be outside these values).

Study 2 finds a relative risk of 2.5 (95% CI 0.9–6.9).

What is the most likely value for the relative risk of asthma in people exposed to air pollution in the second study?

Is it possible that the result could have arisen by chance and there is really no association (i.e., the 'true' population relative risk is 1.0)?

Which of the two studies would give you most concern that air pollution was associated with asthma?

In the second study, the most likely value for the relative risk is 2.5 and the true relative risk could be as high as 6.9; but the confidence interval is very wide, indicating poor precision, and it also includes the value 1.0 (no effect), so it is possible that there is really no association and the result of 2.5 arose by chance. We should certainly not ignore the result just because chance is one possible explanation for our findings; but, on the other hand, our interpretation of the result taken on its own should be cautious, and we should acknowledge the possibility that it could merely reflect the play of chance. Narrow confidence intervals (indicating good precision) are always more informative than wide confidence intervals (indicating poor precision).

Hypothesis testing

When we conduct a study to evaluate the relationship between an exposure and disease we may find an association or we may not. We then have to use the information from the sample of people in the study to infer whether the exposure and outcome are related in the wider population. There are thus four possible outcomes for any study, as shown in Figure 7.2.

If there is really no association between the outcome and exposure then we hope that our study will find just that. Conversely, if the exposure and outcome are truly associated in the population then we want our study to show this association. What we want to minimise are the situations where our study says there is a relationship between exposure and outcome when the truth is that there is none, or our study says there is no association when, in truth, there is. Unfortunately, in practice we can never know for sure whether we are right or wrong.

Could an association have arisen by chance? (type-I error)

When the results of a study suggest that two groups are different, we can carry out a statistical test, known as a hypothesis test. The results of these statistical tests often take the form of a *p-value* and they give us some idea of how likely it is that the groups are really different or, on the contrary, that the results might just be due to random sampling error or *chance*. For example, if a survey of children shows that girls have a higher average BMI than boys, is this difference likely to be real or could it just be chance that the girls in the study sample happened to have a higher BMI than the boys?

STUDY RESULTS (Known)	TRUTH (Unknown)	
	No association	Association
No association	Correct	Type-II error (probability = β)
Association	Type-I error (probability = α)	Correct (probability = $1 - \beta$) = Power

Fig. 7.2 Possible outcomes of an epidemiological study.

In practical terms, the **p-value** from a statistical test tells us the probability that we would have seen a difference as big as (or bigger than) we did if there were really *no difference* between the groups. (The actual definition, which can be found in any standard statistics text, is slightly more complicated than this.) Imagine that the average BMI of the girls in a survey was 20% higher than the average BMI of the boys and that statistical testing gave a *p*-value of 0.01 associated with this difference. We can say from this that, if the average BMIs of boys and girls were really the same, then we would have a 0.01 or 1% probability of seeing an apparent difference of 20% (or more) purely by chance. Conventionally, results are considered to be *statistically significant*, i.e., unlikely to have arisen by chance, if the *p*-value is less than 0.05 ($p < 0.05$); in other words, if the probability that the result could have arisen by chance is less than 5%. We could, therefore, conclude that the 20% difference in BMI between boys and girls was unlikely to have arisen by chance and that, all else being equal, girls probably do have a higher BMI than boys.

Imagine a study finding that, compared with people who exercised regularly, those who did not exercise had a three-fold higher risk of having a heart attack (relative risk = 3.0) and that the *p*-value for this association was 0.005.

What would the relative risk be if the risk of having a heart attack were the *same* for people who exercise and those who do not?

Is it likely that a study would give a relative risk of 3.0 ($p = 0.005$) if there were really no association between exercise and heart attack?

From www.CartoonStock.com

If the risk of having a heart attack were the same regardless of how much a person exercised, i.e., there was *no* association between exercising and having a heart attack, then the relative risk would be 1.0. In the example above the study found a relative risk of 3.0, $p = 0.005$. The small p-value suggests that it is very unlikely that the study would have given a relative risk as big as 3.0 if the true relative risk were 1.0. (With a p-value of 0.005, we would expect this to happen only about 5 in 1,000 times.) The observed association between heart attack and exercise is therefore unlikely to have arisen by chance.

This form of statistical testing is very common, but it is important to note that the conventional distinction between $p < 0.05$ (statistically significant) and $p \geqslant 0.05$ (not statistically significant) is purely arbitrary. However, people tend to believe a result automatically if $p < 0.05$ but not if $p > 0.05$ and this has led to suggestions from some epidemiologists that p-values should not be used. For example, a relative risk of 2.5 ($p = 0.049$) would, by convention, be called 'statistically significant' because 0.049 is less than 0.05. In contrast, a relative risk of 2.5 ($p = 0.051$) would not be classed as statistically significant because 0.051 is greater than 0.05. However, the relative risk is the same in both cases and $p = 0.049$ is so similar to $p = 0.051$ that it is illogical to believe the first result but not the second. P-values are also highly dependent on the size of the study – the bigger the study the smaller the p-value (for the same effect size). Imagine a study with 80 cases and 80 controls that found an odds ratio of 1.7 with a p-value of 0.11. By convention this result would not be statistically significant and we would say that the association could have arisen by chance. If the same study had been twice as big (160 cases and 160 controls) we would have found the same odds ratio (1.7) but now the p-value would have been 0.02, so we would have concluded that the association *was* statistically significant. Hypothesis tests and p-values are tools that can be used to help assess the results of a study, but they should not be used blindly to decide whether or not an association exists. They are aids to judgement, not absolute arbiters.

Could we have missed a true association (type-II error)?

In addition to considering whether an association might have arisen by chance, we should also consider whether we could have *missed* a true relation by chance. Is it possible that an exposure is linked to an outcome but the study was just too small to detect this? To avoid such a situation it is important to ensure that a study is big enough or, in other words, that it has enough *power* to detect with sufficient precision an association that exists. The power of a study is the probability that the study will detect an association of a particular size if it truly exists in the general population. Imagine that an exposure truly causes a two-fold increase in the risk of disease (of course, we can never know this in practice). If a study has 80% power to detect a relative risk of 2.0 between the exposure and outcome then we can say that 80% of the time, or four times out of five, that study would determine that the exposure and outcome were related. It also means that there is a 20% or one in five chance that we would miss the association. There is no hard and fast rule as to how much power a study should have but, in general, most people would probably want a minimum of 80% power and many would aim for 90%.

A major problem in epidemiology is that, for financial or other practical reasons, researchers often cannot conduct as large a study as they would like. However, if they compromise and conduct a small study that shows an association between the exposure and outcome but this is not statistically significant (i.e., poor precision) it is difficult to interpret the results. Is there really no association or might there be an association but the study was just too small to detect it with any certainty? This question is particularly important in the context of clinical trials when it is important to know whether small improvements seen for a new treatment really do represent a benefit that should be passed on to patients or whether the difference could just be due to chance (see Box 7.2).

This raises an important ethical issue that most human research and ethics committees would now consider before giving a study approval to proceed. Is the study big enough to detect the effects the investigators are looking for? If the answer is no then it has to be questioned whether the study should be allowed to go ahead.

Box 7.2 RCTs failed to show a benefit of streptokinase

Between 1959 and 1988, 33 randomised clinical trials were conducted to test whether intravenous streptokinase reduced the risk of death after heart attack. Most of the studies ($n = 25$) found that mortality was lower among the groups given streptokinase but many were small and so their results were not 'statistically significant' (i.e. $p > 0.05$). As a result the benefits of streptokinase were not fully appreciated. In 1992, however, a group combined the results of all the individual streptokinase studies using a technique called *meta-analysis* (we will discuss this further in Chapter 11). This showed that streptokinase was associated with more than a 20% reduction in mortality after heart attack and, because of the large sample size, a total of 36,974 patients when all the studies were combined, this effect was now highly statistically significant ($p < 0.001$) (Lau *et al.*, 1992). Importantly, they also found that, if the results of just the first eight studies, involving a total of only 2,432 patients, had been combined, the 20% reduction in mortality among those given streptokinase would have been apparent back in 1973. The problem was that individually most of the early studies were simply not big enough to detect this effect with sufficient certainty. As a consequence, their results were rarely statistically significant and so were dismissed. If some of these studies had been bigger (or if more emphasis had been placed on the size of the reduction in mortality and less on statistical significance) the beneficial effects of streptokinase would have been discovered much sooner and thousands of lives could probably have been saved.

More about confidence intervals and *p*-values

It is important to understand that the true value of an association is most likely to be somewhere near the point estimate in the middle of a confidence interval; it is much less likely to be near the ends of the interval and even less likely to be outside it completely. Note also that, if a 95% CI *does not* contain the 'no-effect' or 'null' value (1.0 for an RR, OR, etc.) then the *p*-value from a statistical test would be <0.05. Conversely, if the 95% CI *does* include the no-effect value then *p* > 0.05. In the hypothetical asthma studies above, the 95% CI for study 1 does not include the null value. In this situation the corresponding *p*-value would be less than 0.05 and the result would be termed 'statistically significant'. The result of study 2, on the other hand, would not be statistically significant because the 95% CI includes the value 1.0 (and the *p*-value would be >0.05).

Confidence intervals are much more informative than *p*-values. The width of a confidence interval gives an indication of the precision of the estimate and the two bounds tell you both how weak the association might be and also how strong it might be. In contrast, a *p*-value simply gives an indication of whether an observed association could be 'due to chance' and there might really be no effect (i.e., the true RR or OR is 1.0). It effectively focusses on the end of the confidence interval that is closest to the null (does this or does it not include the null value?) and ignores the other end. In recent years there has been a shift away from using *p*-values to reporting of confidence intervals because of the additional information they provide and to reduce the dependence on '*p* < 0.05' which, as you have seen, can be misleading or mean that important results are missed.

Systematic sampling error (selection bias)

Selection bias occurs when there is a systematic difference between the people who are included in a study and those who are not, or when study and comparison groups are selected inappropriately or using different criteria. Unlike random sampling error, we cannot reduce selection bias by simply increasing the size of the study sample – the problem persists no matter how large the sample. Nor are there simple statistical techniques to assess the amount of systematic error in a study and it is not always easy to know what effect it might have on the results.

The issue of selection bias is a major problem in simple descriptive studies such as prevalence surveys. If the sample of people included in the survey is not representative of the wider population the results of the survey can be very wrong, as the Literary Digest found in their biased opinion poll.

Selection bias is also a problem in analytic studies because it can lead to inappropriate comparisons and hence biased measures of association (OR or RR). It is a particular concern in case–control studies because the participants are recruited as two separate groups and it can be difficult to ensure that the final control group makes an appropriate comparison group for the cases. A similar problem can arise in cohort studies when the exposed and unexposed groups are recruited separately, for example when the exposed group comprises workers in a particular occupation or military group and a separate unexposed group has to be identified for comparison.

In a case–control study, it is important to have a clear definition of the population group that you want to study (the target population). This need not be everybody, but could be a specific subgroup of the whole population. Cases and controls should then be selected from the same identifiable group. Ideally all cases in a defined population would be included, but if only a sample is used they should be truly representative of all cases arising in the population. The controls too should then be selected to be representative of this population. (We discussed options for control selection in Chapter 6.)

In cohort studies in which a single group is recruited and then individuals are classified according to their exposure status (as in the Framingham and Nurses' Health studies), the question of how they were recruited is usually less important in terms of the validity of the study results (internal validity), although it can influence the generalisability of the findings since they may apply only to the sorts of people who took part. In some situations, however, selection bias can also influence the effect estimates. As an example, consider a cohort study examining the effect of socioeconomic status of children on risk of injury. If the families in the lowest social group are more likely to refuse to participate, then this group may be under-represented in the total cohort. In this situation, measurement of the risk of injury within the group and comparisons with those of higher socioeconomic status should still be accurate. If, however, those families in the lower socioeconomic group who refuse to take part are also those whose children are at highest risk of injury, then the study will underestimate the true amount of injury in this group. It will then also underestimate the effect of low socioeconomic status on injury risk because the really high-risk children in that group were not included.

As for cohort studies, selection bias is not usually a major issue for internal validity in clinical trials, although it can occur if the allocation process is predictable and the decision whether or not to enter a person into the trial is influenced by the expected treatment assignment. For example, if alternate patients are assigned to receive active drug or placebo, a physician may decide not to enter sicker patients into the trial if he or she thought they were not going to be given the active drug. This selection bias *will* affect the internal validity of the study and this is another reason why the allocation process should be properly concealed.

Some other ways in which selection bias can arise include the following.

Volunteers

It is well known that people who volunteer to participate in surveys and studies (i.e., they spontaneously offer their involvement rather than being selected in a formal sampling scheme) are different from those who do not. In particular, volunteers are often more health-conscious and, as a result, volunteer groups will often contain a lower proportion of, say, smokers than the general population. Advertisements calling for volunteers for a survey or study may also attract people who have a personal interest in the area of the study. The prevalence of various diseases or behaviours in a volunteer group may thus be very different from that in the underlying population because of this self-selection into the study. For this reason, epidemiological research rarely uses groups of volunteers and, if it does, it is advisable to pay close attention to whether the use of volunteers may have biased the results in some way.

Low response rates

What might be thought of as a type of volunteer bias, and one that again is a particular problem in surveys and case–control studies, is the problem of low response rates. People who have a particular disease are often highly motivated to take part in research into that disease. Controls, however, have no such motivation to participate and investigators are finding it increasingly hard to persuade healthy people to take part in studies. It is important to note that, even if potential controls are selected at random, if some do not agree to take part then the remaining group may no longer be a true random sample of the population.

Ascertainment or detection bias

This can occur if an individual's chance of being diagnosed as having a particular disease is related to whether they have been 'exposed' to the factor of interest. An example of this type of bias was seen in early studies of the risk of oral contraceptive (OC) use causing thromboembolism (a condition in which a blood clot develops in the legs and subsequently breaks off and moves to another part of the body, often the lungs). Doctors who were aware of the potential for this risk were more likely to hospitalise women with symptoms suspicious of thromboembolism if they were taking OCs. Early case–control studies, which were hospital-based, then overestimated the risk of thromboembolism associated with OC use. This was because the cases were more likely to be on OCs simply because of the way in which they were selected to be sent to hospital, since in the minds of their doctors this partly determined their diagnosis.

The healthy-worker effect

This is a well-documented type of selection bias that can occur in occupational studies. People who are working have to be healthy enough to do their job, so they tend to be more robust than the general population which also includes

Box 7.3 Differences between responders and non-responders

In a case–control study of the effects of passive smoking on the risk of heart attack or coronary death, the investigators put a lot of effort into trying to achieve a high response rate from controls. Potential controls were initially invited to attend a study centre where they would have blood collected and physical measurements taken as well as completing a risk factor questionnaire. Participants who did not respond to this invitation were sent a shorter questionnaire to complete at home and some people who still did not respond were then visited and interviewed at their homes. There were thus three types of people among the control group: the willing volunteers who replied to the initial invitation, the slightly less willing who replied to the shorter home questionnaire and the even more reluctant who agreed to take part only when visited by an interviewer. The investigators then compared the prevalences of smoking in these three groups (Table 7.1).

Table 7.1 Prevalence of smoking increases with increasing reluctance to take part in a study.

Ease of recruitment	Never smokers (%)	Ex-smokers (%)	Current smokers (%)
Men (age 35–69 years)			
Full participation (willing)	35	40	24
Short questionnaire (less willing)	30	42	28
Home interview (reluctant)	29	42	29
Women (age 35–69 years)			
Full participation (willing)	67	19	14
Short questionnaire (less willing)	66	13	21
Home interview (reluctant)	53	16	31

(Dobson *et al.*, 1991.)

The harder it was to persuade someone to take part in the study, the more likely they were to be a current smoker, especially for women. This suggests that those who refused completely probably had even higher smoking rates. The measured prevalence of smoking in the control group is therefore likely to be an *underestimate* of the true level of smoking in the whole population. Using the study data, the calculated odds ratio for the association between smoking and heart disease in men was 2.3. However, if the *true* proportion of current smokers in the population was actually 3% higher and the proportion of non-smokers 3% lower than in the study controls, then the *true* odds ratio would have been only 1.8. The study would thus have overestimated the strength of the association.

those who are disabled or seriously ill and hence unable to work. As a result, if occupational groups are compared with the general population – which is not uncommon in cohort studies of occupational hazards – they will almost always appear to be healthier overall. Comparisons within a workplace can also be flawed because different types of job often attract different types of people as well as requiring different levels of fitness. Imagine, for example, a cross-sectional study of the effects of heavy physical work on the occurrence of heart disease in which the investigators compared a group of manual labourers with a

Box 7.4 Veteran health

There is concern that men and women who saw active service in conflicts such as the Vietnam war have worse health than those who did not. Studies that have compared mortality rates among Vietnam veterans with those in the general population are hampered by the fact that the veterans had to pass a stringent medical examination at the time of their enlistment and so, at that time, were much more healthy than the average person. An analysis of mortality rates among male Australian Vietnam veterans found that, up until 1979, mortality among the veterans was actually 32% lower than in the general population (Table 7.2). It is highly unlikely that service in Vietnam would reduce a man's subsequent risk of death, so this inverse association is likely to be due entirely to the healthy-worker effect. It is impossible to say how large this effect might be and to assess whether it could actually be masking an underlying increase in mortality in the veterans.

Table 7.2 Standardised mortality ratios (SMRs) and 95% confidence intervals (CIs) for selected causes of death among male Australian Vietnam veterans.

Cause of death and time period	SMR	95% CI
All causes, 1964–1979	0.68	0.63–0.74
All causes, 1980–1994	1.07	1.02–1.12
Cancer, 1980–1994	1.19	1.09–1.30

(Crane *et al.*, 1997.)

In the years from 1980 to 1994, mortality among the veterans was 7% higher overall and 19% higher for cancer. With the increasing time interval since enlistment, the healthy-worker effect will have been wearing off for most causes and it now appears that the veterans do have higher rates of death, particularly from cancer. The question of veterans' health is now a major issue in many countries.

group of people of similar socioeconomic status who had desk jobs. In this situation, subjects who had heart disease might be incapable of doing a manual job. The frequency of heart disease could thus appear to be higher in those with desk jobs, falsely suggesting that heavy work was protective against heart disease. Similar problems can arise in other groups where members are selected on the basis of physical fitness, e.g., the armed forces.

Loss to follow-up

In a case–control study the main concern with subject selection is with regard to who is included in the study. In a cohort study or a clinical trial, selection bias can arise if those who *remain* in a study are different from those who do not, i.e., the issue is selection *out* of the study population rather than selection *in*. This can be a particular problem if more people are 'lost to follow-up' in one exposure group than another and if loss is also related to the outcome of interest. For example, imagine a randomised clinical trial comparing a new drug with the current standard treatment. If the sickest people in the intervention group withdrew from the trial, the people remaining in the intervention group would be healthier than those in the standard treatment group and the new drug would appear to be more beneficial than it really was. The opposite situation would occur if people who were doing well were less likely to return for assessments and thus were more likely to be lost to follow-up.

Control of selection bias

The question of selection bias has to be considered and then eliminated or minimised in the design and conduct of a study. Any error introduced here that leads to inappropriate comparisons is intractable, and cannot be removed in the data analysis. As we have seen, in a case–control study the critical issues are defining the case group clearly, selecting an appropriate control group and then ensuring that high participation rates among both cases and controls are achieved.

A good study will have clearly defined *eligibility criteria* that can be used to determine whether specific cases are included. For example, in a study of myocardial infarction, specific criteria developed by the World Health Organization might be used to define a case or, in a study of cancer, only those patients with histologically confirmed cancer might be included. Then, out of all those who fit the specific case definition, who is actually *eligible* for the study? Are only those cases who are admitted to specific hospitals included or all people with that disease in the community? Are people of any age included or only those within a certain age range? Do people have to be resident in a certain area to be included? Are suspected cases included? Box 7.5 gives eligibility and exclusion criteria for a study of ovarian cancer.

Note that the eligibility criteria describe the target population, i.e., all women who are *eligible* to take part in the study. For practical reasons some eligible women might later be *excluded* from the study. It is important to note that,

Box 7.5 Eligibility and exclusion criteria

Eligibility criteria for cases for a study of ovarian cancer could be as follows:
- A *histologically confirmed diagnosis*: the cancer must be confirmed by a pathologist.
- *Incident*: the woman must have no previous history of ovarian cancer.
- *Primary* ovarian cancer: the cancer must originate in the ovary; metastases (cancers that have spread from another anatomical site) would thus be excluded.
- *Age 18–79*: studies often exclude children for practical reasons and in this case ovarian cancer is very rare in children. Older adults are also commonly excluded, particularly if exposure information is to be collected by questionnaire or interview because the problems of recall increase with age.
- *Resident in a specific geographical area*: women who just happen to be diagnosed with ovarian cancer while visiting that region will be excluded.

Comparable eligibility criteria for the *controls* might then be the following:
- women *aged 18–79*;
- *resident in the same specific geographical area*;
- with *no previous history of ovarian cancer*; and
- with *no history of bilateral oophorectomy* (i.e., they must have at least one ovary and so be at risk of developing ovarian cancer).

Exclusion criteria might include the following:
- *women who are unable to give informed consent* (for example they have dementia);
- *women too sick to take part* (this decision might be made by the treating doctor); and
- *women who do not speak English* (if the main study documents are all in English it might not be financially viable to translate them into other languages).

if large numbers of women are excluded, regardless of how good the reasons for this, then the resulting study sample might no longer be representative of the whole population. For example, the exclusion of very sick women might mean that cases of advanced cancer are under-represented in the study group. If advanced cancers differ somehow from early cancers in terms of their aetiology then this might affect the overall results.

Once a study has been conducted, all we can do is consider whether any bias is likely to have made the association appear stronger (further from the null) or weaker (closer to the null) than it really is (see Figure 7.3). Any such consideration

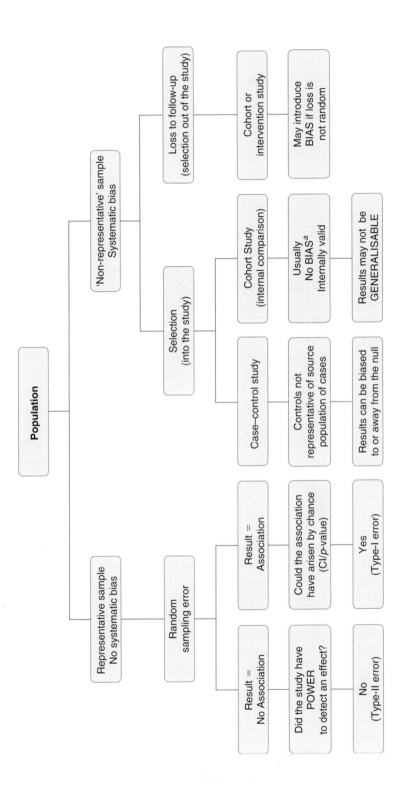

a The same cannot be said for cohorts with an external comparison group, where factors like the healthy-worker effect can introduce bias at this stage

Fig. 7.3 An overview of the types of selection error and their consequences for effect estimation.

can only be based on informed guesswork and the results of any case–control study with low participation rates (particularly among controls) or of a cohort study or trial with high loss to follow-up are likely to be viewed with suspicion because of the possibility that some unaccounted-for bias could explain the results.

Measurement or information error

No measurement of exposure is likely to be perfect and there may also be errors in the measurement of outcome. These measurement errors may lead to misclassification of participants with respect to their exposure status and/or outcome (disease). In other words, someone may be labelled as 'exposed' (or as a 'case') when they were actually 'unexposed' (or a 'non-case'). This can then lead to bias in the results of the study. Some error can and will creep in whenever we measure or collect information from or about study participants and, as in the process of subject selection, this error (and any resulting misclassification) can be either random or systematic.

Many biological parameters, such as blood pressure, vary on a day-to-day, hour-to-hour and even minute-to-minute basis. Assuming that the blood pressure measuring system we are using is accurate, and that our participant has not, for example, just run up a flight of stairs, then any variation will be random. Depending on when we take our measurements, we will obtain different readings that will vary around the patient's *usual* blood pressure. We will over-estimate some people's blood pressure and we will under-estimate it for others. This type of *random variation* can be minimised by taking readings on more than one occasion and using the average value in the study.

In addition to natural variation in what we are trying to measure, there will also be some imprecision inherent in the measuring system that we are using. As we discussed above, no measuring device will give exactly the right results 100% of the time; but, if the device is accurate, any error in the measurements will again be random. As with biological variation, we can reduce random measurement error by taking repeated measurements on one subject and using the average value in the study. However, if the device is not 100% accurate then there may also be some *systematic error* in the measurements. Unlike random error, systematic error cannot be reduced by taking repeated measurements.

Suppose that you were conducting a study looking at some aspect of diet (something that is notoriously difficult to measure) and wanted to classify people by the amount of fruit they ate – high or low. Even with this crude separation, you would inevitably end up with some people in the wrong groups. This **misclassification** could result from either imprecise or inaccurate measurement of fruit consumption (refer back to Figure 7.1). If the measurement is imprecise (*random error*), some 'high' fruit eaters will end up in the 'low' fruit group and some 'low' fruit eaters will end up in the 'high' group. This would have the effect of diluting any difference between the groups and making them more similar than they really were. Alternatively, if the measurements were inaccurate and, for example, everyone tended to over-estimate the amount of fruit they ate, perhaps because fruit is perceived as being 'good' for you, then we would also have *systematic error*. Similarly, when asked about how much they smoke and drink, people may tend to underestimate the true amounts because smoking and excessive alcohol consumption are often perceived as undesirable behaviours.

From www.CartoonStock.com

"...then we add a smidgin of this – that's less than a dollop,
but more than a pinch..."

The effects of measurement error

The effects of both biological variation and measurement error mean that measurements will never be perfect – even if there is no systematic error there will always be some degree of random error. If something is measured on a continuous scale (for example height in centimetres or weight in kilograms) then **random error** will not lead to any bias in estimates of the average height or weight of the study population. This is because, although the height of some people will be overestimated and the height of others underestimated, if these errors are truly random, the overestimates and underestimates will cancel each other out when we calculate the average height. Similarly, if we classify people into groups, for example above and below the average height, the consequence of any measurement error will be that people are classified into the wrong groups. If the error is random, then the resulting misclassification will also be random and overall we will still have the correct proportion of people in each group. However, the same cannot be said for **systematic error**: if people systematically underestimate their weight then their average weight will be an underestimate of the true average for the population. Likewise, the resulting misclassification will be systematic, with too many people classified into the lower weight groups and too few into the heavier groups.

Both random *and* systematic errors create problems when, instead of simply looking at the distribution of exposure in a population, we are interested in the association between exposure and outcome. *Both random and systematic misclassification will introduce bias into measures of association such as odds ratios and relative risks.*

When assessing the likely effects of measurement error and misclassification, the most important consideration is whether the errors are likely to be *the same* or *different* in the various study groups. In a case–control study we are usually concerned about whether errors in *exposure* measurement for cases and controls are the same. In a cohort study or a clinical trial we are often more concerned about whether the *outcome* measurement may have differed between the exposed and unexposed groups, although exposure measurement may also be an issue.

Non-differential misclassification

When measurement error and any resulting misclassification occur equally in all groups being compared, they are described as being *non-differential* (because they are the same or 'not different' in all study groups). For example, non-differential error occurs when the amount and type of error in exposure measurement for cases and controls are the same in a case–control study; or error in measurement of outcome is the same for the exposed and unexposed groups in a cohort study.

Imagine a case–control study in which everything is measured perfectly, with no error. The hypothetical results of this study are shown in Table 7.3.

Non-differential random misclassification

Now imagine that the instrument used to measure exposure (this could be a biological test of some sort, a measuring device or a questionnaire) is not perfect. As a result, 10% of all people who are exposed are misclassified as unexposed and 10% of all unexposed people are misclassified as exposed. (Note that this is the same as saying that the instrument has 90% sensitivity and specificity; it correctly identifies 90% of those who are exposed (sensitivity) and 90% of those who are unexposed (specificity). We will discuss sensitivity and specificity in more detail in Chapter 14.) The key point here is that the misclassification is *non-differential*, namely it affects everyone in the study. In this situation 10% or 30 of the 300 exposed cases and 25 of the 250 exposed controls will be misclassified as unexposed. In addition, 10% or 10 of the 100 unexposed cases and 15 of the 150 unexposed controls will be misclassified as exposed. This means that, instead of obtaining the true picture shown in Table 7.3, we would find results that looked like Table 7.4.

Table 7.3 The 'true' results of a hypothetical case–control study with no measurement error.

	Cases	Controls	Total
Exposed	300	250	550
Unexposed	100	150	250
Total	400	400	800

$$OR = \frac{300 \times 150}{100 \times 250}$$
$$= 1.80$$

Table 7.4 The effect of non-differential random measurement error: 10% of all cases and controls are misclassified with regard to their exposure status.

	Cases	Controls	Total
Exposed	300 − 30 + 10 = 280	250 − 25 + 15 = 240	520
Unexposed	100 − 10 + 30 = 120	150 − 15 + 25 = 160	280
Total	400	400	800

$$OR = \frac{280 \times 160}{120 \times 240}$$
$$= 1.56$$

Because we have randomly misclassified some of the cases and controls, we have obtained an odds ratio of only 1.56 instead of the true odds ratio of 1.80. This makes the association seem weaker than it really is; i.e., the effect estimate, in this case an odds ratio, is biased towards the null. Note that some complex exposures, particularly things like diet, are particularly hard to measure and levels of misclassification are likely to be much greater than 10%. In this situation any measures of relative risk would be biased even closer towards 1.0 and real effects can disappear completely. For example, if the level of misclassification in the above example had been 20% instead of 10%, the odds ratio would have been 1.37 ((260 × 170) ÷ (140 × 230)); with 30% misclassification it would have been only 1.23 ((240 × 180) ÷ (160 × 220)).

Non-differential systematic misclassification

Now imagine the same study but this time the instrument used to measure exposure *systematically* overestimated people's exposure. As a result, 20% of all unexposed people, both cases and controls, were misclassified as exposed. Note that this misclassification is again non-differential because it affects both cases and controls.

How many of (a) the 100 unexposed cases and (b) the 150 unexposed controls would have been misclassified as exposed?

So, in total, how many (a) cases and (b) controls would have been classified as exposed and how many as unexposed?

Table 7.5 The effects of non-differential systematic measurement error: 20% of unexposed cases and controls are misclassified as exposed.

	Cases	Controls	Total
Exposed	300 + 20 = 320	250 + 30 = 280	600
Unexposed	100 − 20 = 80	150 − 30 = 120	200
Total	400	400	800

$$OR = \frac{320 \times 120}{80 \times 280}$$
$$= 1.71$$

What would the odds ratio have been?

Would it have been an underestimate or an overestimate of the true odds ratio?

In this situation, 20% or 20 of the 100 unexposed cases and 30 of the 150 unexposed controls will be misclassified as exposed. This means that we would obtain results that looked like Table 7.5 and we have again underestimated the true odds ratio of 1.80.

The same effects can occur in a cohort study. The hypothetical results of a cohort study in which everything is measured correctly are shown in Table 7.6.

Now imagine that at the start of the study 30% of *all* exposed people are misclassified as unexposed (i.e., the misclassification is systematic but non-differential, as we would expect in a cohort study). In this situation 3,000 of the exposed people will be misclassified into the unexposed cohort and, because the cumulative incidence of disease in the exposed group is 2%, there will be an extra 60 cases (2% of 3,000) in the unexposed cohort. This means that our results would look like Table 7.7 and again the relative risk is an underestimate of the true association. If there had been the same level of random misclassification (i.e., it occurred in both directions) then we would have observed a relative risk of only 1.31.

Table 7.6 The 'true' results of a hypothetical cohort study with no measurement error.

	Total	Cases	Cumulative incidence (%)
Exposed	10,000	200	2.0
Unexposed	10,000	100	1.0
Total	20,000	300	1.5

$$RR = 2.0 \div 1.0$$
$$= 2.00$$

Table 7.7 The effect of non-differential measurement error in a cohort study: 30% of all exposed participants are misclassified as unexposed.

	Total	Cases	Cumulative incidence (%)	
Exposed	10,000 − 3,000 = 7,000	200 − 60 = 140	2.0	RR = 2.0 ÷ 1.2
Unexposed	10,000 + 3,000 = 13,000	100 + 60 = 160	1.2	= 1.67
Total	20,000	300	1.5	

The effects of non-differential misclassification

In the presence of non-differential misclassification, either random or systematic, estimates of the association between exposure and outcome will almost always be underestimates of the true effect. In other words, the odds ratio or relative risk will be biased towards the null. This means that, if a study gives a relative risk of 2.0, but there is likely to be non-differential misclassification, then the true association is likely to be even stronger than that observed (i.e. >2.0). Similarly, if a study gives a relative risk of 0.8 in the presence of non-differential misclassification, then the true relative risk is likely to be lower than this (i.e <0.8), again making the real association stronger than that observed. (Box 7.6 shows an example of an unusual situation in which non-differential error does *not* bias a result towards the null.)

Differential misclassification

When the measurement error and resulting misclassification occur to a greater extent in one group than another they are described as being **differential**. The effects of differential misclassification are generally harder to predict than those of non-differential misclassification.

Differential random misclassification

Imagine that all of the cases in a case–control study had their blood pressure measured by a single doctor at the local hospital but that, for practical reasons, the controls had their blood pressure measured by their local doctor. In this situation it is likely that there would be less random error in the blood pressure readings for cases that came from a single doctor than in those for controls that came from a number of different doctors. Similarly, because they are affected by the disease of interest, cases might think harder about past exposures that could have caused their disease and so might simply provide more precise information than controls who would have no such incentive to recall information.

If, in the hypothetical case–control study from Table 7.3, the measurement of exposure among cases was perfect but 20% of exposed controls were misclassified

Box 7.6 When non-differential misclassification does not bias towards the null

If an exposure has more than one level then misclassification between two of the groups will make those two groups look more similar than they really are. In a case–control study of smoking and respiratory disease, for example, participants might be classified as non-smokers, light smokers and heavy smokers. The distinction between smoker and non-smoker is likely to be fairly clear (and for simplicity we will assume that it is perfect), but there will inevitably be some misclassification between the light and heavy smoking groups. If the non-smokers form the reference group, the misclassification will make the odds ratios for light and heavy smokers more similar than they should be. The effect of this will be to bias the odds ratios for the highest group (heavy smokers) towards the null again but the odds ratio for the *middle group* (light smokers) will now be biased away from the null (Table 7.8). Overall, however, the net result is that the association is weakened.

Table 7.8 Non-differential misclassification can bias away from the null when there are more than two exposure groups.

	Cases	Controls	Odds ratio
Truth			
Non-smokers	150	200	1.0
Light smokers	120	125	1.3
Heavy smokers	130	75	2.3
20% of light smokers misclassified as heavy smokers and vice versa			
Non-smokers	150	200	1.0
Light smokers	122	115	1.4
Heavy smokers	128	85	2.0

as unexposed and vice versa, we would obtain the results shown in Table 7.9. In this situation, 20% or 50 of the 250 exposed controls will be misclassified as unexposed and 20% or 30 of the 150 unexposed controls will be misclassified as exposed.

Now, because we have random misclassification just among the controls, we have a higher odds ratio of 2.22, making the association seem stronger than it really is. (Note that, if we had randomly misclassified 20% of cases instead of controls, the odds ratio would have been (260 × 150) ÷ (140 × 250) = 1.11, i.e., less than 1.80.) Differential random misclassification can therefore make an association look either weaker or stronger than it really is.

Table 7.9 The effect of differential random measurement error: 20% of controls are misclassified with regard to their exposure status.

	Cases	Controls	Total
Exposed	300	$250 - 50 + 30 = 230$	530
Unexposed	100	$150 - 30 + 50 = 170$	270
Total	400	400	800

$$OR = \frac{300 \times 170}{100 \times 230}$$
$$= 2.22$$

In practice, random error is usually non-differential because it is an inherent property of the exposure being measured or the measuring device and affects everyone in the study. Differential random error is likely to be a problem only if different measuring systems are used in different study groups. *The best way to avoid differential random error and any consequential misclassification is thus to ensure that exactly the same instruments and methods are used in all of the different study groups.*

Differential systematic misclassification

In contrast to random error, systematic error is often differential. It is a particular problem in standard case–control studies in which cases already have the disease of interest when the exposure information is collected or measured. As a result, it is possible for measurements of exposure to be influenced by the disease status (case or control) of the participants. For example, the cases in a case–control study of respiratory disease might overestimate the amount of passive smoking they had been exposed to because they thought that this might have caused their disease. The controls, however, would have no such reason to overestimate their exposure. (This type of error is known as **recall bias**.) This might make it look as if passive smoking was associated with respiratory disease even if there was really no difference between the cases and controls.

Imagine that, in the hypothetical study above, the exposure in cases was overestimated and, as a result, 20% of unexposed cases were systematically misclassified as exposed, but controls were not affected. This would mean that, in the example, 20% or 20 of the 100 unexposed cases would be misclassified as exposed and, instead of the true picture shown in Table 7.3, we would obtain results that looked like Table 7.10.

We have now overestimated the true odds ratio of 1.80, making the association seem much stronger than it really is. If the misclassification had gone the other way and exposed cases had been misclassified as unexposed, or unexposed controls had been misclassified as exposed, then the bias would have gone in the opposite direction and we would have underestimated the effect.

Table 7.10 The effects of differential systematic misclassification: 20% of unexposed cases, but *not* controls, are misclassified as exposed.

	Cases	Controls	Total
Exposed	300 + 20 = 320	250	570
Unexposed	100 − 20 = 80	150	230
Total	400	400	800

$$OR = \frac{320 \times 150}{80 \times 250}$$

$$= 2.40$$

The effects of differential misclassification

If there is misclassification, either random or systematic, in a study and this occurs *to a different extent in the two study groups* (cases and controls or exposed and unexposed) then the study results can be biased either up or down, towards or away from the null value, and it is often impossible to know which way the bias would have gone or how large the effect might be. This type of misclassification can be very difficult to deal with because, unless you have some idea of how much misclassification is occurring and where it is occurring, you cannot work out what the true results should have been.

Sources of measurement error

As you will have gathered, almost every study will be subject to some degree of measurement error. One common but easily avoidable source of bias is the use of different instruments or measuring systems for different study groups or parts of groups. Examples of this include the use of different laboratories to analyse biological specimens, different locations for interviews of cases and controls (e.g., hospital versus home) and different interview methods (face-to-face versus telephone interview or postal questionnaire). Other particularly troublesome sources of error are the possibilities of recall bias and interviewer or observer bias.

Recall bias

Some degree of error is inevitable in any epidemiological study that requires participants to recall their past exposures. If this error is random and if, in a case–control study, it occurs in both cases and controls (i.e., it is non-differential) then the effects will usually be to bias the effect estimates towards the null. What can be more problematic is **recall bias**, a type of differential measurement error that can occur in case–control studies and cross-sectional studies. It arises when cases (or those with disease in a cross-sectional study) are more likely to overestimate or underestimate their exposure than controls. If an exposure is thought to cause disease, then cases might be more likely to recall or to exaggerate their past exposure than controls, leading to overestimation of the effect of that exposure on disease (as in the passive smoking example above). The opposite effect would occur if cases tended to underestimate their exposure because they feel guilty about it. This could occur, for example, in a study of the effects of sunburn in childhood on the occurrence of childhood skin cancer. If mothers are asked whether their children have ever been sunburnt, the mothers of children with cancer might tend to underestimate (or under-report) the occurrence of sunburn in their children because they feel guilty about admitting they allowed their children to become burned when they were young. This could lead to falsely low estimates of the frequency of sunburn in cases and consequently a weakened association between sunburn and skin cancer.

It is obviously difficult to know, even qualitatively, the extent to which such bias may operate in any given study, so much effort is put into designing information collection systems to limit the likelihood of it occurring. For example, through the use of highly structured questionnaires, standard prompts and so forth.

An equivalent bias has occasionally been seen in cohort studies when information about outcomes has been obtained from the participants themselves. In this situation the problem arises when members of the exposed group are more (or less) likely to recall having had the outcome of interest than are those in the unexposed group. For example, in a telephone follow-up ascertaining self-reported diagnosis in US veterans, those who had served in Vietnam (the *exposure* of interest) reported higher rates of a variety of conditions than did non-Vietnam veterans; but when a sub-set of the veterans was examined more thoroughly, there was little real difference between those who had and had not served in Vietnam (CDC, 1988).

Interviewer or observer bias

Differential error may also occur if data collectors ask questions or record information in a different way for cases and controls (or for exposed and unexposed groups in a cohort study). For instance, an interviewer who knows the case/control status of a subject may probe more deeply with the cases than with the controls, resulting in differences in the quality of exposure data obtained for the two groups. Similarly, if in a cohort study or trial the observers know whether or not a person is exposed or unexposed (or treated/untreated), they may be more or less likely to diagnose the outcome of interest. A logical way to avoid these possibilities is to blind the interviewers/observers to the subject's status, although this is often not possible. Again, the use of objective criteria for outcome assessment, structured questionnaires and interview schedules, training and tape-recording interviews for quality control all help minimise **interviewer bias**.

Control of measurement error

It is difficult to get rid of measurement error once it has occurred and so it is important to minimise the potential for error at the design stage of the study.

Whether you are conducting your own research or reading the reports of others, some important things to consider include the following.

Definitions

Everything that is measured in a study needs to be carefully defined. If the exposure is smoking, what makes someone a smoker? Anyone who has ever smoked a cigarette? 10 cigarettes? 100 cigarettes? A cigarette a day for six months? In practice most people probably try a cigarette at one time or another, so to classify them all as smokers would not be sensible. Common definitions that have been used are that someone should have smoked at least 100 cigarettes in their lifetime or that they should have smoked at least one cigarette a day for a defined period, usually a few months.

In addition to the important distinctions of exposed/unexposed (and of case/non-case in a cohort study or trial), it is also essential to have clear definitions of the co-factors being measured. These are other factors that may influence (or 'confound' – see Chapter 8) the results of a study, e.g., age, socioeconomic status and smoking.

Choice of instrument

Instruments in epidemiological studies can range from sophisticated laboratory tests through questionnaires to simple observations. Inevitably the means of measurement used will influence the degree of error in the data. A set of scales that weigh to the nearest 100 g would be more accurate than scales that weigh to the nearest kilogram. Ideally the instrument used should be that which minimises both *random* and *systematic* error. Consideration should also be given to the circumstances of time and place of use of the instrument, since these may also affect the results obtained. For example, a face-to-face interview with a trained interviewer might elicit more reliable information than a questionnaire completed by the study participants themselves, but it would also be more expensive.

Quality control

Whatever measuring devices are used, they need to be standardised. Instruments need regular calibration against a standard value and interviewers need training in a standard approach to obtaining data. Structured questionnaires help here, too. If the study continues for some time, consistency should also be monitored and maintained.

Assessment of measurement error

The two main issues in measurement are (i) is the instrument accurate (i.e., no systematic error) and (ii) is it precise (minimal random error)? The accuracy and precision of an instrument can be assessed by conducting validation and repeatability studies.

Fig. 7.4 An overview of the types and consequences of measurement error.

Assessing accuracy

In some situations accurate measuring devices or tests are available but too complex or costly to use on everyone in the study, so the investigators have to use a simpler or cheaper and less accurate tool. In this situation it is good practice to conduct a *validation study* in which both the accurate expensive ('gold standard') test and the simpler, potentially less accurate test are used on a subset of people in the study and the results are compared. In this situation it may then be possible to 'correct' the results of the study for any inaccuracies in the cheaper test (we will not consider the mechanics of this here).

Assessing precision

Another desirable way to test how well a measuring device performs is to measure its 'repeatability' or precision. If the same thing is measured on two different occasions or by two different people, how well do the two measurements compare? This might simply be a case of repeating laboratory tests on some samples or it might involve asking some study participants to complete a study questionnaire twice on two different occasions to see how well their answers agree. In a cohort study that has repeated measures over time (such as the Nurses' Health Study) it is sometimes appropriate to average the values to give better precision.

Assessment of the likely effects of error on the results of a study

Epidemiological studies are fraught with difficulties because, unlike a laboratory scientist, an epidemiologist cannot fully control the participants in their studies.

This means that all studies are likely to have some degree of error and the important thing is to assess the likely impact of any such error on the results of the study (Figures 7.3 and 7.4). Is it possible that an observed association is entirely due to error, or would the association still exist (and perhaps be even stronger) if the error could be eliminated?

Selection bias

Participation rates in studies are rarely 100%, so are those who did not take part likely to differ from those who did and, if so, how would this affect the results? This is often difficult to know because, if people did not agree to take part in a study, then of course there is no information about them.

External comparisons

Although it might not be possible to obtain information about the non-responders in a study, it is often possible to acquire some information about the wider target population. In this situation it is possible to compare the actual study population with the wider population to see whether there are any differences. For example, many countries have cancer registries, so in a case–control study of cancer it might be possible to find some basic information such as the age and stage (extent of disease) distribution of the cancer patients diagnosed in a particular region at the time of the study. By comparing the cases who took part in the study with these routine statistics it is possible to see whether the people who did not take part differed in some way from those who did, e.g., they might tend to be older and sicker. Similarly, it may be possible to extract information about possible risk factors such as smoking and alcohol consumption from a national health survey. It is then possible to compare, for example, the smoking habits of the study population with those of the general population. If there are fewer smokers among the controls in a case–control study than in the general population then it is possible that the study may have overestimated the strength of the association between smoking and disease.

Sensitivity analysis

It is also possible to estimate the possible effects of bias on the results of a study by conducting what is known as a 'sensitivity analysis'. If there is loss to follow-up in a cohort study or clinical trial, then imagine the worst-case scenario (Box 7.7) that everyone lost from one group developed the outcome of interest and nobody lost from the other group did. How would that have affected the results of the study? What if the loss had been the other way around or if only half of the people lost had developed disease? How bad would the loss have to have been to explain the whole association? If there is still an association after such worst-case assumptions then the association cannot be an artefact due

Box 7.7 The worst-case scenario

Imagine a study that compared a new anti-arrhythmic drug (drug A) with an older drug (drug B) for the prevention of sudden death. The results of this hypothetical study are given in Table 7.11.

Table 7.11 Results of a hypothetical study comparing two anti-arrhythmic drugs.

Drugs	Number of patients randomly allocated	Number of sudden deaths	Mortality per 100 people
Drug A	860	36	4.2
Drug B	842	72	8.6

From these results, drug A appears to reduce the risk of sudden death by about half (RR = 4.2 ÷ 8.6 = 0.49) compared with drug B. However, what if we find that some patients were lost to follow-up: 32 from group A and 16 from group B. The worst-case scenario (if we are hoping to find evidence in favour of drug A) would be if all the patients lost from group A had actually died from an arrhythmia while all those lost from group B were alive and feeling so well that they had decided not to return for follow-up. We can then recalculate the mortality for drug A on the basis of this scenario (the mortality for drug B will not change):

Mortality in group A if the 32 patients lost to follow-up died due to an arrhythmia = (36 + 32) ÷ 860 = 7.9 per 100 people

Drug A is still found to give a benefit compared with drug B, although the reduction in risk of mortality is now less than 10%. In practice it is highly unlikely that all participants lost to follow-up from group A had met an untimely arrhythmia-related death whereas none of those taking drug B had. The true reduction in risk for drug A is therefore likely to be greater than 10% and in this situation we might be happy to conclude that, even in the presence of the loss to follow-up, drug A was more useful than drug B.

entirely to bias. (Note that this does not imply that the association is real, it could also be due to confounding, which we will discuss in Chapter 10.)

Measurement error and misclassification

There will always be some degree of random measurement error in a study and, as a result, if subjects have been classified into different exposure groups there will always be some misclassification. The degree of misclassification will depend on the variable being measured and the tool being used to measure it. Things like age and height do not change (or change predictably) and can be measured fairly easily. In contrast we have alluded to the fact that something like diet is very hard to measure and so will be associated with a lot more mis-classification. On top of this there may also be systematic error such as recall bias.

When looking for associations between exposure and outcome, the central issue is whether any error and resulting misclassification is likely to be differential or non-differential; i.e., is it likely to have occurred to the same extent in all study groups or to a differing extent in different groups? As you have seen, the likely effects of **non-differential misclassification** (either random or systematic) are to bias the estimates of effect (RR or OR) towards the null, making associations look weaker than they really or, in some situations, masking them altogether (see Figure 7.4). In contrast, **differential misclassification** can bias estimates upwards or downwards, towards or away from the null. In a survey the key question is whether the error is random or systematic.

If information from a validation study is available it may be possible to make a correction to the results of a study to allow for the fact that the measurements were not perfect. However, any such correction will also not be perfect. **Sensitivity analysis** involves repeating the data analysis using different assump-tions in the same way as we did to assess the effects of loss to follow-up above. If a proportion of subjects had been misclassified, what effect would this have had on the results?

At the very least, it is essential to assess the likely degree of measurement error and/or misclassification and then make some judgements as to how this might have affected the results (Table 7.12).

- If the error or misclassification is non-differential, how bad is it likely to be? If the study found an association then, in all probability, the real association is even stronger. If the study did not find an association, is it possible that there was so much error that a real association could have been missed? (Note that non-differential misclassification is very unlikely to make it appear that an association exists when in reality there is none.)

- If the error or misclassification is likely to be differential, is it possible to pre-dict what the differences might have been? For example, are cases more or less likely to have over-reported exposure? Could the observed association be due to misclassification? Or might the real association be stronger than that observed? (Note that, as well as making associations look weaker or stronger than they really are, differential misclassification can make an association appear where there is none, it can make it seem that there is no association when in reality there is one and it can even make a positive association look like an inverse association and vice versa.)

Table 7.12 The likely effects of misclassification on the results of a case–control study.

Type of error/misclassification	True odds ratio (OR)	Study results	Type of bias
Non-differential	2.0	≥1.0 but <2.0	Result biased towards null but not below
	1.0	1.0	No effect if there is no association
	0.5	>0.5 but ≤1.0	Result biased towards null but not above
Differential – cases overestimate (or controls underestimate) exposure	2.0	>2.0	Result biased upwards with no upper limit. An inverse association (OR < 1.0) could appear to be a positive association (OR > 1.0)
	1.0	>1.0	
	0.5	>0.5	
Differential – cases underestimate (or controls overestimate) exposure	2.0	<2.0	Result biased downwards with no lower limit. A positive association (OR > 1.0) could appear to be a inverse association (OR < 1.0)
	1.0	<1.0	
	0.5	<0.5	

Summary

No epidemiological study will be perfect, the important thing is to minimise errors and then evaluate the likely effect of any remaining error. Errors can be **random** or **systematic** and can relate to **subject selection** or **measurement** of exposure and/or outcome. Random sampling error can be assessed from a confidence interval, but systematic selection bias is a major problem in surveys and can be a problem in case–control studies, particularly with regard to selection of the control group. In cohort studies or clinical trials, selection bias is more likely to occur when people are **lost to follow-up**.

In a survey, systematic measurement error is a bigger problem than random error. In analytic studies, the important distinction is between **non-differential** error (it occurs equally in all study groups), which will almost always bias the study results towards the null, and **differential error** (it occurs to a different extent in the different study groups), which can bias the study results either towards or away from the null.

Questions

1. Imagine that a research team wanted to estimate the prevalence of vegetarianism in the community by means of a short questionnaire distributed with a

women's health magazine. Would this give an accurate picture of the percentage of people who were vegetarians?

2. In a case–control study of liver disease and alcohol consumption, all patients in a community who had newly been diagnosed with liver disease were recruited as cases and people without liver disease were selected at random from the community to act as controls. All of the cases and controls were then asked about their alcohol intake. Only 25% of the controls selected from the community agreed to take part in the study.

   (a) Do you think that people with a high alcohol intake would be more or less likely to agree to take part in the study than average?

   (b) Is alcohol consumption in the controls likely to be higher, the same as or lower than in the whole community?

   (c) What effect would this have on the estimate of the association between alcohol and liver disease?

3. The authors of a study report a RR of 1.8 (95% CI 1.6–2.0) for the association between alcohol intake and cancer. The authors of a second study report an OR of 1.8 (95% CI 0.7–3.5) for the association between caffeine intake and the same cancer. What do the results of these studies tell us about risk factors for the cancer?

4. Imagine that, in the hypothetical study shown in Table 7.3, cases underestimated their exposure and, as a result, 20% of exposed cases were falsely classified as unexposed, but that the classification of controls was not affected.

   (a) Is this type of misclassification random or systematic? Is it differential or non-differential?

   (b) What effect would it have had on the results of the study?

   (c) Compare your answer to (b) with that in Table 7.10, where cases systematically *overestimated* their exposure.

REFERENCES

CDC (Centers for Disease Control). (1988). Health status of Vietnam veterans. II. Physical health. *Journal of the American Medical Association*, **259**: 2708–2714.

Crane, P., Barnard, D., Horsley, K. and Adena, M. (1997). *Mortality of Vietnam Veterans: The Veteran Cohort Study. A Report of the 1996 Retrospective Cohort Study of Australian Vietnam Veterans*. Canberra: Department of Veterans' Affairs.

Dobson, A. J., Alexander, H. M., Heller, R. F. and Lloyd, D. M. (1991). Passive smoking and the risk of heart attack or coronary death. *Medical Journal of Australia*, **154**: 793–797.

Herbst, A. L., Ulfelder, H. and Poskanzer, D. C. (1971). Adenocarcinoma of the vagina. Association of maternal stilbestrol therapy with tumor appearance in young women. *New England Journal of Medicine*, **284**: 878–881.

Lau, J., Antman, E. M., Jimenez-Silva, J. *et al.* (1992). Cumulative meta-analysis of therapeutic trials for myocardial infarction. *New England Journal of Medicine*, **327**: 248–254.

Muddied waters: the challenge of confounding

Box 8.1 Are university admissions biased towards men?

Table 8.1 shows that in one year a prestigious university admitted 52% of male applicants compared with only 45% of female applicants, suggesting that there was a bias in favour of men. When quizzed about this, the two main faculty heads said that it couldn't be true, they had both admitted a higher proportion of women than men: the success rate in arts was 38% for women and only 32% for men and that in science was 66% for women compared with only 62% for men. How can this be?

Table 8.1 University admissions.

Faculty	Men			Women		
	Applicants	Admitted	Percentage	Applicants	Admitted	Percentage
Arts	4,100	1,300	32	8,250	3,150	38
Science	8,200	5,100	62	2,900	1,900	66
Total	12,300	6,400	52	11,150	5,050	45

This is an example of *Simpson's paradox* and it arises because, in the example, women were more likely to apply to arts courses, for which applicants had a lower overall success rate.

(Based on an analysis of graduate admissions data conducted at the University of California, Berkeley (Bickel *et al.*, 1975).)

In the previous chapter we considered two reasons why the results of a study might not be the truth, namely chance and error or bias. In this chapter we will consider the third possible 'alternative explanation' – confounding.

Confounding refers to a mixing or muddling of effects that can occur when the relationship we are interested in is confused by the effect of something else. It is a major problem that has to be addressed in all non-randomised research (and in some randomised trials as well, especially if they are small). The following hypothetical case–control study of alcohol and lung cancer illustrates how easily the problem can arise and how it can be diagnosed. It also suggests how confounding can be dealt with and we will discuss this in more detail later in the chapter.

Is alcohol a risk factor for lung cancer?

Imagine a (very small) case–control study with 20 cases (people with lung cancer ☹) and 20 controls who do not have lung cancer (☺). Is drinking alcohol associated with the risk of lung cancer? If all the cases and controls were asked about their alcohol consumption we could classify people as 'drinkers' (☹, ☺) or 'non-drinkers' (☹, ☺) and calculate an odds ratio to estimate the strength of the association between alcohol and lung cancer (Figure 8.1).

What is the odds ratio for the association between alcohol and lung cancer?

Can we conclude that alcohol consumption is associated with lung cancer?

As Table 8.2 shows, the odds ratio for the association between alcohol and lung cancer is 3.0, suggesting that alcohol drinkers have a three times greater risk of lung cancer than non-drinkers.

Fig. 8.1 A hypothetical case–control study of alcohol and lung cancer (blue = drinkers, black = non-drinkers).

Table 8.2 Calculation of the odds ratio for the association between alcohol and lung cancer.

	Cases	Controls
Alcohol drinkers	10	5
Non-drinkers	10	15

$$\text{Odds ratio} = \frac{a \times d}{b \times c}$$
$$= \frac{10 \times 15}{5 \times 10} = 3.0$$

What about smoking? We know that smokers are more likely to develop lung cancer and it is possible that they are also more likely to drink alcohol than non-smokers. Could this explain the finding? To investigate this we need to separate the smokers from the non-smokers and look at the 'alcohol' effect in each group. Figure 8.2 shows that 12 of the 16 smokers were also alcohol drinkers compared with only 3 of the 24 non-smokers.

Now calculate the odds ratio for alcohol and lung cancer separately for (i) smokers and (ii) non-smokers. (Hint: first draw up the appropriate 2 × 2 tables.) Is alcohol associated with lung cancer among smokers? Among non-smokers? How do you explain the change in the pattern of the alcohol–lung cancer relationship?

The odds ratio for the association between alcohol and lung cancer among smokers is 1.0. Fewer of the non-smokers drink alcohol but again the odds ratio is 1.0 (see Table 8.3). This process in which we divide or *stratify* the study participants into two or more separate groups (*strata*) is known as **stratification**.

So, although there appeared to be an association between alcohol and lung cancer in the whole study population, it disappears when we consider smokers

Fig. 8.2 Separating smokers and non-smokers (blue = drinkers, black = non-drinkers).

Table 8.3 Calculation of the odds ratio for the association between alcohol and lung cancer, stratified by smoking status.

		Cases	Controls
Smokers	Alcohol drinkers	9	3
	Non-drinkers	3	1
Non-smokers	Alcohol drinkers	1	2
	Non-drinkers	7	14

$$\text{Odds ratio} = \frac{9 \times 1}{3 \times 3} = 1.0$$

$$\text{Odds ratio} = \frac{1 \times 14}{2 \times 7} = 1.0$$

and non-smokers separately. We could then go on to combine the odds ratios in smokers and non-smokers to calculate a *pooled* odds ratio that is *adjusted* for the effects of smoking. In this example the adjusted odds ratio is also 1.0. (We will not discuss the methods for calculating an adjusted odds ratio here, but a common method, that developed by Mantel and Haenszel (1959), is shown in Appendix 5.)

The apparent (**crude**) overall relationship we saw between alcohol and lung cancer arose because of **confounding** by smoking. While those with lung cancer were indeed more likely to drink alcohol than those without lung cancer, alcohol and smoking go together so they were also more likely to be smokers than those without lung cancer. The increased risk of lung cancer among alcohol drinkers was in fact due entirely to their smoking.

This situation, in which an apparent relationship between an exposure and an outcome is really due, in whole or in part, to a third factor that is associated both with the exposure and with the outcome of interest is known as **confounding**. In the example, smoking is said to be a **confounder** of the alcohol–lung cancer link. Confounding is a *mixing of effects* because the effect of the exposure we are interested in (e.g., alcohol) is mixed up with the effect of some other factor (e.g., smoking). To look at the real effect of the exposure we have to deal with the effect of the confounder in some manner.

Criteria for a confounder

For something to be a confounder it must
- be a risk factor for disease among those who are not exposed to the factor of interest,
- be associated with the exposure of interest (in the source population or among the controls in a case–control study) and
- not be an intermediate between exposure and the outcome (i.e., it must not lie on the causal pathway).

Look back to Figure 8.2 and check that smoking fulfils the criteria for a confounder in the alcohol and lung cancer example.
- *Among non-drinkers* what proportion of (i) cases and (ii) controls smoked?
- *Among the controls* what proportion of (i) smokers and (ii) non-smokers drank alcohol?
- Is alcohol likely to *cause* smoking? (That is, could smoking lie on a causal pathway between alcohol and lung cancer?)

In the alcohol example, smoking was a confounder for the following reasons.
(1) *It was associated with lung cancer*: among people who did not drink alcohol, 3 out of 10 cases were smokers (30%) compared with only 1 of 15 controls

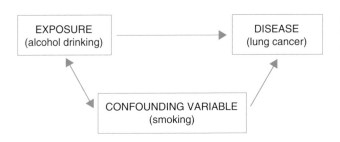

Fig. 8.3 Confounding (e.g., alcohol, smoking and lung cancer).

(7%). That is, among non-drinkers, the cases were more likely to smoke than were the controls.

(2) *It was associated with alcohol among the controls*: 3 out of 4 controls who smoked also drank alcohol (75%), compared with only 2 out of 16 controls who did not smoke (12.5%). That is, among the controls, smokers were more likely to drink alcohol than were non-smokers.

(3) *It is not on a causal pathway between alcohol and lung cancer*: although alcohol and smoking often go together, alcohol does not 'cause' someone to be a smoker.

An example of the third criterion is seen in the association between obesity and heart disease. High blood pressure is related both to obesity (the exposure) and to heart disease (outcome) and could, therefore, be a potential confounder of this association. However, since raising blood pressure is part of the causal path through which obesity acts to increase the risk of heart disease (obesity → increased blood pressure → heart disease), it would be misleading to adjust for this, since it would remove part of a real causal effect.

Figure 8.3 illustrates these criteria, showing how a confounder is related both to the exposure and to the outcome of interest. If an exposure is related to a confounding variable and this is, in turn, related to disease, the exposure itself may appear to be related to the disease even when it is not.

The effects of confounding

In the example above, the apparent effect of alcohol on lung cancer was entirely due to the effect of smoking, but confounding does not necessarily create an apparent effect where really there is none. Confounding can lead to either overestimation or underestimation of the size of a real effect, it can completely hide a real association that exists and in very extreme situations it can even reverse the direction of an effect, making it appear that a cause of a disease actually protects against it. (This is known as *Simpson's paradox* and it explains the apparent contradiction in the university admissions data in Box 8.1 at the start of the Chapter).

Age, sex and socioeconomic status (SES) are common confounders. As an example, many diseases occur more frequently in older people. If the exposure

Table 8.4 Results of a hypothetical case–control study of high energy intake and heart disease, stratified by level of physical activity.

Energy intake	Total		High physical activity		Low physical activity	
	Heart disease	Controls	Heart disease	Controls	Heart disease	Controls
High	730	600	520	510	210	90
Low	700	540	100	150	600	390

of interest also occurs more commonly in the elderly, e.g., a poor diet, then the confounding effects of age would have to be considered.

Confounding in a case–control study

Authors of early studies that looked at the relation between diet and heart disease found that the more a person ate the lower their risk of heart disease. This apparent association was all the more surprising because we know that obesity is a risk factor for heart disease. However, one factor that the studies did not take into account was physical activity and, on average, people who are physically active eat more than those who are inactive. Could this have affected the results of the studies? The results of a hypothetical case–control study evaluating the association between energy intake and heart disease are shown in Table 8.4.

What is the odds ratio for the *crude* association between high energy intake and heart disease?

What is the odds ratio for the association between high energy intake and heart disease in people with (i) high and (ii) low levels of physical activity?

Is the association between high energy intake and heart disease confounded by the level of physical activity?

The crude odds ratio for the association between high energy intake and heart disease in this study is (730 × 540) ÷ (700 × 600) = 0.9, i.e., those with high energy intake appear to have a 10% *lower* risk of coronary heart disease (CHD). When we stratify by physical activity the odds ratio is (520 × 150) ÷ (100 × 510) = 1.5 among the physically active and (210 × 390) ÷ (600 × 90) = 1.5 among the inactive. Thus, when we remove the confounding effects of physical activity by stratification, high energy intake is associated with a 50% *higher* risk of CHD (OR = 1.5). In this example the confounding had reduced the odds ratio (from 1.5 to 0.9).

Table 8.5 Results of a hypothetical cohort study of high energy intake and heart disease, stratified by level of physical activity.

Energy intake	Total		High physical activity		Low physical activity	
	Person-years	Developed heart disease	Person-years	Developed heart disease	Person-years	Developed heart disease
High	60,000	720	50,000	500	10,000	220
Low	55,000	700	15,000	100	40,000	600

Confounding in a cohort study

Now imagine that, instead of a case–control study, we had conducted a cohort study to look at the effects of high energy intake on heart disease. The results of this study are shown in Table 8.5.

What is the crude rate ratio for the association between high energy intake and heart disease?

What is the rate ratio for the association between high energy intake and heart disease in people with (i) high and (ii) low levels of physical activity?

Is the association between high energy intake and heart disease confounded by the level of physical activity?

The overall incidence rate of heart disease among those with a high energy intake is $720 \div 60,000 = 12.0/1,000$ person-years (py) and the incidence rate among those with a low energy intake is $700 \div 55,000 = 12.7/1,000$ py, giving a *crude* rate ratio of 0.9 ($12.0 \div 12.7$). However, when we stratify by level of physical activity we see a different picture:

- in the active group, the incidence rate of heart disease among those with a high energy intake is $500 \div 50,000 = 10.0/1,000$ py, whereas that among those with a low energy intake is $100 \div 15,000 = 6.7/1,000$ py, giving a rate ratio of 1.5;
- in the inactive group, the incidence rate of heart disease among those with a high energy intake is $220 \div 10,000 = 22.0/1,000$ py, whereas that among those with a low energy intake is $600 \div 40,000 = 15.0/1,000$ py, again giving a rate ratio of 1.5.

As in the case–control example above, when we remove the effects of physical activity the true association between a high energy intake and heart disease is stronger (RR = 1.5) than when we did not allow for the effects of physical activity. Confounding is just as much a problem in cohort studies (or any other non-randomised follow-up studies, including non-randomised clinical trials) as it is in case–control studies.

Table 8.6 Characteristics of women at time of recruitment into a cohort study of oral contraceptive use and coronary heart disease.

	Oral contraceptive use	
	Yes	No
Percentage aged		
20–29 years	60%	30%
30–39 years	40%	70%
Percentage of low SES	50%	40%
Percentage smoking >15 cigarettes/day	17%	12%
Mean body-mass index (weight (kg)/height (m)^2)	26.5	27.0
Percentage with a history of		
Hypertension	1%	1%
Stroke	0.03%	0.3%
Venous thromboembolism	1%	8%

(Figures adapted from Vessey and Lawless 1984.)

So how can we tell if an association is confounded?

If when you stratify or adjust for a potential confounder the effect estimate changes then confounding is present. In the lung cancer example at the start of the chapter the odds ratio dropped from 3.0 to 1.0 when we adjusted for smoking, indicating that smoking was a strong confounder. In the heart disease example the estimate increased from 0.9 to 1.5 when we adjusted for physical activity, so again this was confounding the association. A general rule of thumb is that, if when you adjust for a potential confounder the crude and adjusted effect estimates differ by 10% or more, then the crude estimate is confounded to some degree and it is more appropriate to present the adjusted value.

When will a possible confounder actually be a confounder in practice?

There are many things that could confound an association between exposure and outcome but in practice they might not actually do so.

Table 8.6 shows the characteristics of a group of women at the time of recruitment into a cohort study of oral contraceptives (OCs) and coronary heart disease (CHD).

Assume that all the factors are known risk factors for CHD. Which of them might be confounders of the OC–CHD relationship? Why?

For something to be a confounder it has to be associated both with the exposure of interest (OC use) and with the outcome of interest (CHD). All of the above factors are known risk factors for CHD, so they are all associated with CHD. Some

Table 8.7 Likely effects of potential confounders in a cohort study of oral contraceptive (OC) use and coronary heart disease (CHD) when the true RR = 3.0.

	Oral contraceptive use		Likely observed RR[a]
	Yes	No	
Percentage aged			
20–29 years	60%	30%	2.5
30–39 years	40%	70%	
Percentage of low SES	50%	40%	3.2
Percentage smoking >15 cigarettes/day	17%	12%	3.3
Mean body-mass index (BMI)			
(weight (kg)/height (m)^2)	26.5	27.0	2.9
Percentage with a history of			
Hypertension	1%	1%	3.0
Stroke	0.03%	0.3%	2.9
Venous thromboembolism	1%	8%	2.4

[a] Estimated RR for OC use and CHD, assuming that the RRs for the associations between the potential confounders and CHD are 2.0 for age, 2.0 for SES, 4.0 for smoking, 4.0 for BMI, 10.0 for stroke and 5.0 for venous thromboembolism.

are also associated with OC use – we can see from Table 8.6 that, compared with non-users, OC users are

- twice as likely to be under the age of 30 as non-users (60% versus 30%),
- slightly more likely to be of low SES (50% versus 40%),
- slightly more likely to be current smokers (17% versus 12%),
- 10 times less likely to have had a stroke (0.03% versus 0.3%) and
- 8 times less likely to have had a venous thromboembolism (1% versus 8%).

So do these factors confound the association between OC use and CHD?

In practice, it turns out that only the large differences in age and in the proportions of women with a history of thromboembolism are likely to affect the results appreciably. If OC use truly increased the risk of CHD, say the true RR = 3.0, then this much confounding by age might reduce the observed RR to about 2.5 (Table 8.7). Since CHD increases with age, the rate in the OC users will be lower simply because they are younger, thus reducing the (real) difference between the OC users and non-users. Similarly, the eight-fold difference between the OC users and non-users in terms of their history of thromboembolism, a strong risk factor for CHD, will also bias the observed RR downwards to about 2.4.

This contrasts strikingly with the confounding influence of a history of stroke. Theoretically this looks sure to be an important confounder, given the 10-fold difference between OC users and non-users in terms of their past stroke experience and the very strong known link between stroke and heart disease.

Table 8.8 Results of a hypothetical case–control study of high energy intake and heart disease, stratified by level of physical activity (present in only 6% of the population).

Energy intake	Total		High physical activity		Low physical activity	
	Heart disease	Controls	Heart disease	Controls	Heart disease	Controls
High	472	231	52	51	420	180
Low	1210	795	10	15	1200	780
Odds ratio	1.3		1.5		1.5	

However, because stroke is so rare in young women this imbalance affects only a tiny proportion of the total study group, and so has a trivial effect on the crude RR, biasing it downwards by only about 3%, from 3.0 to 2.9. Even if a history of stroke had been five times more common in the study groups (0.015% and 1.5%), the RR would have been biased downwards by only about 10%, from 3.0 to 2.7.

More predictably, strong independent risk factors for CHD such as smoking and low SES also fail to confound when their distributions in the groups being compared are reasonably similar. So for something to be a confounder in practice it must be not only quite prevalent in the population but also associated quite strongly *both with the exposure and with the outcome.*

As another example, consider the case–control study of energy intake and heart disease shown in Table 8.4. In this study the prevalence of the confounder (physical activity) in the population was very high – 660 of the 1,140 controls or 58% were physically active. What would have happened to our analysis if the population had been much less active? Table 8.8 shows results from a similar study for a population in which only 6% of controls were physically active. (To obtain these numbers we have just divided the numbers in the physically active group by 10 and multiplied the numbers in the inactive group by 2.) The stratum-specific odds ratios are unaffected but the crude odds ratio is now 1.3 instead of 0.9; i.e., there is much less confounding because physical activity is much less common.

We can summarise this by saying the following.

- If the association between a potential confounder and *either* the exposure *or* the outcome is weak then it is unlikely to have much effect on the results of a study.
- If a potential confounder is either *rare* or almost *ubiquitous* then it is unlikely to have much effect on the results of a study because these will be driven by the large number of people who are not exposed to the rare confounder (or those who are exposed to the ubiquitous confounder).

The most important confounders are therefore those that are both *relatively* common and strongly related to exposures and disease outcomes. The typical confounders that we mentioned above – sex, age and SES – fulfil all of these criteria. Another common confounder is smoking, which is strongly associated with many other lifestyle factors, including high alcohol and coffee consumption, a less healthy diet (less fresh fruit and vegetables) and low levels of physical activity, and is also a major risk factor for many diseases. There are also many other disease-specific confounders: sun-exposure is a major confounder in studies of other risk factors for skin cancer, obesity is a confounder in studies looking for causes of type-2 diabetes and so on.

Control of confounding

There are two strategies for dealing with confounding. The first is to try to prevent it from occurring in the first place and this can be done at the study design stage by *randomisation, restriction* or *matching*. The alternative is to deal with it when it occurs by using analytic techniques such as stratification and statistical modelling. The effectiveness of all of these strategies except randomisation depends on the ability to identify and measure any confounders accurately.

Control of confounding through study design

Confounding occurs when a confounding variable is distributed unevenly across our study groups (e.g., in the lung cancer example at the start of the chapter, cases were more likely to be smokers than controls). One way to avoid confounding is therefore to design a study so that all groups are similar with respect to any potential confounders.

Randomisation

The most effective approach to prevent confounding is *random allocation* of people to the different study groups. Clearly, this is possible only in an intervention study. When a trial is large enough, random allocation will generally ensure a balanced distribution of all characteristics between the intervention (exposed) and control (unexposed) groups. *However, even randomisation cannot guarantee the absence of confounding, especially with smaller studies,* so it must always be looked for. The analysis must then include all participants in the groups to which they were originally randomised (regardless of whether they actually received the intervention). This is known as '*intention to treat*' analysis and we will discuss this further in Chapter 14.

A major advantage of randomisation over other forms of control of confounding is that it deals not only with confounders that we know and can measure, but also with other unrecognised or unmeasurable confounders. These too will, on balance, be evenly distributed by the randomisation process. Such *unknown confounders* (e.g., aspects of personality that affect complex lifestyle patterns) cannot be dealt with by any other method.

Box 8.2 Confounding by indication

If in a trial the participants are *not* randomly allocated to the various treatment groups then confounding is still a major problem, particularly what is often called ***confounding by indication*** (Miettinen, 1983). This arises because, even among a group of people who all have the same medical condition, those who choose to take or who are prescribed a particular medication may well differ from those who do not take it or who are not prescribed it. Those who take the drug might tend to have more (or less) severe disease than those who do not take it and they should certainly not have any of the other conditions/exposures that are contra-indications to use of that drug. As a result the outcomes of those who take the drug may well differ from the outcomes of those who do not in a way that has nothing to do with the treatment itself. The obvious solution to this problem is a randomised trial in which people are allocated to the various treatment groups at random.

Restriction

Since randomisation is not possible in the majority of epidemiological studies, are there any alternatives? One option is to *restrict* the study sample to people with or without the confounding characteristic. This can be done by restricting a study to a particular age or socioeconomic group, thereby removing confounding by age or SES, or by restricting a study to non-smokers if smoking is a potential confounder. For example, we know that infection with human papillomavirus (HPV) is a major factor (potentially a *necessary cause*, see Chapter 10) in the development of cervical cancer and we also know that HPV infection is strongly associated with a number of other lifestyle factors such as smoking and use of oral contraceptives. This makes it very difficult to evaluate the association between smoking and cervical cancer because it is hard to be sure that any association observed is not simply due to confounding by HPV infection. (Smokers are more likely to be HPV-positive than non-smokers, so this could explain why they are more likely to develop cervical cancer.) By restricting a study to include only HPV-positive women, any confounding by HPV status is removed and it is possible to evaluate the effects of other co-factors, such as smoking. Restriction is, however, of limited practical value when it is necessary to control for more than one or two likely confounders.

Matching

The third possibility is to select study subjects so that major known confounders are evenly distributed across the study groups. This is achieved by *matching* subjects on the presence or absence of the confounding variable(s). This is most often done in case–control studies in which controls are selected to match the cases in some predetermined way, e.g., by age and sex. It can also be used in the same way in cohort studies, but this is uncommon and we will not consider this further. Matching can be done on an individual basis, with one or more controls matched to each case so that, for instance, each control is matched by year of birth to a specific case. Alternatively, *frequency matching* aims to select controls to match the general distribution of the confounding variable in cases. For example, if one-quarter of cases were female and three quarters were male, controls would be selected to ensure that there was a similar ratio of males to females. If, in this situation, the cases and controls were not frequency matched by sex and controls were simply selected as a random sample of the population, it is likely that about half would be female and half male. There would therefore be many more female controls than female cases but fewer male controls than male cases. Sex would be a potential confounder in the analysis (because it is associated with the disease), but any adjustment for sex would be statistically inefficient because of the large sex imbalance between cases and controls.

While it may seem tempting to match cases and controls on as many factors as possible in the hope of removing all possible confounders, this can lead to *overmatching* and greatly decreases the efficiency and increases the cost of a study. It is much harder to find a suitable control who matches a long list of criteria than it is to find someone who is only the same age and sex as the case (and even that is not always as easy as it sounds).

Finally, *it is essential that any matching factors are accounted for in the analysis*. The process of matching does not itself remove confounding – it can actually introduce different confounding, which must then be allowed for. If the matching factor is associated with the exposure of interest then, even if it is *not* associated with disease and so is not a true confounder (see criteria for a confounder above), the fact that cases and controls have been matched for that factor *will make it a confounder in the study*. In general, if a matching factor is positively associated with the exposure, the matching process will make cases and controls look more similar than they should. This means that, if the matching is not taken into account in the analysis, the calculated odds ratios will underestimate the true association between exposure and disease (it will be closer to 1.0). If frequency matching has been used it is sufficient to treat the matching factors as normal confounders (see 'Control of confounding' below), but there are special techniques for analysing individually matched data (see Box 8.3). The only exception to this rule is that if, in practice, it turns out that a matching factor is *not* associated with exposure in a case–control study. In this situation matching cases to controls on that factor will not have introduced any additional confounding and the factor need not be allowed for in the analysis.

Matching was a primary technique for control of confounding in the early decades of the modern case–control study (from the mid twentieth century until

Box 8.3 Analysis of individually matched data

To analyse the data from a simple matched case–control study you have to compare each case with their matched control (or controls if more than one control is selected for each case). In Table 8.9 the numbers no longer represent individual people but 155 matched pairs of cases and controls so there are 40 pairs for which both the case and the control are exposed, 25 pairs for which only the case was exposed and so on.

Table 8.9 Analysing data from an individually matched case–control study.

	Controls	
Cases	Exposed	Unexposed
Exposed	40	25
Unexposed	10	80

Matched odds ratio = 25 ÷ 10 = 2.5

If a case and their matched control are both exposed (or both unexposed) that pair (or set) cannot tell us anything about the association between exposure and disease. The interesting case–control pairs are those for which one member is exposed and the other is unexposed. The matched odds ratio is calculated by simply dividing the number of pairs for which the case was exposed and the control unexposed by the number of pairs for which the control was exposed and the case unexposed:

$$\text{Matched OR} = \frac{\text{No. of pairs for which the case was exposed and the control unexposed}}{\text{No. of pairs for which the control was exposed and the case unexposed}} \qquad (8.1)$$

Note that, if we had not taken the matching into account in the analysis, we would have said that 65 (40 + 25) out of the 155 cases were exposed and 90 (10 + 80) were unexposed compared with 50 (40 + 10) exposed and 105 (25 + 80) unexposed controls, giving an unmatched odds ratio of $(65 \times 105) \div (90 \times 50) = 1.5$, which is considerably less than the matched value of 2.5.

the 1980s). The ready availability now of flexible and reasonably straightforward computing packages that allow effective control for confounding at the stage of data analysis (either by stratified or multivariable analysis) has lessened its importance, although it continues to be used to increase efficiency in a variety of situations.

Does increasing the size of a study help?

In any observational epidemiological study increasing the size of the study will not make any difference to the amount of confounding. (To convince yourself of this, go back to one of the earlier examples and try doubling the numbers of people in each group. This will not alter the odds ratios or rate ratios and will not get rid of the confounding.) The only time study size does matter is in the context of a randomised controlled trial. The bigger a randomised trial is, the more likely it is that any confounders (known and unknown) will be balanced across the study groups and the less likely it is that there will be any confounding.

Control of confounding in data analysis

If you have designed a study using restriction or matching to reduce the effects of confounding, it is no longer possible to study the effects of the confounding variables. For example, if you have restricted your study to people aged between 60 and 70 years, or have matched cases and controls for age, it would no longer be possible to look at the direct effects of age on disease. This means that it is often preferable to collect information on potential confounders and then to control for these in the analysis. The aim of the analysis is exactly the same as the design options mentioned above, namely to ensure that the confounders are balanced across the groups, and in practice this is achieved by comparing exposure–disease patterns within narrow ranges of one or more confounders. These approaches apply equally to case–control and cohort studies and also to clinical trials if they are not randomised or if, in a randomised study, the randomisation did not lead to an equal balance of important confounders across the study groups.

Stratification

This is the method that we used in the alcohol and lung cancer example where we stratified by smoking status and the steps are shown in Figure 8.4. Study subjects are split into groups, or strata, based on levels of the confounding variable. The association between the exposure and outcome of interest is then measured separately in each stratum. If the people in each stratum are homogeneous (the same or similar) with respect to the confounding variable, there can no longer be any confounding by that factor. An analysis could be done separately for men and women to remove confounding by sex, for different age groups, for smokers and non-smokers (as in the example of alcohol and lung cancer) and so on.

In practice it is rarely possible to remove all confounding so we will be left with some **residual confounding**. For example, in a study of US health professionals the crude RR (0.56; 95% CI 0.38–0.84) suggested that men who consumed high levels of fruit and vegetables had almost half the risk of lung cancer of those who ate little fruit and vegetables (Feskanich *et al.*, 2000). When the authors adjusted their analysis for a simple measure of smoking status (never, past, current smoker) the RR increased to 0.86 (95% CI 0.58–1.29), suggesting that the crude

Fig. 8.4 A scheme for
identifying and dealing with
confounding and effect
modification.

RR was confounded by smoking. When they also adjusted for more detailed measures of smoking, including time since stopping and current amount smoked, the RR increased still further to 1.07 (95% CI 0.71–1.61). This shows convincingly that the simple adjustment for smoking status was not sufficient to remove all of the confounding by smoking and there was considerable residual confounding. If they had not adjusted for the additional smoking variables the results would have left some room for optimism that improving diet might confer some benefit, whereas the fully adjusted result suggests that unfortunately this is not the case.

Note that, although stratification can also be used for studies in which cases and controls have been frequency matched, it is generally not appropriate for individually matched studies. These should be analysed using a special 'matched' analysis as described above or using special modelling techniques (see below).

In the examples above, the stratum-specific odds ratios were exactly or almost exactly the same, but this is rarely the case in practice. If the stratum-specific estimates are similar then it is reasonable to assume that the small differences between them are simply due to chance. If instead they are quite different then there may be *effect modification* or in other words the 'effect' (the association between exposure and outcome) may be different in the different strata. For example, regular physical activity might reduce the risk of a particular disease among people who are overweight but it might confer no benefit for those of normal weight. In this situation obesity *modifies* the effect of physical activity on disease and it would be inappropriate to treat obesity as a confounder (see Figure 8.4). In practice, however, there is always some variation between the odds ratios in different strata and it can be very difficult to know whether this indicates a meaningful difference or is just random variation. There are statistical tests (tests for heterogeneity) that can be used to help decide whether the variation could just be due to chance. However, these are not very powerful and are unlikely to detect variation unless the difference is very great (in which case it would be apparent without a statistical test) or the study is very large.

If, however, the stratum-specific estimates are similar, it is then possible to combine the estimates from each separate stratum to summarise the overall effect in the whole group. There are several ways to do this and the effect is then said to be 'adjusted' for the confounder (see Appendix 5). (Note: this process is analogous to the standardisation that you met in Chapter 2.)

If, when we adjust for something, the adjusted measure of association is *different* from the original crude measure, then we know that the crude association was confounded. In the alcohol and lung cancer example the crude OR was 3.0 and the adjusted OR was 1.0, showing that the crude OR was heavily confounded by smoking. As we discussed above, however, it is rarely possible to control for *all* confounding and there is always likely to be some residual confounding. This means that, if adjustment changes an observed odds ratio quite markedly, e.g., it reduces it from 5.4 to 2.6, then it is likely that, if we could have controlled for the confounding perfectly, the true odds ratio would have been even less than 2.6. We then have to decide whether we think that there is a *true* association between the exposure and disease or whether all the *observed* association could be due to confounding. However, if the control for confounding only changed the odds ratio from 5.4 to 5.1 then it is likely that, even if we could have controlled completely for confounding, the true odds ratio would still have been about 5.0, suggesting that it is more likely to be a real association.

Multivariable modelling

Stratification may be impractical when a study is small or you need to control for several confounders simultaneously, because you are likely to end up with small numbers in any one stratum. If, for example, you wanted to control for sex, age with five 10-year age groups (20–29, 30–39, 40–49, 50–59 and 60–69) and smoking (non-smoker versus smoker), you would end up with 20 different strata (five age groups for smokers and five for non-smokers for each sex). On average, each stratum will contain only 5% of your study population and, with small numbers, it can be difficult to obtain precise estimates of the association in each. An alternative is to use statistical modelling techniques to estimate the strength of the relationship of interest while controlling for all of the potential confounders. The most commonly used multivariable approach for unmatched (or frequency-matched) case–control studies is *multiple logistic regression*. (Individually matched case–control data can be analysed by a variation of this called *conditional logistic regression*, which takes the individual matching between cases and controls into account.) A common technique used to analyse person-time data from a cohort study is *Cox proportional hazards regression*. (Note that this generates what are often called *hazard ratios*, although they are essentially the same as incidence rate ratios.) We will not discuss the details of these procedures here – they can be found in any standard medical statistics text. A word of caution, however: multivariable modelling can be performed very easily with modern statistics software but it is important to know what you are doing. The models can be complex and they are based on a number of underlying assumptions. If you are not familiar with the techniques it is wise to seek advice from a statistician before diving in. Furthermore, it is important to be familiar with your data before starting any modelling and nothing can replace simple stratified analyses, as outlined above, for this.

Confounding: the bottom line

- Confounding is almost ubiquitous in practice and almost any paper that reports associations between two factors will say that they have 'adjusted' for this, that and the other to control for confounding.
- Unlike the problem of bias, for which, as we discussed in the previous chapter, it can be hard to know what effects it might have on the results of a study, *known* confounders can be identified and addressed *if information about the confounders has been collected.*
- Even if an analysis has 'adjusted for confounders' there is likely to be *residual confounding* either by measured confounders or by unmeasured/unknown confounders.

  Known confounders: a big difference between the unadjusted and adjusted measures suggests that there may be considerable residual confounding; a small difference suggests that residual confounding is not a big problem.

  Unknown/unmeasured confounders: unless we are talking about a randomised trial we will not know anything about the likely effects of these, but if we see a strong association between exposure and outcome then the confounding would have to be enormous (very strong associations between the confounder and both the exposure and the outcome) to explain the whole association. In practice we might hope that we would know about such strong confounders!

Questions

Table 8.10 shows some data from a study of injuries involving moped riders in Spain. The authors obtained information from the Spanish Registry of Traffic

Table 8.10 Results of a study of head injury and helmet use.

	Driver		Passenger		Total	
	Head injury	Other injury	Head injury	Other injury	Head injury	Other injury
No helmet	17,869	51,900	3,052	12,522	20,921	64,422
Helmet	7,342	86,212	485	7,971	7,827	94,183
Total	25,211	138,112	3,537	20,493	28,748	158,605

(Lardelli-Claret *et al.*, 2003.)

Crashes regarding 187,353 moped riders injured in traffic accidents between 1990 and 1999. They then compared the group with head injuries (cases) with those with other types of injury (controls).

1. What is the crude odds ratio for the association between not wearing a helmet (exposed) and head injury?
2. What is the odds ratio for the association between not wearing a helmet and head injury among (i) moped drivers and (ii) moped passengers?
3. Was the crude association between not wearing a helmet and head injury confounded by position on the moped?
4. Does the position of the rider (driver or passenger) on the moped affect their chances of sustaining a head injury? (Hint – first calculate the crude odds ratio for the association between moped position and head injury and then consider whether this could be confounded by helmet use.)

REFERENCES

Bickel, P. J., Hammel, E. A. and O'Connell, J. W. (1975). Sex bias in graduate admissions: data from Berkeley. *Science*, **187**: 398–404.

Feskanich, D., Ziegler, R. G., Michaud, D. S. *et al.* (2000). Prospective study of fruit and vegetable consumption and risk of lung cancer among men and women. *Journal of the National Cancer Institute*, **92**: 1812–1823.

Lardelli-Claret, P., Luna-del-Castillo, J. D. D. and Jimenez-Moleon, J. J. (2003). Position on the moped, risk of head injury and helmet use: an example of confounding effect. *International Journal of Epidemiology*, **32**: 162–164.

Mantel, N. and Haenszel, W. (1959) Statistical aspects of the analysis of data from retrospective studies of disease. *Journal of the National Cancer Institute*, **22**: 719–748.

Miettinen, O. S. (1983). The need for randomization in the study of intended effects. *Statistics in Medicine*, **2**: 267–271.

Vessey, M. P. and Lawless, M. (1984). The Oxford Family Planning Association contraceptive study. *Clinical Obstetrics and Gynaecology*, **11**: 743–757.

9

Bringing it together: reading and writing papers in practice

In Chapters 6–8 we have looked at the different epidemiological study designs and examined the various misfortunes that can befall them. In practice you will almost certainly have to read individual papers and reports and, if you are involved in research, you may write some of your own. Both activities demand a very practical approach and this is what we will focus on here. We will emphasise the perspective of the reader, but the writer should be thinking about exactly the same things, since good writing demands that the readers' needs and perspectives are kept firmly in mind.

Good studies are difficult to design and implement, and interpretation of their results and conclusions is not always as straightforward as we might hope. How, then, can we make the best use of this information? The central question we have to answer when we read a study report is '*Are the results of the study valid?*' If the authors report an association between exposure and outcome, is it real? If they find nothing, do we accept this? Or could there be an alternative explanation for the results, namely chance, bias and/or confounding?

Frank and Ernest

© 1990 Thaves. Reprinted with permission. Newspaper dist. by NEA, Inc.

Much of the following discussion will pick up and integrate the core epidemiological issues covered in the previous chapters. Some quite detailed sets of guidelines for 'critical appraisal' of the health literature exist already and we do not intend to add to this list (although we do offer a flowchart for more general guidance). Instead we will focus on the essence of our challenge: what are the practical effects of the ways in which subjects were selected and information collected, and the likely influence of confounding and chance on the results we see?

To extract the maximum information from a paper we need a systematic approach to identifying its strengths and weaknesses. The general strategy we propose and examples we use are most directly relevant to analytic population research (seeking causes), but the principles hold true much more widely, as we show later for descriptive studies. While the elements are universal, the approach can (and should) be tailored to suit your own personal style.

The research question and study design

When reading a paper, the first step is to identify the *research question* that the authors set out to answer and then the strategy they used to attempt to answer that question. Was the *study design* appropriate to answer the question posed? This involves consideration of what the *ideal* type of study would be and also what would be *practical* in that particular situation.

As you have seen, the *ideal* study to answer a question of cause and effect would often be some sort of randomised trial, but in many situations this would be impossible for numerous ethical and/or practical reasons. Next best would generally be a cohort study in which exposure is measured prior to the development of disease, but again the resources, time and money required to conduct a large enough study often make it unfeasible. So, from a practical viewpoint the key question should be 'Was the research design the best that could have been done in the circumstances to answer that particular question?' If it was not the best, can it still provide useful information? Are there existing studies addressing the same issue that were of better design against which the findings of the current study can be compared?

Many studies are conducted not because they will provide the strongest possible evidence for a causal association between exposure and outcome, but because they can answer a range of other questions of interest. For example, the results from the ecological study of *Helicobacter pylori* infection and stomach cancer rates in China shown in Figure 6.3 cannot directly answer the question 'Does *H. pylori* infection cause stomach cancer?' We can, however, answer the question 'Are stomach cancer rates higher in areas where *H. pylori* infection is more common?' Trials, and to a lesser extent cohort studies and case–control studies, can address issues of causality more directly, whereas other types of study provide more circumstantial evidence, but if the results are valid each can increase our understanding of the relation between an exposure and outcome. As an example, ecological and migrant studies conducted across countries with widely differing levels of solar ultraviolet (UV) radiation have consistently revealed an association between sun exposure in childhood and melanoma rates. In contrast, case–control studies, which have generally been conducted within a single country or region with a narrow range of UV exposures, have not given consistent results (Whiteman *et al.*, 2001). In this particular situation ecological studies with their wide variety of exposure levels can provide better information than the case–control studies.

So how do we decide whether the results of a study are valid? We have to consider the three main alternative explanations: bias – both the *selection of participants* for the study and the *information* that was *measured* or collected from or about them – confounding and chance.

The study sample: selection bias

Who was included in the study, how were they selected and are there possible sources of selection bias? Specific questions to ask when reading a paper include those below.

- *Is the comparison group appropriate?*
  In a case–control study are the controls really representative of the population from which the cases arose? If in a cohort study the comparison cohort was recruited separately from the exposed cohort, are the two groups really comparable?
- *What proportion of eligible participants actually took part in the study and, if appropriate, what proportion was lost to follow-up?*
  Participation or follow-up rates less than 90% (some would say 80%) may be cause for some concern. If the rates are lower than this, could participation (or loss to follow-up) be related to either the exposure or the outcome of interest? That is, could those who refused to take part (or who were lost to follow-up) have differed in some way from those who did take part? If so, might this have led to an overestimation or underestimation of the level of exposure and/or outcome? Most importantly, could this have differed between study groups?
- *Finally, what is the likely effect of any selection bias on the results of the study?*
  Ideally the authors of the paper will have considered all of these issues in their discussion, but if they have not then it is up to the reader to decide whether bias might be present and, if so, what effect it may have had on the results. In practice there will almost certainly be some potential for selection bias. Participation rates are never 100% and in many developed countries it is becoming increasingly hard to persuade people to take part in research, especially when they see no benefit to themselves. This is a major issue in case–control studies when the motivation for a 'case' to take part may be much greater than that of an unaffected 'control'. Also, people are becoming increasingly mobile, so follow-up in a cohort study that runs for more than a few years is never likely to be 100%.

If we were to reject all studies with less than 100% participation or follow-up rates, we would be left with nothing to review. In practice, participation or follow-up rates greater than 80% or 90% are generally considered to be good, but rates lower than this do not necessarily invalidate the findings. The challenge for both investigator and reader is to think practically and to decide whether any potential biases related to selection might have compromised the study results (the **internal validity**) and, if so, how and to what degree the results might be biased. It is often impossible to quantify this, but *sensitivity analyses* making various assumptions about the size and direction of possible bias can be informative.

Example 1: case–control studies of blood transfusion and Creutzfeldt–Jakob disease

In five case–control studies of Creutzfeldt–Jakob disease (CJD) the controls were more likely to report having had a blood transfusion than cases (Riggs *et al.*, 2001). Does this tell us that blood transfusions might protect against CJD (a finding contrary to the causal hypothesis)? If we consider the control groups, we find that in three of the five studies they were selected from among hospitalised patients and in another study more than 12,000 telephone calls were made in order to recruit just 784 controls. The use of hospital controls and the very low participation rate should ring alarm bells. People who are in hospital are more likely to have had a blood transfusion than those who are not; and in addition, given the publicity surrounding 'mad cow disease', people who have had a blood transfusion may well be more likely to agree to take part in a study of CJD. Furthermore, in the same four studies approximately 20% of controls reported having had a blood transfusion – an improbably high proportion, probably due at least in part to these selection pressures. So what can we conclude about the association between transfusion and CJD from these studies? Not much. The high transfusion rate in controls almost certainly overestimates the base rate in the population from which the cases came. We have no idea whether the true background rate is similar to that in cases (i.e., there is no association) or lower than in cases (a positive association). Our next example shows how external information can help resolve such dilemmas.

Example 2: a case–control study of ovarian cancer and smoking in Australia

In the Australian ovarian cancer study mentioned in Chapter 6 the authors also considered the relation with smoking. In this study approximately 90% of eligible cases but only 73% of selected controls agreed to participate – a reasonable percentage these days, but less than ideal. The authors found that smoking rates were higher among cases than controls (OR = 1.5; 95% CI 1.2–1.9), but could this be due to selection bias?

If smokers were less likely to take part the prevalence of smoking in the control group would be *lower* than that in the general population. This would exaggerate the difference between cases and controls and so increase the odds ratio, making it look as if smoking is associated with ovarian cancer when in reality it might not be. To address this issue the authors compared the prevalence of smoking among the controls with that in the National Health Survey conducted at about the same time. There was no difference between the proportions of smokers in the two samples, suggesting that the study results were not seriously biased (Green *et al.*, 2001).

Measuring disease and exposure: measurement bias

We then have to consider the information collected from or about the people in the study – particularly the measurement of 'outcome' and 'exposure' but also measurement of other factors that might be important confounders. Attention to unbiased measurement of *outcome* is crucial for cross-sectional, cohort and intervention studies. It is of relatively less importance in a case–control study, in which cases are selected because they have already experienced the outcome of interest (although a clear definition of what constitutes a case is still essential). Accurate measurement of *exposure* is important in every study, and in a case–control study it is critical to ensure that there are no systematic differences in measurement between cases and controls. Good measurement of *confounders* is often overlooked, but this is also essential to enable optimal control of confounding in the analysis (see comments on residual confounding in Chapter 8).

Some questions to ask when reading a paper are the following.
- *Were the outcome/exposures/confounders clearly defined, and how were they measured?*
- *Have all relevant outcomes and/or exposures and/or confounders been included and, if not, how important are those omitted?*
- *Were the same definitions and methods of measurement used in all of the study groups?*
- *Is measurement error likely to be a problem and, if so, could there be **non-differential misclassification**?*

No measurement is perfect and some measurements are very poor. The effect of the ubiquitous random error and consequent non-differential misclassification must always be considered. The practical implication of this is that effects (OR, RR) estimated in the face of equal measurement error in the compared groups will usually appear *weaker* than they truly are. Thus a finding of a positive association, despite poor measurement, should not be dismissed because of this – the true association is likely to be more impressive. On the other hand, a null finding or a very weak effect in the presence of non-differential misclassification is uninformative since it may reflect the imprecise measurement (thereby masking a true association) or there may truly be no effect.

- *Is the extent of any measurement error likely to differ between groups (e.g., could there be **recall** or **interviewer bias** in exposure measurement in a case–control study) and so could there be **differential misclassification**?*

Differential misclassification can bias results in either direction. It is particularly important to consider this possibility in cross-sectional and case–control studies when exposure is measured after the outcome has occurred. In analytic research it is generally easier to distinguish clearly between outcome states (diseased versus non-diseased) than it is to measure exposures precisely, but the avoidance of differential outcome assessment is central to the integrity of cohort studies and trials, and again for cross-sectional studies.

- *Finally, what practical effects might any measurement bias (outcome or exposure) have had on the results of the study?*

Example 3: a case–control study of body-mass index (BMI) and asthma in Mexico

A significant association between asthma and obesity (defined as BMI $\geqslant 30\,\mathrm{kg/m^2}$ based on self-reported weight and height) was observed among women (adjusted OR = 1.7; 95% CI 1.1–2.7), with a weaker non-significant association (adjusted OR = 1.3; 95% CI 0.6–2.9) seen among men (Santillan and Camargo, 2003); but how reliable are self-reported data on body size and could measurement error have affected the results? The authors specifically addressed this question by weighing and measuring all of the participants. They found that, on average, people tended to report that they were taller and lighter than they really were, particularly the men. As a result, the *true* prevalence of obesity based on measured BMI was higher than that based on self-reported BMI and the difference was somewhat greater for cases (40% versus 24% for men and 44% versus 38% for women) than for controls (28% versus 22% for men; 24% versus 23% for women). Assuming that the measured BMI values are correct, is the *true* association between obesity and asthma likely to be stronger or weaker than that seen for self-reported obesity?

In this example there is *differential* error since cases, particularly men, were more likely to underestimate their weight and overestimate their height than controls. The effect of these errors was to reduce the association seen: for men the true prevalence of obesity is 40% in cases versus 28% in controls compared with a difference of only 24% versus 22% for self-reported obesity. As a result the association between asthma and *measured* obesity (adjusted OR = 2.5, 95% CI 1.1–5.9 for men and OR = 2.3, 95% CI 1.5–3.8 for women) is stronger than that based on self-reported BMI. (Note that, although the OR based on measured

Box 9.1 Sensitivity analysis: kangaroos and Ross River virus (RRV) infection

Authors of a case–control study found an odds ratio of 4.3 (95% CI 0.9–21) for the association between seeing kangaroos in the backyard and risk of RRV infection, possibly because kangaroos provide a host for the mosquitoes that spread RRV. However, information was missing for a number of cases and controls, so the authors performed a sensitivity analysis.

If they assumed that all cases and controls for whom exposure data were missing had seen kangaroos, the OR was 1.9 (95% CI 0.7–5.1); if they assumed that none had seen kangaroos the OR was 3.5 (0.9–14.1). If they assumed that cases were more likely to remember exposure than controls (i.e., there is recall bias) and, therefore, that cases with data missing had not seen kangaroos whereas controls had seen them, then the association disappeared completely (OR = 1.0, 95% CI 0.4–2.8). This analysis raised questions about the validity of the observed association between sighting of kangaroos and RRV infection.

(Harley *et al.*, 2005)

BMI is likely to give a more accurate estimate than that based on self-reporting, even this may be an underestimate of the 'true' effect since there is still likely to be some *non-differential* random misclassification.) Validation studies such as this can provide valuable insights into the accuracy of study results as can sensitivity analyses (Box 9.1).

Confounding

The next major issue to consider is that of confounding.
- *Have the authors considered all important confounders and controlled for them in their analysis?*
- *Could there be residual confounding by variables that have not been considered or because of incomplete adjustment for factors that have?*
- *If so, what effect might this have had on the study results?*

Again, the important thing is to think practically: in which direction is any residual confounding likely to operate? If when the authors adjusted for confounding the association became *stronger* (i.e., the confounding had originally biased the effect towards the null) then, if there is residual confounding, the real effect is likely to be even more extreme than that observed. Conversely, if the adjustment brought the estimate *closer* to 1.0 (i.e., the confounding had biased the estimate away from the null) then the true result may be even closer to the null than that reported. In the latter situation our confidence in the value of a positive effect estimate would decrease, unless it was very large. A large effect is less likely to be wholly due to confounding because, to explain away a very strong RR (e.g., 10.0), the confounder itself would have to be an even stronger risk factor for the disease. If it is such, it is unlikely not to be known already, and hence should have been measured and controlled for.

Example 4: a cross-sectional study of risk factors for depression in the UK

Among 14,217 adults aged over 75 years, the risk of depression appeared to be somewhat higher among women than among men (crude OR = 1.3, 95% CI 1.1–1.5) (Osborn *et al.*, 2003). After adjustment for potential confounding factors including age, marital status, living alone, smoking and alcohol consumption, the adjusted OR was 1.1 (95% CI 1.0–1.3). The adjustment has reduced the OR, bringing it closer to 1.0. It is also likely that there is further residual confounding, which might bring the true OR even closer to 1.0, suggesting that sex is not associated with depression (at least in this study).

Example 5: a cohort study of statin use and atrial fibrillation in the USA

A cohort of patients with coronary artery disease was followed for a minimum of 12 months to document the incidence of atrial fibrillation (AF); 263 of the patients were using statins (cholesterol-lowering drugs) and 186 had never used them (Young-Xu *et al.*, 2003). (Note that this was an observational study, not a randomised trial.) Overall, the rate of AF was lower among the group taking statins, giving a crude relative risk of 0.5 (95% CI 0.3–0.8). When the authors adjusted for potential confounding factors including age, systolic blood pressure, alcohol consumption, history of heart failure and total serum cholesterol level, the RR was 0.4 (95% CI 0.2–0.8).

Assuming that there are no important selection or measurement errors, what conclusions can we draw about the association between statin use and AF?

It appears that there was some confounding by the other factors such as age since the RR dropped from 0.5 to 0.4 after adjustment, indicating that the real effect of statin use was even stronger than the crude RR suggested. However, doctors prescribe treatment partly on the basis of prognostic judgements, which are difficult to measure. There may thus be other unknown and unmeasured confounders that have not been controlled for, so we would still need to be cautious about this particular result. (Large, well-conducted RCTs remove this potential problem of 'confounding by indication'; see Chapter 8.)

Chance

Finally, it is important to consider the role of chance. Have the authors included confidence intervals for their estimates? How narrow (good precision) or wide (poor precision) are they? If an association is seen, how likely is it that there is really no effect (i.e., the association arose by chance)? If there is no clear association (e.g., if the confidence limits are very wide and include 1.0), is it possible that there is a real effect but the study was simply too small to detect it? Is the study useful or are the results inconclusive? As well as *statistical significance* it is also important to consider whether the results are *socially* or *clinically* significant. We will return to this issue in Chapter 11.

Study validity

Once we have considered all of these aspects (summarised in Figure 9.1) we can make an overall judgement of the *validity* of the study results. There are two separate issues here. The first and most important, often called **internal validity**, is the extent to which the results of a study reflect the true situation *in the study sample* in the absence of any alternative explanations. These alternative explanations, namely chance, bias and confounding, have been the focus of this and the previous chapters. *The prime objective of study design, implementation, analysis and interpretation is to maximise the internal validity of a study*. The second issue is one of **generalisability** or **external validity**. Are the results of a study applicable to populations other than the study population?

Internal validity

Have the authors discussed the limitations of their study? What conclusions do they draw with respect to the research question? Are these conclusions justified? Does the study appear to be internally valid or could the results be due to chance, bias or confounding? It is important to remember that in public health we are dealing with real people and complex exposures that are often difficult to measure and/or impossible to control adequately and we are, quite rightly, constrained as to what we can do by codes of ethics. Any study is thus likely to fall short of perfection and it is important to realise this. Research should be appraised in the light of what it has been able to achieve – there will be deficiencies but, given the particular circumstances, could things realistically have been improved? The evidence reported in a research paper might not always be strong but, if it is the best that is likely to be available, we should not discount it because of the flaws. Rather we should draw from it what information we can that bears on the question in hand.

External validity

It is important to remember that the aim of the 'causal arm' of epidemiology is to discover general scientific truths about cause and effect. Can the results of a

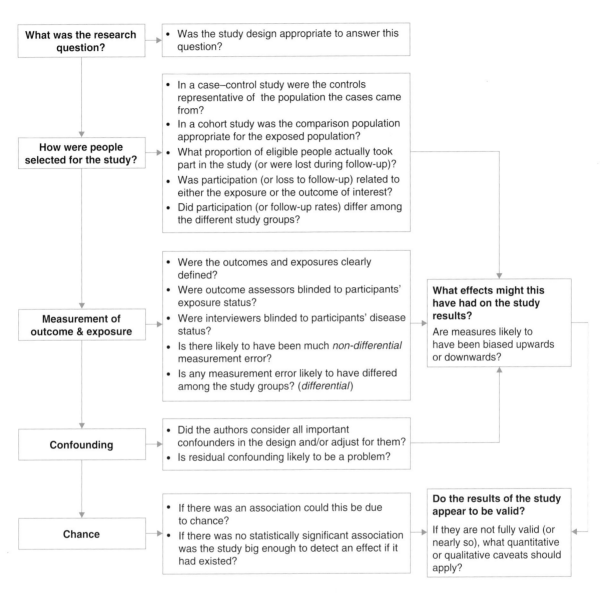

Fig. 9.1 Issues to consider when reading epidemiological papers.

study of, for example, American men aged 50–65 be generalised to older or younger men? Women? Non-Americans? (Note that such a question presumes the internal validity of a study: *if a study is not internally valid, then the results should not be applied to anyone.*)

There are no firm rules to help with generalising from a study to the wider population. In case–control comparisons population-based studies are the ideal in order to reduce the possibilities of selection bias and, as a result, it might not require such a leap of faith to extrapolate the results from one population to another. However, the process is not simply a matter of statistical representativeness, but is more fundamentally one of biological insight. The question then is 'How relevant (biologically) is a result for a given population?' Can a study in a very select population (e.g., Japanese cities, Czech women, Brazilian men) inform us about disease causation more generally? Well, we certainly hope so. As an example, careful follow-up of the survivors of the atomic bomb blasts in Hiroshima and Nagasaki, Japan, has yielded volumes of information regarding the relation between exposure to ionising radiation and subsequent risks of mortality, cancers and other rare diseases. While this information comes only from the Japanese, no one would argue that radiation would not have similar effects in other nationalities and we certainly do not want to see this 'unnatural experiment' repeated. While this generalisation is perhaps easier than many because of the magnitude and timing of the effects and the well-understood physical and biological properties of ionising radiation, the principle is identical for other abstract causal speculation.

Generalising from clinical and other trials raises additional issues. For practical reasons, many clinical trials are conducted on highly selected groups of people who are almost certainly not representative of the general population. This can make the results of the specific trials easier to interpret (internal validity), but means that they can be harder to generalise to other groups (see Chapter 11).

Descriptive studies

The discussion above has focussed on papers evaluating associations between exposure and outcome and that, therefore, address the 'Why?' of epidemiology. It is equally important to evaluate the results of descriptive studies that provide the 'Who?', 'Where?' and 'When?' information that is essential to make a community diagnosis. In practice this requires us to consider exactly the same issues: selection and measurement error, confounding and chance.

- How was the survey sample selected? Is it representative of the wider population?
- How was the factor of interest measured? Is it likely to be over- or under-reported?
- If we are making comparisons, are we comparing like with like or is there a need for standardisation (to remove confounding by, e.g., differences in the age structure of populations)?
- Could any observed excesses (or deficits) of disease in different populations, in different places or at different times be due to chance? For example, it is unlikely that several cases of a rare disease would occur in the same small community (what is known as a 'cluster' – see Chapter 12), but it is not impossible for this to occur by chance. Similarly, rates of disease (particularly rare

diseases) will naturally vary from year to year, so could an apparent increase or decline just be due to chance?

It is also important to note that, although *representativeness* is not the primary issue in studies of aetiology, it is crucial for applying the results of a descriptive study to a wider population. If a sample of people is surveyed to identify the health needs of an area then, if those participating do not represent the whole population, the results could be very misleading. If, for example, they were unusually healthy then the needs of the population might be greatly underestimated, and vice versa.

Writing papers

We have focussed on the information that you need to look for when reading a paper and, as we suggested at the start of this chapter, it goes without saying that this is also the information that you need to provide when writing a paper. To improve the reporting of experimental research, some journals now require that authors follow the checklist of points contained in the Consolidated Standards of Reporting Trials or CONSORT statement (Moher *et al.*, 2001). This document has since been modified to give the TREND (Transparent Reporting of Non-randomised Designs) checklist for reporting results of studies of behavioural and public health interventions with non-randomised designs (Des Jarlais *et al.*, 2004). Similar guidelines for observational studies are being developed (e.g. Tooth *et al.*, 2005).

Questions

We have not included any questions for this chapter, but the Epidemic Intelligence Service of the US Centers for Disease Control and Prevention has developed an excellent exercise 'Cigarette smoking and lung cancer' that draws on many of the issues covered in this and the previous chapters. This and other similar exercises are freely available from http://www.cdc.gov/eis/casestudies/casestudies.htm.

REFERENCES

Des Jarlais, D. C., Lyles, C., Crepaz, N. and the TREND Group. (2004). Improving the reporting quality of non-randomized evaluations of behavioral and public health interventions: the TREND statement. *American Journal of Public Health*, **94**: 361–366.

Green, A., Purdie, D., Bain, C., Siskind, V. and Webb, P. M. (2001). Cigarette smoking and risk of epithelial ovarian cancer (Australia). *Cancer Causes and Control*, **12**: 713–719.

Harley, D., Ritchie, S., Bain, C. and Sleigh, A. C. (2005). Risks for Ross River virus disease in tropical Australia. *International Journal of Epidemiology*, in press.

Moher, D., Schultz, K. F. and Altman, D. G. for the CONSORT Group. (2001). The CONSORT statement: revised recommendations for improving the quality of reports of parallel-group randomised trials. *Lancet*, **357**: 1191–1194.

Osborn, D. P. J., Fletcher, A. E., Smeeth, L. *et al.* (2003). Factors associated with depression in a representative sample of 14,217 people aged 75 and over in the United Kingdom: results from the MRC trial of assessment and management of older people in the community. *International Journal of Geriatric Psychiatry*, **18**: 623–630.

Riggs, J. E., Moudgil, S. S. and Hobbs, G. R. (2001). Creutzfeld–Jakob disease and blood transfusions: a meta-analysis of case–control studies. *Military Medicine*, **166**: 1057–1058.

Santillan, A. A. and Camargo Jr, C. A. (2003). Body mass index and asthma among Mexican adults: the effect of using self-reported versus measured weight and height. *International Journal of Obesity*, **27**: 1430–1433.

Tooth, L., Ware, R., Dobson, A., Purdie, D. and Bain, C. (2005). Quality of reporting of observational longitudinal research. *American Journal of Epidemiology*, in press.

Whiteman, D. C., Whiteman, C. A. and Green, A. C. (2001). Childhood sun exposure as a risk factor for melanoma: a systematic review of epidemiologic studies. *Cancer Causes and Control*, **12**: 69–82.

Young-Xu, Y., Jabbour, S., Goldberg, R. *et al.* (2003). Usefulness of statin drugs in protecting against atrial fibrillation in patients with coronary artery disease. *American Journal of Cardiology*, **92**: 1379–1383.

10

Who sank the boat?
Association and causation

Box 10.1 Who sank the boat?

As the story goes, there were five animals living by the sea, a cow, a donkey, a sheep, a pig and a mouse. One fine day they decided to go rowing on the bay.

First the cow got into the boat, it rocked a bit but she settled herself down comfortably at the back. Then the donkey got in carefully and sat down at the front to balance the boat. Next the pig climbed in, clutching her umbrella – the boat is low in the water by now. Then the sheep climbed in carrying her knitting and she sat down opposite the pig.

The boat is still afloat, but only just. Finally the little mouse jumped aboard and – disaster! The boat capsized and the animals had to swim to the shore.

(*continued*)

Box 10.1 (*continued*)

So who sank the boat?

(Storyline (adapted) and pictures from '*Who Sank the Boat?*' (Allen, 1983),
reproduced with permission from Penguin Books Australia Ltd.)

The search for the causes of disease is an obvious central step in the pursuit of better health through disease prevention and Box 10.1, abstracted from a wonderful children's picture book, illustrates perfectly the complexity of assigning causality. In the previous chapters we have looked at how we measure health (or disease) and how we look for associations between exposure and disease. Being able to identify a *relation* between a potential cause of disease and the disease itself is not enough, though. We need to go one step further and decide whether this relation is causal.

What do we mean by a cause?

It is tempting to think that a cause is a single condition or event that inevitably leads to a particular effect or outcome; i.e., that there is a one-to-one relationship such that wherever or whenever the cause occurs the effect will follow. If we consider this more closely, it quickly becomes apparent that things are not so simple and that everyday causal phenomena are rather more complicated than they might seem at first. For example, while it might appear that all we need to do to turn on a computer is press the 'on' button, we know better: what if the wiring is faulty, there is no power supply or the hard drive has died an untimely death? To 'cause' the computer to come on we need power, good wiring, a functioning hard drive and relevant software in addition to the pressure of our finger on the button. We could describe each of these separate requirements as **component causes**, since they are all part of the one **sufficient cause** that will inevitably lead to the effect – in this case the computer turning on. In this situation they are also **necessary causes** because in the absence of just one of these things the computer will not work.

In the same way, disease rarely occurs as the result of a single event or exposure. Even though it might seem that an infectious agent would be a sufficient cause in its own right, not everyone develops disease following exposure to a particular bug. The real-life food-poisoning example in Chapter 1 made this clear – although people who ate the cold chicken were 3.8 times more likely to suffer from food poisoning than those who did not, almost one quarter (23%) of those who ate the cold chicken suffered no ill effects. Whether someone does become ill depends both on their susceptibility to the agent and on the dose they receive. For tuberculosis (TB), for example, a person's susceptibility reflects whether they have been infected before and are now immune and their overall level of health at the time. The infectious agent, the tubercle bacillus, is only a component of the total or sufficient cause that will lead to TB. It is, however, a **necessary cause** in that, by definition, TB cannot occur without it. We will look at causation and infectious diseases in more detail in Chapter 12.

Some definitions

There are many definitions of a cause but the following, from Rothman (1986; p. 11), is appealing because of the brevity with which it captures the concept:

a cause is *'an event, condition or characteristic* [or a combination of these factors] *that plays an essential role in producing an occurrence of the disease'*

There are also many ways in which such entities (causes) can be classified, but the following subdivision serves well.
- A **sufficient** cause is a factor (or more usually a combination of several factors) that will inevitably produce disease.
- A **component** cause is a factor that contributes towards disease causation but is not sufficient to cause disease on its own.
- A **necessary** cause is any agent (or component cause) that is required for the development of a given disease (for example the specific infectious agent).

In terms of working out 'who sank the boat' we can say that each one of the animals was a **component** cause and that together they created the **sufficient** cause

Fig. 10.1 A conceptual scheme for the causes of a hypothetical disease. (*From:* Rothman, Causes, *Am. J. Epidemiol.,* 1976; 104, p. 589, by permission of the Society for Epidemiological Research.)

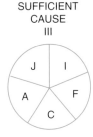

that caused the disaster. Probably none was actually **necessary** to sink the boat – any group of similarly sized animals would have had a similar effect. The ordering of the events, i.e., whether the mouse got in first or last, also did not matter; it was the sum of the weights that caused the boat to sink. This may also be true in much disease causation, but sometimes the component causes will have to occur in a specific order or they will have to be present at the same time. For example, TB infection will occur only if the individual is susceptible at the time they are exposed to the infection; and thrombosis (blood clotting) in an artery leading to a heart attack or stroke rarely occurs unless the blood vessel is already damaged or partly blocked.

A useful model for considering causal mechanisms is the 'pie' diagrams used by Rothman (1976) and shown in Figure 10.1. In this scheme

- I, II and III are three different **sufficient causes** for a disease;
- A is a **necessary cause** for the disease because it is present in all three sufficient causes; and
- A, B, C, D, E, F, G, H, I and J are component causes.

So, for example, if 'A' were the cow, 'B' the donkey, 'C' the pig, 'D' the sheep and 'E' the mouse, we would have sufficient cause I while the other 'pies' show that different combinations of animals or other objects would also have led to the boat overturning.

In practice, when considering causes of disease we mostly find ourselves dealing with what we are calling *component* causes. Aside from something like a major disaster such as an earthquake or nuclear explosion, it is hard to imagine identifying a single factor that is truly necessary and sufficient to cause disease. We also have to accept that, other than for something like an injury, we are unlikely to know either the precise nature of any sufficient cause or many of the possible component causes of disease. This need not matter – we do not have to eliminate all components of a particular cause in order to prevent disease due to that cause. If any one of them is identified and removed (e.g., B in the example above), then we will prevent cases of disease due to sufficient causes that contain component B (i.e., I and II). Some disease will still occur, however, as a result of sufficient cause III.

The causes of many diseases, and especially those like cancer that develop over many years, are going to be complex and we may never identify all their components. It is thus encouraging to know that by just identifying one or two we may still prevent a large proportion of the disease. If we could have stopped any one of the animals, even the mouse, from getting into the boat then it would not have turned over at that point in time. However, if the wind blew up or a wave came along once they had pushed off then they may have sunk later: a different sufficient cause leading to a similar outcome. Searching for modifiable causes that are associated with a large population attributable risk, i.e., ones which cause a large number of cases of disease, will give the greatest benefit in terms of public health. (We will take this up again in Chapter 13.)

Look back to Table 5.4. The attributable risks for diarrhoeal disease sum to more than 100%. Why is this so? Is it a problem?

If we assume that each of the causes of diarrhoeal disease shown can be represented by one of the letters in Figure 10.1 (for example, if unsafe water were cause 'A', being underweight were cause 'B' and vitamin A deficiency were cause 'C'), we can immediately see that the total amount of disease attributable to each component cause will be much greater than 100%. Ensuring that everyone had access to clean water (i.e., removing cause 'A') would prevent all disease due to sufficient causes I, II and III. However, if we have already removed the problem of being underweight (cause 'B') and so prevented disease due to sufficient causes I and II, then the extra benefit of providing clean water could only prevent the extra disease due to sufficient cause III. Similarly, although ensuring vitamin A sufficiency would prevent some disease on its own, once we have provided clean water and removed the problem of being underweight it would have little extra benefit.

In thinking about how component causes might act together, we need to keep in mind that in no sense need they be similar: one component might be the absence of a protective factor and another the presence of a quite different harmful factor. For instance, if we consider the underlying causes of lung cancer we would probably find that cigarette smoke is a component in most sufficient causes. However, since not all smokers develop lung cancer we can surmise that smoking is not a sufficient cause on its own but also requires other factors (for example weakened DNA-repair capacity) to complete a sufficient cause. Similarly, since lung cancer can develop in the absence of smoking, we can presume that there is at least one sufficient cause that does not have personal smoking as a component cause.

Association versus causation

In preceding chapters we have considered how we can determine whether a particular exposure is *associated* with the outcome of interest. The next stage is to determine whether such an association may be causal. Just because a particular exposure is associated with the development of a disease does not automatically imply cause and effect. We must attempt to draw appropriate causal inferences explicitly from our data, in the light of other evidence.

In London during the cholera epidemics of the nineteenth century one common belief, the 'miasma' theory, was that cholera was caused by noxious vapours in the air. While John Snow was conducting his pioneering work implicating contaminated water, William Farr, director of the Office of the Registrar General, was also interested in the transmission of cholera. He had noticed that cholera mortality seemed to be higher in lower-lying areas and so collected mortality data for a number of districts in London at different elevations. This revealed a dramatic inverse relation between elevation and mortality and Farr was able to calculate a formula that could accurately predict the mortality rate for any given elevation. Figure 10.2 shows a graph of actual cholera death rates for various levels of elevation above the River Thames as well as the death rates predicted by Farr's theory. These data were taken as strong evidence in favour of the miasma theory, under which it was felt that the vapours would be most concentrated and, therefore, most dangerous at lower elevations.

However, like most ecological research (the graph compares rates of cholera in areas at various elevations, not individual data), these observations provide weak evidence for a true causal association, and we must consider whether other differences between people living at different elevations could explain them. As it happened, people living closest to the river were also more likely to be exposed to contaminated water than their neighbours in the higher areas. This confounding factor could explain the apparent association between elevation and cholera mortality entirely, and today it is John Snow, not William Farr, whom we recognise

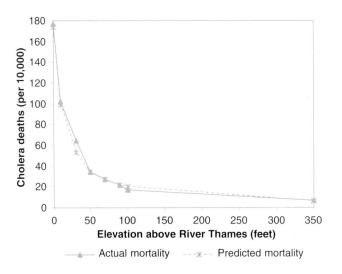

Fig. 10.2 Actual (——) and predicted (-----) cholera death rates at various levels of elevation above the River Thames in London, England, 1849. (*Data source:* Farr, 1852.)

as having solved the mystery of cholera. Ironically, in trying to prove his own 'air-borne' theory, Farr also provided much of the crucial evidence that ultimately supported Snow's theory of contaminated water.

This example highlights the necessity of not accepting the results of any study, however exciting, at face value. There are two substantial steps to be taken before we can reasonably promote an exposure–disease relation as warranting serious attention with respect to disease control. We must first thoroughly consider alternative non-causal explanations for an association: could it be an artefact due to chance, bias or confounding? We need to apply the approach outlined in Chapter 9 to decide whether the results we are looking at (our own or those reported by someone else) are believable. In the cholera example we have postulated that confounding by water supply is the most likely explanation for the close association seen in Figure 10.2, and that the relation with elevation is an artefact. If, however, the answer to the question 'Is it real?' is at least a qualified 'yes' then we can move on to the next step – a formal evaluation of whether the observed relation could be causal.

Evaluating causation

How should we do this? The nature of causation has been a central theme of philosophy for centuries (see Box 10.2) and in recent times has been given a fair bit of attention by epidemiologists. This has given a useful perspective on thinking about how we operate, but epidemiologists are fundamentally pragmatic and seek practical tools. Unfortunately, in the causal realm our tools are not as precise as we might like and views on how to apply them differ somewhat.

Various sets of guidelines have been proposed to assist our causal evaluations. There are many similarities among them, and arguably the best known – certainly the best written – were set forth by a British statistician, Sir Austin Bradford Hill, in an after-dinner speech. He put forward a list of nine aspects of an association to be considered when assessing whether it was likely to be causal (Hill, 1965). He was adamant that these should serve only as '*aids to thought*' and were not absolute requirements to be met before an exposure could be considered to cause a disease. Various modifications of this list have been suggested, and many of the elements remain cornerstones of judgement on whether an exposure really does cause a disease, or whether an intervention is effective in preventing or treating disease. These elements are discussed below.

Temporality

For an exposure to cause a disease it must precede the development of the disease. This might seem obvious, but in some instances, say for a condition like cancer that is often present for many years before diagnosis, it can be difficult to decide whether an exposure really did occur before the true origin of disease. If we find

Box 10.2 Some potted philosophy

Do we learn about the world from observation and experience or by reason? This was the major tension in Western causal thinking for many centuries. Broadly speaking, observation or learning from our own experience (*induction*) gradually replaced more abstract reasoning about how the world worked (*deduction*). The practical inductive approach fits pretty well with public health and epidemiology – we collect facts, decide what they mean and then act accordingly – but, of course, it is not perfect. Starting with David Hume in eighteenth-century Scotland, many philosophers have demonstrated that induction can never *prove* a cause-and-effect relationship (this became known as Hume's problem). Just because we observe that the computer turns on the first 99 times we press the button does not mean that it will turn on again the 100th time (we are all familiar with this phenomenon). Final proof is thus unobtainable by this process. In Europe in the middle decades of the twentieth century, Karl Popper in a sense turned Hume's problem around and said that, although induction based on supportive observations could never finally *confirm* a hypothesis, contrary data could be used to *refute* one. Consider the statement 'all swans are white'. We may see only white swans but can never prove that this statement is true – it just takes one black swan to disprove it. The hypothesis can stand only until we see that one black swan.

 We will never know anything with absolute certainty and this is something we must learn to live with comfortably. You will note that the subsequent guidelines to causal reasoning incorporate both judgement and probabilistic elements – implying that we do not demand certainty. If we did we would

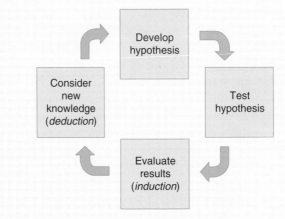

Fig. 10.3 An integrated cycle of causal reasoning.

(*continued*)

Box 10.2 (*continued*)

never act, the antithesis of the remit of public health. In pursuit of making good judgements on how and when to act, epidemiologists have long sought to bring good evidence to bear on a question. In the past decade or so this has come into sharper focus with research increasingly aiming to test critical elements of causal belief or hypothesis along the lines proposed by Popper and his followers last century. This has led to an integrated cycle of causal reasoning that essentially combines both induction and deduction (Figure 10.3).

that people with stomach cancer have lower levels of vitamin C in their blood than those without stomach cancer, can we be sure that the low levels of vitamin C really preceded the growth of the cancer? Or might the lower vitamin C levels be a result of the disease process? These questions can frequently be answered only by performing follow-up studies and, even then, it may be difficult to establish the order of exposure and effect with certainty. Of all Bradford Hill's factors this is the only one that is an absolute requirement.

Strength of association

The stronger an association is (usually as described by the relative effect, OR or RR), the less likely it is to be due solely to either bias or confounding. A strong association is thus more suggestive that the effect is real. However, just because a relation is weak does not mean that it cannot be causal: only that it is harder to eliminate study error as a possible explanation for the apparent effect.

What constitutes a 'weak' or a 'strong' effect? There is no universal agreement on this but we would generally consider an effect (OR, RR) greater than 2.0 to be moderately strong and an effect greater than 5.0 to be strong. Note, however, that a small effect observed consistently in many studies, especially if these are of different designs and performed in different settings, may well give stronger evidence of causality than an effect that is strong in one or two studies but not found in others (see '*Consistency*' below, and Chapter 11). It is important not to be too dismissive of 'weak' effects, since these can be of great public health importance when the exposure is common and the consequences severe.

Consistency

An effect found consistently across a range of studies of different types and/or in different populations gives some reassurance that it is not an artefact. For example, the Australian ovarian cancer case–control study discussed in Chapter 5 gave an association between higher egg consumption and ovarian cancer (Pirozzo *et al.*, 2002). This seemed unlikely to be a real effect until it was discovered that the authors of four previous population-based studies that had evaluated the relation between eggs and ovarian cancer had also reported an increase in risk of ovarian cancer among women who ate more eggs (Figure 10.4).

Figure 10.4 summarises the data neatly and accurately. If we look first at the square boxes that represent the relative risks, we see that, while there is some variability, all are greater than 1.0 and in four the association is statistically significant (i.e., their 95% confidence intervals do not cross 1.0). When the data from all five studies were combined the overall 'pooled' RR was 1.9 (95% confidence interval 1.5–2.3), suggesting that there was an almost two-fold increase in risk among women who ate the most eggs. The results are, therefore, very consistent and so increase belief that the association between eggs (or some component of, or contaminant in, eggs) and ovarian cancer might be causal.

However, lack of consistency does not in itself rule out causality. Differing results could reflect variation in study design or quality, or an exposure could have a different effect in people with a different genetic make-up. Thoughtful consideration of reasons for varying findings (heterogeneity) among studies is a crucial element of any good review of a topic (Chapter 11).

Dose–response relationships

If a factor does cause a disease, then the risk of developing the disease is likely to be related to the amount or 'dose' of exposure. This is often a function of both level and duration of exposure. Figure 10.5 shows some data from the first eight years of follow-up of the US Nurses' Health Study. The investigators calculated the age-adjusted relative risk that a woman would develop type-2 diabetes on the basis of her body-mass index (BMI; weight/height^2) and found that the risk of diabetes increased dramatically with increasing body size, particularly for women with a BMI greater than $25\,\mathrm{kg/m^2}$ (the upper limit of what is usually considered to be 'normal'). Among the heaviest women, those with BMI of

Fig. 10.4 The relation between higher egg consumption and ovarian cancer risk in five population-based studies. The squares represent the relative risk, with the size of the square being proportional to the size of the study, and the horizontal lines represent the 95% confidence intervals. The open diamond represents the relative risk and 95% confidence interval from all five studies combined.

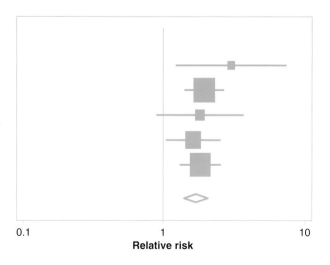

Relative risk

$35\,\text{kg/m}^2$ or greater, the risk of diabetes was almost 60 times that of women with BMI less than $22\,\text{kg/m}^2$. Similarly, we saw that the risk of lung cancer increases sharply with increasing numbers of cigarettes smoked (Figure 1.1). Patterns of relative risk like these add weight to the idea that an association is causal. Note, however, that measurement of dose is not always straightforward. Doll and Hill used a simple measure of dose of smoking, namely 'average number of cigarettes smoked per day'. This clearly worked very well, but does not capture other important information such as the number of years that someone has smoked. These days this additional information would almost always be included in any assessment of effects of smoking, often in a combined variable called 'pack-years', where one pack-year is equivalent to smoking 20 cigarettes a day for 1 year (or 10 cigarettes a day for 2 years, etc.).

Of course, some genuine cause-and-effect relationships will not give such a regular pattern. For instance, there may be a 'threshold' effect, whereby any exposure above a certain level will lead to disease. A dose–response relationship can therefore add weight to an evaluation of causality but its absence need not count against making a causal link.

Biological plausibility

A causal hypothesis should obviously be viewed in the light of its plausibility. If there is a likely biological mechanism through which an exposure might cause the disease, this can add substantial weight to a causal argument. Lack of plausibility does not necessarily rule out causality, because increasing knowledge of disease mechanisms may make an association appear more credible in time. (The characteristic of plausibility is also tempered by the realisation that scientists are ingenious by nature and can probably come up with a plausible-sounding hypothesis in most situations if they believe an association to be causal.)

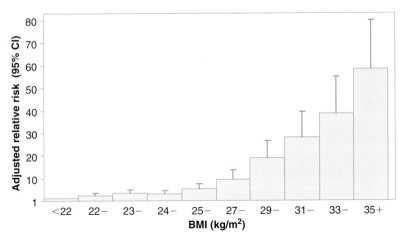

Fig. 10.5 Age-adjusted relative risks and 95% confidence intervals for type-2 diabetes in relation to body-mass index. (From Colditz *et al.*, Weight as a risk factor for clinical diabetes in women. *Am. J. Epidemiol.*, 5, 1990; 132: 505, reprinted by permission of the Society for Epidemiological Research.)

Specificity

Bradford Hill presented this concept somewhat less clearly than the others on his list – he suggested that, if an association were limited to a specific outcome, then this would argue in favour of causation. He went on to say that this characteristic should not be over-emphasised because factors could cause more than one disease and diseases might have more than one cause. This concept was crudely interpreted as 'one cause – one disease' in attempts to argue that cigarette smoking did not cause lung cancer: cigarettes were linked to many different diseases, therefore their effects were not specific, therefore they caused none of them.

When we recall that many diseases are based on similar underlying pathologies (e.g., vascular diseases of the brain, heart and other organs frequently stem from atherosclerosis) it is hardly surprising that a single exposure (e.g., a high-fat diet) can be linked to a variety of different conditions. Nonetheless, we would still not expect an exposure to be linked to *all* outcomes; thus there must be some degree of specificity that we can use to inform an evaluation of causality (Weiss, 2002). For example, bicycle helmets would be expected to reduce the risk of head injury but not of other types of injury (specificity of outcome). If results of studies suggested that helmet use did indeed reduce the risk of injuries to the head only, then this would strengthen belief that it was a causal (or in this case protective) association. An association seen only for one particular type of analgesic (as in the Phenacetin study described in Chapter 6) could again strengthen belief in causality (specificity of exposure). Similarly, individuals might be susceptible to an exposure only if they have a particular genetic make-up, so, if the relation is seen only for those with the specific genotype (specificity of susceptibility), then belief in causality is again strengthened.

Pulling it all together

Bradford Hill also suggested that consideration should be given to any **experimental data** – these could come from studies in animals or other organisms or from intervention studies in humans. Such evidence is crucial to assessing the benefits of interventions. The final two characteristics that he put forward are sensible but of less direct help than the others: **coherence** – a cause-and-effect interpretation should not conflict with the known facts; and **analogy** to existing known causal associations. An additional aspect to consider is that, if a relation is causal, then removal of the exposure should lead to a reduction in the effect – as was seen in the time trends of cigarette sales and lung cancer mortality in Figure 6.2.

Consideration of these issues can help us decide whether an association is likely to be causal. Sometimes the decision may be clear cut, but it is equally likely to be controversial, and in this situation there can be no 'right' answer. It is important to remember that these elements do not provide an infallible checklist that will lead to the correct decision. Rather, they provide a framework for an evaluation of causality.

Bradford Hill (Hill, 1965) summarised the questions that should guide a consideration of causality as follows:

Is there any other way of explaining the set of facts before us, is there any other answer equally, or more likely than cause and effect?

Evaluating causality in practice: does *H. pylori* cause stomach cancer?

You have seen in earlier chapters that there appears to be a link between infection with *H. pylori* (a bacterium that infects the stomach) and stomach cancer rates. Now let us consider whether this relation might be causal. Many case–control studies have been conducted to evaluate this, but these are fraught with problems, in particular because people with stomach cancer may test negative for *H. pylori* even if they have been infected in the past. As a result there is the potential for differential misclassification of cases as *H. pylori*-negative, thereby biasing the odds ratio towards the null. Cohort studies are impractical because of the logistics of testing thousands of cohort members for *H. pylori*. The best evidence therefore comes from well-designed *nested case–control studies* (see Chapter 6) in which blood samples were collected prior to the diagnosis of cancer. In 2001, a group pooled the data from all 12 such studies to evaluate this association (*Helicobacter* and Cancer Collaborative Group, 2001). (We will discuss *pooled* studies further in Chapter 11.) In all of the studies the cases and controls were matched for age and sex and there were no other major confounders; there were also no obvious sources of selection or measurement bias. Authors of all 12 studies reported an increased risk of stomach cancer associated with infection, which was statistically significant (i.e., unlikely to be due to chance) in nine. The odds ratio from all 12 studies combined was 2.4 (95% CI 2.0–2.8).

So could the relation be causal? The association is quite *strong* and also *consistent* across these better studies. In all of them the blood samples used for testing for *H. pylori* were collected before diagnosis of cancer, suggesting that infection does indeed *precede* cancer. Since, by and large, someone is either infected or not infected, it is not possible to look for a *dose–response* relationship, but the association appears to be fairly *specific* for stomach cancer and laboratory studies have shown that some types of *H. pylori* may be more carcinogenic than others. Further *experimental evidence* comes from studies that have shown that *H. pylori* infection induces cancer in some animal models. A relation is also biologically *plausible* because the bacterial infection directly affects the stomach, which is where the cancer occurs. Taken together, there is thus good evidence for the conclusion, now widely accepted, that *H. pylori* infection is indeed a cause of stomach cancer.

And then what?

Once a cause-and-effect association has been established beyond any reasonable doubt, action can be taken to change public policy, legislation, health education, clinical practice or the direction of research. Thalidomide is no longer given to women during pregnancy because it causes birth defects; diethylstilboestrol is no longer prescribed to prevent miscarriage because it can cause vaginal cancer in the women's daughters; dietary advice and drugs are used to lower cholesterol levels to prevent heart disease; the hazards of smoking are publicised, and legislation restricting smoking in public has been enacted in many countries; seat-belt wearing is becoming ubiquitous internationally – the list goes on.

It is worth noting that it has taken a long time, decades even, to establish causality for some of these associations. Although wholly reliable criteria for truly establishing causality do not exist, modern society often demands rapid 'proof', increasingly for legal rather than social or health reasons. This tension between the desire for full knowledge and the social need for action is a given in public health. The clearer our insight into the evidence the better our judgements will be. Remember, however, that we are all fallible and absolute proof is impossible.

So, to conclude, if we had stopped the mouse from jumping into the boat (i.e., removed one component cause) it would not have overturned at that precise point in time (we would have prevented that particular outcome). But who is to say what would have happened if the other animals had ventured out into the rougher water in the middle of the lake . . .

REFERENCES

Allen, P. (1983). *Who Sank the Boat?* Thomas Nelson Australia. Republished by Penguin Books Australia Ltd., 1998.

Colditz, G. A., Willett, W. C., Stampfer, M. J. *et al.* (1990). Weight as a risk factor for clinical diabetes in women. *American Journal of Epidemiology*, **132**: 501–513.

Farr, W. (1852). Influence of elevation on the fatality of cholera. *Journal of the Statistical Society London*, **15**: 155–183.

Helicobacter and Cancer Collaborative Group. (2001). Gastric cancer and *Helicobacter pylori*: a combined analysis of 12 case–control studies nested within prospective cohorts. *Gut*, **49**: 347–353.

Hill, A. B. (1965). The environment and disease: association or causation? *Proceedings of the Royal Society for Medicine*, **58**: 295–300.

Pirozzo, S., Purdie, D., Kuiper-Linley, M. *et al.* (2002). Ovarian cancer, cholesterol and eggs: a case–control analysis. *Cancer Epidemiology Biomarkers and Prevention*, **11**: 1112–1114.

Rothman, K. J. (1976). Causes. *American Journal of Epidemiology*, **104**: 587–592.

(1986). *Modern Epidemiology*. Boston: Little Brown & Co.

Weiss, N. S. (2002). Can the "specificity" of an association be rehabilitated as a basis for supporting a causal hypothesis? *Epidemiology*, **13**: 6–8.

11

Assembling the building blocks: reviews and their uses

While it is important to be able to read and interpret individual papers, the results of a single study are never going to provide the complete answer to a question. To move towards this we need to **review** the literature more widely. There can be a number of reasons for doing this and some require a more comprehensive approach than others. If the aim is simply to increase our personal understanding of a new area then a few papers might provide adequate background material. Traditional *narrative reviews*, which give less emphasis to complete coverage of the literature and tend to be more qualitative, retain value for exploring areas of uncertainty or novelty, but are less readily scrutinised for flaws. In contrast, a major policy decision might require a *systematic review* of all the relevant literature. We will focus on the systematic approach here, but this can of course be tailored according to need.

Like a primary research paper, an epidemiological review should aim to produce a helpful synthesis of primary data – looking for patterns but not hiding differences – and it should normally offer a formal causal interpretation. Although its primary data units are whole studies rather than individuals, the review process should have the same rigour as its component studies. A **systematic review** should be a response to a clearly formulated question and involve the identification of *all* relevant primary research studies that address that question. Each study found should be included or excluded according to predetermined selection criteria, and critically appraised. The findings should then be summarised and appropriate conclusions drawn. In some situations this process can be taken one step further by combining the results of the component studies in a **meta-analysis**. An even more rigorous approach, known as a **pooled analysis** or **re-analysis**, is to obtain the original data from all relevant studies and re-analyse them as a single large study.

It follows from this that such a review should be structured in the same way as a primary paper: an *introduction* to show why the research question is of interest; a *methods* section to explain how studies were identified, included/excluded and appraised, and how the data were abstracted; the *results* where patterns are highlighted and differences assessed; and, finally, a *discussion* where the results are interpreted, threats to validity considered and conclusions drawn.

So how should we go about conducting a systematic review? We stress that what follows is an overview of principles and methods; more detailed 'how to' manuals are fairly widely available (e.g., Glasziou *et al.*, 2001.). The following summary focusses on the various stages of the review process as a guide to both reading and writing a systematic review.

Identifying the literature

The first challenge when conducting a systematic review is to identify all of the relevant literature. The potential sources of data are numerous. MEDLINE is probably the most commonly used source for epidemiological papers, but only about one third of the approximately 10 million medical articles on library shelves are indexed in the MEDLINE database (which is freely available through the US National Library of Medicine search engine PubMed at www.nlm.nih.gov). Another valuable database, particularly for systematic reviews of trials of the effects of healthcare interventions, is that of the Cochrane Collaboration (www.cochrane.org). There are also many other electronic databases that may be valuable sources of literature depending on the question you are researching (e.g., CANCERLIT and PSYCHLIT each have an obvious specialised focus).

No electronic literature search is ever likely to be complete, so it is important to use multiple strategies. Once several relevant articles have been identified, it can help to check the papers that they cite, and also to look in the other direction, i.e., for papers that have cited them (e.g., using the Science Citation Index). Other sources include personal communication with experts in the field who may know of additional published articles (and unpublished material); international registers of trials or other research (e.g., the IARC Directory of Ongoing Research in Cancer Prevention available online at www.iarc.fr); theses, seminars, internal reports and non-peer-reviewed journals (sometimes described as the 'grey literature'); and other electronic information including topic-specific internet databases.

Publication and related biases

When searching the literature it is important to bear in mind that studies with positive and/or statistically significant findings are more likely to be published than those without significant results. This **publication bias** is related not only to selective acceptance by journals but also to selective submission to journals by researchers who may decide not to submit reports from research that either finds no association at all (i.e., a null finding) or in which the results are not statistically significant.

Closely related to publication bias are the problems of preferential detection of articles in English and studies with overlapping publications on the same topic. For an English speaker there are several barriers to the inclusion of non-English studies in a review, including the difficulties associated with translation and the fact that non-English articles may be published in local journals that are not indexed by major bibliographic databases. This is more likely to be the case for less exciting findings. A less recognised problem is that of multiple but apparently unrelated publications from one study with (usually) positive results. Such a study is more likely to be identified than those published only once (or with all papers clearly from the one source) and, if included as separate studies in the review, could lead to overestimation of an association.

Different types of study

The amount and types of literature generated by a search will vary enormously depending on the subject area. For a review of a specific treatment the studies may all be clinical trials, whereas an aetiological review is likely to include observational studies of all types from case reports to cohort studies, with few or no trials. As you have seen, different types of study answer different types of questions, or may be subject to different biases when answering the same question, so it is sensible to group them separately, at least to start with. This grouping may then provide a logical framework to help organise the data within the review.

A common approach to grading the quality of individual studies has been to classify study designs according to a hierarchy such that those at the top are considered to provide stronger evidence of an effect than those further down the scale (Table 11.1). You will notice that this ranking puts randomised trials at the top of the pile. (Variations of this scheme include yet another layer at the top for systematic reviews of randomised controlled trials as the 'ultimate' evidence.) While a classification of this type may be appropriate in the clinical context where RCTs are the norm, a ranking based largely on evidence from trials is often not much help for an aetiological review. Even more important is the disregard for the quality of individual studies inherent in this approach. A well-designed

Table 11.1 A system commonly used to classify levels of evidence.

Level	Evidence
I	Evidence from at least one properly randomised controlled trial
II-1	Evidence from well-designed controlled trials without randomisation
II-2	Evidence from well-designed cohort or case–control studies, preferably from more than one centre or research group
II-3	Evidence from comparisons over time or between places with or without the intervention; dramatic results in uncontrolled experiments could also be regarded as this level of evidence
III	Opinions of respected authorities, based on clinical experience, descriptive studies and case reports, or reports of expert committees

(Harris *et al.*, 2001.)

and properly conducted cohort or case–control study could provide better evidence than a small or poorly conducted trial, but this rigid hierarchy would rate the evidence from the trial more highly. The need to move away from such a rigid approach has been well documented both for clinical research (Glasziou *et al.*, 2004) and for health services research in general (Black, 1996).

A preferable approach, adopted by decision-making bodies around the world such as the US Preventive Services Task Force (USPSTF) and the Canadian Task Force on Preventive Health Care (CTFPHC), is not to classify studies purely on the basis of their *design* but also according to the *quality of the evidence* they provide. As its name suggests, the USPSTF regularly reviews the evidence for and against a wide range of preventive interventions. They rate studies according to specific criteria for that design (based on the key questions of subject selection and measurement that we discussed earlier). A 'good' study would generally meet all of the specified criteria, a 'fair' study does not meet them all but is judged not to have a fatal flaw that would invalidate the results and a fatally flawed study is classified as 'poor' (Harris *et al.*, 2001). We have examined specific quality issues for the various designs in earlier chapters (Chapters 6–9), and Box 11.1 considers the value of randomised and non-randomised designs in health-care evaluation in a bit more detail. (An additional marker of better study quality that appealed to us was the inclusion of an epidemiologist (or statistician) among the authors of a research paper (Delgardo-Rodriguez *et al.*, 2001)!)

Study inclusion, appraisal and data abstraction

Studies should be selected for inclusion in the review on the basis of pre-defined criteria. Depending on the research question, it might be appropriate to restrict

Box 11.1 Randomisation versus observation

Most generic lists rank RCTs first in terms of study quality. For appropriate questions, i.e., about the effects of various interventions, this is reasonable, as you have seen. However, even for such questions caveats need to be applied. If a randomised trial is not competently conducted, or is too small, then its theoretical advantages disappear, and it can give misleading results (Schultz *et al.*, 1995). There are also many situations in which a trial would be unfeasible, unethical, undesirable or unnecessary (Black, 1996), and they are generally irrelevant for questions related to frequency or measurement validation (e.g., of the performance of a screening or diagnostic test).

Estimates of the effects of treatment may differ between randomised and non-randomised studies, but when direct comparisons have been made neither method has consistently given a greater effect than the other (McKee *et al.*, 1999). Overall, it seems that dissimilarities between the participants in RCTs and non-randomised studies explain many of the differences; the two methods should therefore be compared only after patients not meeting the RCT eligibility criteria have also been excluded from the non-randomised study. Not surprisingly then, treatment effects measured in randomised and non-randomised studies are most similar when the exclusion criteria are the same and where potential prognostic factors are well understood and controlled for in the non-randomised setting. It is also important to consider the stability (precision) of the RCT effect estimates – some are based on so few endpoints (especially when death is the outcome of interest) that chance differences from the true underlying effect are quite likely. (For an example of these issues from studies comparing the effectiveness of various interventions to unblock coronary arteries see Britton *et al.* (1998).)

The generalisability of the results of RCTs can also be questionable, given the highly selected nature of the participants: patients excluded from randomised controlled trials tend to have a worse prognosis than those included (McKee *et al.*, 1999). When both randomised and non-randomised studies have been conducted and estimates of treatment effect are reasonably consistent for patients at similar risk, it allows more certain generalisation to the broader target populations of the non-randomised studies.

the review to specific research designs, for example only randomised trials, or to those with specific methodological features. Such features might include

- the study size (e.g., only those studies with more than a certain number of cases),
- the participants (e.g., a specific age range or sex),
- a specific outcome or the way in which outcome was measured (e.g., histological or serological confirmation),

- the way in which exposure was measured or classified (e.g., a specific blood test to measure an infection, more than two levels of alcohol intake) and
- the duration of follow-up (e.g., more than 12 months).

The validity of studies that meet the criteria should then be evaluated as outlined in Chapter 9 and key information on design, conduct, potential for error and results abstracted onto purpose-designed forms. In an ideal world the appraisers should be blinded to the authors and the study results since this knowledge has been shown to influence judgements about validity. In practice this is not always possible, since the reviewers may already be too familiar with the literature. Rigorous systematic reviews of clinical interventions, such as those conducted through the Cochrane Collaboration, will often specify the need for multiple assessors to reduce the potential for bias, but this level of rigour is less common (and of limited added value) for aetiological reviews.

Summarising the data

The next step in any review is to draw the data together to simplify their interpretation and to assist in drawing valid conclusions. It is important to look both for consistency of effects across studies (homogeneity) and for differences between studies (heterogeneity). Could differences be due to chance variation or can they be explained by features of the studies or the populations they were conducted in? Graphs can be used to summarise the results of many studies in a simple format and in some situations the technique of *meta-analysis* can be used to combine the results from a number of different studies.

Graphical display of results

One way to display the results of a number of different studies is in a figure called a *forest plot*. Figure 11.1 shows a forest plot from a systematic review of the relation between weight/BMI and ovarian cancer risk (Purdie *et al.*, 2001). It shows the results of all 23 case–control studies whose authors had reported data on this association, ordered with the most recent study at the top and the oldest at the bottom. The odds ratio for each individual study is represented by the black square, with the size of the square indicating the size (or 'weight' – see *Meta-analysis* below) of that particular study. The horizontal bar through each box shows the 95% confidence interval for the odds ratio and the vertical line indicates the point where there is 'no effect', i.e., an odds ratio of 1.0. When the confidence interval crosses this line (i.e., it includes the null value) it indicates that the result is not statistically significant (i.e., $p > 0.05$). (Note the use of the logarithmic scale, which balances positive and inverse relative effects visually

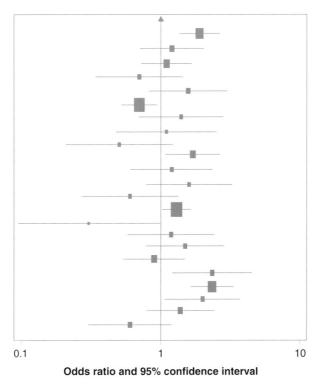

Fig. 11.1 Diagrammatic representation of the results of 23 case–control studies evaluating the relation between extremes of weight/BMI and risk of ovarian cancer (Purdie *et al.*, 2001).

Odds ratio and 95% confidence interval

around the null; i.e., an OR of 2.0 would be the same distance from 1.0 as an OR of 0.5 in the opposite direction.)

Assessing heterogeneity

In this example the results of the 23 studies are scattered both sides of the null, and they show no obvious pattern. The next step should be to evaluate this *heterogeneity* in more detail. Are there any differences between the studies that could explain some of the variation in their results?

One major methodological difference between the studies in this example is subject selection: some were population-based and others were hospital-based. We touched on some of the problems inherent in hospital-based studies in earlier chapters – could this difference explain any of the variation in the study results? (Other possibilities to consider might include the geographical areas where the research was done – for example, separating high and low-risk countries, and the ages of the participants.) In this case, if we separate the hospital- and population-based studies (Figure 11.2) we start to see some regularity. In each of the 11 population-based studies at the bottom of Figure 11.2, the OR is

Fig. 11.2 Diagrammatic
representation of the results of
12 hospital-based and 11
population-based case–control
studies evaluating the relation
between extremes of weight/
BMI and risk of ovarian cancer
(Purdie *et al.*, 2001).

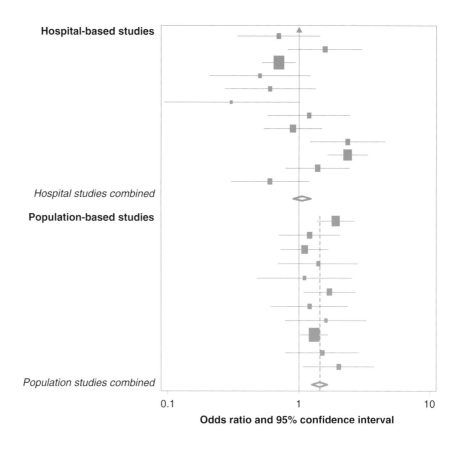

Fig. 11.2 Diagrammatic representation of the results of 12 hospital-based and 11 population-based case–control studies evaluating the relation between extremes of weight/BMI and risk of ovarian cancer (Purdie *et al.*, 2001).

greater than 1.0 (although many of the individual results are not statistically significant), suggesting that obesity/higher weight is associated with an increased risk of ovarian cancer. In contrast, the results of the hospital studies still vary widely. In this situation it was felt that using hospital-based controls might not be appropriate, since their use might lead to overestimation of the prevalence of obesity in the population and thereby lead to underestimation of the obesity–cancer association.

Meta-analysis

Meta-analysis is a powerful technique that allows the results of a number of different studies to be combined. Each study is assigned a weight based on the amount of information it provides (e.g., the inverse of the standard error of the OR) and in general larger studies have greater weight. A weighted average of the individual study results can then be calculated. The assumption underlying this analysis is that all of the studies are estimating the same underlying effect and any variation between their results is due to chance. If their results are very different (i.e., they are *heterogeneous*), as in the hospital-based studies of BMI above, then this assumption need not be true and it might not be appropriate to combine the results.

The diamond at the bottom of Figure 11.2 represents the combined odds ratio for the 11 population-based studies; the centre indicates the point estimate and the ends show the 95% confidence interval. In this case, it indicates that being overweight increases the risk of ovarian cancer by 40% (pooled OR = 1.4; 95% CI 1.2–1.6). Notice that the diamond does not overlap the 'no-effect' line (i.e., the confidence interval does not include 1.0), so the pooled OR is statistically significant. If we draw a dotted line vertically through the combined odds ratio, it passes through the 95% confidence interval of each of the individual studies. This is an indication that the results of the studies are fairly *homogeneous*, but it is certainly not definitive. In this case a formal test for heterogeneity gives a *p*-value of 0.63, which is well away from being statistically significant and so supports the 'eyeball' finding that the results are all fairly similar.

In contrast, if we combine the results of the 12 hospital-based studies, we find a combined OR of 0.9 (95%CI 0.9–1.2), but a line through this point would not pass through the confidence intervals of the individual studies. This suggests that the results of the hospital-based studies are heterogeneous, and this is confirmed by a statistical test for heterogeneity, which gives $p < 0.001$, which is highly statistically significant. In this situation it is inappropriate to combine the results into a single estimate of effect.

As we discussed in Chapter 5, absolute measures of effect such as the attributable risk, absolute risk reduction and number needed to treat can provide a better sense of the practical impact or clinical importance of an exposure–outcome relation than a relative measure does. Combining these absolute measures from studies conducted in very different populations can, however, be problematic, since they will usually depend on the baseline risk in a population, and this may vary widely. For this reason, relative effect measures (OR or RR) are usually used to summarise the evidence, and then applied to the relevant baseline rate to show the predicted absolute difference.

Finally, a word of caution: the ability of meta-analysis to provide unbiased summary estimates has been seriously debated. Combining the results of a number of studies usually generates an estimate with narrow confidence limits, thereby giving a sense of precision and accuracy that may be illusory. As you have seen, there are numerous ways in which bias can occur and the old adage still holds true: 'rubbish in–rubbish out'. Combining results cannot get rid of bias or undetected confounding and, although a combined odds ratio from several poor studies may look good, it will not compensate for problems in the individual studies.

Pooled analysis

A pooled analysis goes one step further than a meta-analysis. Instead of combining the summary results (OR or RR) from a number of different studies, the investigator obtains a copy of the raw data from the original studies for relevant variables and re-analyses them as a single large dataset. Pooled analyses remain relatively uncommon: the effort involved to obtain the original data, clean, recode and re-shape each dataset to a common standard, conduct a new analysis and write the paper, all the while maintaining full approval of all contributing investigators, is monumental. Nonetheless, some dedicated teams have done this very successfully and made seminal contributions to advancing knowledge and resolving controversies. An excellent example is the Oxford-based Collaborative Group on Hormonal Factors in Breast Cancer which, since the mid 1990s, has been producing reports based on analyses of over 50,000 women with breast cancer and 100,000 without, from data provided by more than 50 separate studies. The collaboration's first paper showed with great precision the very low absolute risk of breast cancer conferred by the majority of patterns of oral contraceptive pill use (Collaborative Group on Hormonal Factors in Breast Cancer, 1996). This report removed a great deal of the uncertainty that remained about this relation, despite many prior publications from individual studies.

Practical versus statistical significance

Randomised controlled trials evaluating the drug finasteride for treatment of lower urinary tract symptoms in men have shown that there is a *statistically significant* improvement in symptom score from 2.5 to 2.8 in men treated with finasteride (Hirst and Ward, 2000). However, for men to experience a subjective change in quality of life, their symptom score has to change by at least three points. An increase of 0.3 points, although a 12% improvement, is therefore not *clinically significant*.

You will recall from Chapter 7 that narrower confidence limits come with larger sample sizes, as do 'small' or statistically significant p-values. By combining the results of a number of studies in a meta-analysis or pooled analysis we effectively increase the sample size and consequently reduce the play of chance in the summary odds ratio. This makes it crucial that we consider how meaningful the result of an intervention is in practical terms (social, preventive, biological or clinical significance), and we can use the confidence interval to help judge this.

This is illustrated in Figure 11.3, which shows the results of four hypothetical reviews of interventions (the same arguments apply to individual studies too). In review (a) the result is both practically important and statistically significant because the point estimate falls beyond the '*minimum practically important difference*' line and the confidence interval does not include the value 1.0 (in fact, even the lower bound is above the minimum important difference line). The tightness of the confidence interval around the RR also gives reassurance of its precision. In review (b) the result is again practically important but not statistically significant, since the confidence interval is wide and does include 1.0.

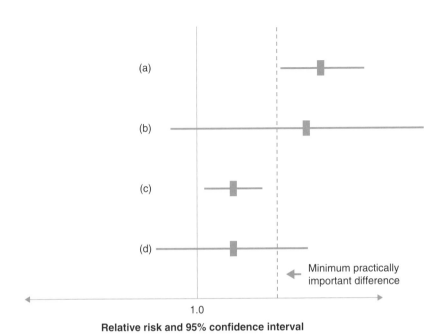

Fig. 11.3 Statistical and biological significance: point estimates and confidence intervals from four hypothetical reviews.

The width of the confidence interval suggests that there have been few studies, leaving imprecision and therefore some uncertainty about the role of chance. The finding could be important but we really need more data for a confident judgement. (Although we are thinking here primarily of additional epidemiological data to include in the meta-analysis, this could be complementary information from, say, ecological research or biology.) In contrast, the results shown for (c) are statistically significant but not important, as in the finasteride example above. The narrow confidence interval tells us that our estimate is fairly precise (i.e., there are plenty of data). Finally, the results of review (d) are neither statistically significant nor practically important. This provides little useful evidence about the benefit of the intervention – the very wide confidence interval that spans well across the null shows that this is a very poor test of the original hypothesis.

In summary, *statistical significance* is evident on looking at the *p*-values from appropriate statistical tests and from the confidence intervals around the point estimates; and the extra information the latter give as to the *precision* of an effect estimate is valuable. In health research where we are looking to improve outcomes through preventive, clinical or other interventions, we often have a fair idea of how big an effect needs to be for it to be *clinically or practically significant*. This might be a certain percentage improvement (i.e., a relative effect) or an absolute increase (as in the finasteride example above) and this might also have to be weighed against any adverse effects of the therapy. In observational (aetio-logical) epidemiology, however, there is no clear rule as to how big an effect should be for it to be meaningful. A relative risk greater than 2.0 would probably be considered fairly strong and thus, by implication, *practically significant*. An RR less than this would not, however, immediately be dismissed because, as you saw in Table 5.5, the *absolute* risk may still be large.

Assessment of causality

Systematic reviews and particularly meta-analyses and pooled analyses can con-tribute directly to an assessment of causality. Reviews that generate combined effect estimates across studies provide more precise summary measures of the *strength* of an association and sometimes of the *dose–response* relationship. Our discussion above of the homogeneity (or otherwise) of study results addresses the concept of *consistency* in practice. We do not require that effect estimates be near-identical across studies to meet this criterion: simply showing that most are positive (or negative) and reasonably similar with respect to their confidence intervals (i.e., the 95% CIs are overlapping) may suffice. Also, if more extreme heterogeneity can be shown to be due to differing methodology or degrees of study error, and results among the better studies are reasonably consistent, then the review has again allowed extraction of helpful causal information (Weed, 2000). The causal argument of the review should then be fully developed along the lines presented in Chapter 10.

Assessing the quality of a systematic review

A principal feature of a modern systematic review is that it must have a compre-hensive methods section. The authors should have detailed their literature-searching strategy and the processes of study selection and appraisal and data extraction. Box 11.2, which shows a condensed excerpt from the methods sec-tion of a review of the benefits of a low fat diet for weight loss (Pirozzo *et al.*, 2003), gives a sense of the comprehensive approach required.

Table 11.2 outlines the key criteria for appraising the validity of a systematic review. As for the reporting of individual trials, a set of guidelines has been estab-lished to improve the reporting of meta-analyses. This 'Quality of Reporting of Meta-analyses' or QUOROM statement (Moher *et al.*, 1999) was developed specifically for reporting meta-analyses of randomised controlled trials, but most of the guidelines apply to the reporting of all types of meta-analysis. Omitted from some such lists, but always central to making a comprehensive judgement, is a consideration of the logic and insight of the review, especially its treatment of error, heterogeneity, causality and practical importance.

Box 11.2 Should we recommend low-fat diets for obesity?

Research question

To determine the effectiveness of low-fat diets in achieving sustained weight loss in obese or overweight people.

Search strategy

The following sources were included in the literature-searching process: The Cochrane Library (Issue 2, 2001), MEDLINE, EMBASE, the Science Citation Index, bibliographies and handsearching. The original searches of MEDLINE and EMBASE were conducted from the beginning of each database until January 2001. The search was updated in February 2002. The references of all relevant studies were searched in the Science Citation Index to identify any additional trials.

Trial selection

The titles and abstracts of the records identified were independently screened by two investigators. Articles were rejected if the reviewers determined from the title and abstract that the study (a) was not a report of a randomised controlled trial, (b) did not address a low-fat diet, (c) did not have a follow-up period that was at least 6 months in duration, or (d) concerned persons less than 18 years old. When a title/abstract could not be rejected with certainty, the full text of the article was obtained for further evaluation. The full text of all selected articles was examined independently by two investigators to identify all relevant trials. Differences in opinion were resolved by consensus.

Quality assessment of trials

The trials were assessed independently by two investigators using specific quality criteria related to the following aspects of study methodology:
(1) randomisation and concealment of allocation;
(2) blinding of caregivers, participants and, in particular, outcome assessors; and
(3) follow-up and intention-to-treat analysis.
Trials were categorised according to the extent to which they met the quality criteria:

   A = all criteria met,

   B = one or more criteria only partially met and

   C = one or more criteria not met.

Data extraction

Three reviewers independently extracted data from the studies, with any differences resolved by the fourth reviewer. A specially developed data-extraction form was used. This form incorporated general trial information, trial characteristics, details of the intervention, patient-selection procedures and characteristics of sample, study outcomes and results.

(Excerpted from Pirozzo et al., 2003.)

Table 11.2 Guidelines for appraising the validity of a systematic review.

Criteria	What to look for	Comments
Focussed research question	The main research question should be clear from either the title or the abstract. The exposure, such as a risk factor or therapy, and the outcome(s) of interest should be expressed in terms of a simple relationship	If the review addresses multiple questions it is likely a general introduction to the area and may have limited sources of evidence for the conclusions drawn. Statements may be made with few citations and limited in-depth analysis of studies. Caution should be exercised in accepting conclusions from this type of review
Inclusion and exclusion criteria	The eligibility criteria used to select studies should be stated and should specify the participants, exposures and outcomes of interest and, in some cases, the study design	If the eligibility criteria are not clearly stated you have no way of knowing whether studies were included (or excluded) solely on the basis of their results, which could bias the conclusions of the review
Comprehensiveness of search strategy	A detailed search strategy indicating that the authors have searched all the relevant bibliographic databases with a variety of appropriate search terms. Other strategies such as handsearching and snowballing[a] may be used	It is possible to evaluate the thoroughness of the search strategies only if the methods used by the authors are made explicit. If there is no methods section then you should be cautious in accepting any of the results
Assessment of included studies	Statements that indicate whether individual included studies are scientifically sound as measured against established criteria	The criteria for appraising the individual studies should reflect the study design. For example, for a review based on a therapy the criteria should relate primarily to RCTs
Reproducibility of assessments[b]	Statements that the appraisals were conducted independently by at least two reviewers and any differences resolved by consensus or by a third person	Since appraisal of studies involves judgement calls, decisions based on these appraisals are subject to random errors or mistakes and systematic errors or bias. Having two independent reviewers should minimise these
Similarity of results of included studies	Detailed reporting of the results of individual studies with some measure of the differences (heterogeneity) between them	If the results are very different, it might not be appropriate to combine them in a meta-analysis. Instead there should be some assessment of the reasons for the differences (different populations, different study methods, etc.)
Overall logic and insight	Discussion of how error and heterogeneity have been handled, also causality and practical importance	These issues are central to making a comprehensive judgement

[a] Snowballing refers to the iterative process of searching whereby the results of the initial search are used to identify missed papers either through a search of the reference list at the end of the identified paper or by using the Science Citation Index to see who has cited the identified paper.
[b] Multiple assessors are used in rigorous systematic reviews of clinical interventions such as those conducted through the Cochrane Collaboration, but this level of rigour is less commonly used for aetiological reviews. This need not invalidate the results as long as the criteria used to include and exclude studies are clearly specified.
(Adapted from Oxman et al., 1994.)

Making judgements in practice

Primary epidemiological data (from individual studies) and secondary data (from reviews) are not ends in themselves. They aim to tell us about the healthiness of populations, what we might need to change to improve their condition, and how we might go about this. Judgements about need are primarily the remit of health departments and organisations (local, regional and global), using appropriate descriptive data. In contrast, identification of causes and preventive factors comes largely from academic research, and in addition a wide variety of professional, community and government groups have interests in specific topics. The aim of the whole enterprise is to take action to improve health. This is not a modern phenomenon and, as you have seen, many advances in public health pre-dated epidemiology. The strong call to base all such actions on good evidence is, however, quite recent, and has spread rapidly from clinical medicine to public health. Much effort is spent these days on collating knowledge to answer practical questions as to what interventions might work, and a common starting point is a review. An existing review can be useful, but often one will need to be commissioned to address the precise question being asked. Newly emerging issues will sometimes not have been studied adequately, which leaves reviewers, planners and decision-makers in something of a quandary. This book is not primarily about how to make action decisions under conditions of uncertainty, but the logic of epidemiology can certainly help. As one of the seminal figures in health services research said;

The absence of excellent evidence does not make evidence-based decision making impossible; what is required is the best evidence available not the best evidence possible (Muir Gray (1997))

A systematic epidemiological review, then, is often an early response to a question about the effects of an intervention, but may also be used practically (as opposed to academically) to support broad overviews of causation aimed at informing and influencing health policy. Approaches vary depending on the specific purpose of the review, and we conclude this chapter with descriptions of how some influential national and international bodies engaged in disseminating helpful judgements and interpretations operate.

The US Preventive Services Task Force (USPSTF)

The USPSTF was convened by the US Public Health Service in the 1980s to assess the merits of preventive activities in clinical practice. It aims to provide simple practical guidelines for clinicians regarding the utility of preventive interventions that they might use in their practice (over 200 to date). Many of the interventions assessed relate to early detection of a wide range of conditions, counselling to change behaviour and primary chemoprevention (e.g., aspirin to prevent cardiovascular disease). Topic teams assigned by the task force prepare systematic reviews of the evidence according to a standard protocol. The *evidence* for a particular preventive service is classified as good, fair or poor and then combined with a judgement of the *net benefit* of the service (substantial, moderate, small or zero/negative). The USPSTF assesses the reviews centrally and then makes formal recommendations with specific ratings (AHRQ, 2004; Harris *et al.*, 2001), examples of which are given below.

A The USPSTF *strongly recommends* screening for cervical cancer in women who have been sexually active and have a cervix. The USPSTF found *good evidence* . . . that screening with cervical cytology reduces incidence of and mortality from cervical cancer . . . The USPSTF concludes that the *benefits of screening substantially outweigh potential harms* (January 2003).

B The USPSTF r*ecommends* structured breastfeeding education and behavioural counselling programmes to promote breastfeeding. The USPSTF found *fair evidence* that programmes combining breastfeeding education with counselling are associated with increased rates of initiation of breastfeeding . . . (2003).

C The USPSTF makes *no recommendation* for or against routine osteoporosis screening in post-menopausal women younger than 60. The USPSTF found fair evidence that screening women at lower risk can identify women who may be eligible for treatment but it would prevent a small number of fractures. The USPSTF concludes that the *balance of benefits and harms of screening and treatment is too close* to make a general recommendation for this age group (September 2002).

D The USPSTF *recommends against* the use of beta-carotene supplements for the prevention of cancer or cardiovascular disease. The USPSTF found good evidence that beta-carotene supplementation provides no benefit in the prevention of cancer or cardiovascular disease in middle-aged and older adults . . . The USPSTF concludes that beta-carotene supplements are *unlikely to provide important benefits and might cause harm* in some groups (June 2003).

I The USPSTF concludes that the *evidence is insufficient to recommend for or against* behavioural counselling in primary care settings to promote physical activity. The USPSTF could not determine the balance of benefits and harms . . . (August 2002).

A parallel activity for community prevention is conducted under the aegis of the Centers for Disease Control and Prevention (CDC) by the Task Force on Community Preventive Services (http://www.thecommunityguide.org).

The World Cancer Research Fund

The World Cancer Research Fund (WCRF) International aims to raise awareness and develop and strengthen scientific knowledge on food, nutrition and the prevention of cancer. In 1997 the WCRF and the American Institute for Cancer Research jointly published a comprehensive review of nutrition and cancer

(WCRF and AICR, 1997) and in 2001 the WCRF commissioned a second report to incorporate new evidence that had accumulated since 1997. It has contracted out a series of reviews to international teams of experts on various cancers. Their very detailed methodological plans for the review are critiqued by others and refined before the reviews are conducted, much as outlined above. These reviews (including a biological perspective) are themselves further evaluated and combined into a single report by a central scientific committee. While these reviews are not directly linked to policy, the aim is to provide good scientific evidence that can be used by policy makers, research scientists, health professionals and community groups around the world. To this end the final chapter of the review assesses policy implications directly. Over 30,000 copies of the first report have been disseminated.

The International Agency for Research on Cancer (IARC): monographs programme

Three times a year the IARC convenes a working party of experts to review the literature relating a specific exposure or exposures to cancer. This process is one of the most comprehensive conducted anywhere since, in addition to studies in humans, the working parties also include experts on the exposure itself (chemists, toxicologists, physicists, etc.), on animal studies and on molecular biology. The IARC secretariat performs comprehensive literature searches and sends the material to the individual scientists who are asked to summarise the literature in a particular area. During a week-long face-to-face meeting sub-groups of the working party (exposure data, human studies, animal studies and laboratory data) discuss and finalise the drafts and prepare a summary for their section. The full group then comes together to reach a final consensus. The human and animal data are first classified separately as providing *sufficient*, *limited* or *inadequate* evidence of carcinogenicity or, occasionally, evidence suggesting a lack of carcinogenicity. These data are then combined with the exposure data and molecular information to make a more formal assessment of causality, classifying agents as (http://monographs.iarc.fr)

- carcinogenic to humans,
- *probably* carcinogenic to humans,
- *possibly* carcinogenic to humans,
- *not classifiable* regarding carcinogenicity to humans or
- *probably not* carcinogenic to humans.

As of April 2004 they had classified 90 agents as clear carcinogens with another 64 classified as probable and 236 as possible carcinogens, reflecting the general lack of certainty when dealing with evidence of this type. (Only one compound has been classified as probably not carcinogenic!) A further 496 agents were found to be not classifiable because there was just insufficient evidence to make any judgement.

Box 11.3 Should women under the age of 50 be offered routine mammographic screening?

The debate surrounding this question highlights the difficulties of interpreting evidence. In 1993, an expert panel at the US National Cancer Institute (NCI) concluded that there was no evidence for a benefit of mammographic screening for women aged 40–49 years and the NCI withdrew their recommendation for screening in this age group. In response, the American Cancer Society reaffirmed their recommendation *for* screening, which was based on the view of a separate expert panel. The publication of additional data in 1996 opened up the question again and the NCI responded by convening a consensus conference in 1997. The independent experts at the conference again concluded that there was insufficient evidence to recommend routine mammography for women under the age of 50 years. This conclusion led to such a public outcry that the NCI was forced to reconsider their position. The question went back to the National Cancer Advisory Board, a presidentially appointed committee, who voted 17 to 1 in favour of recommending mammographic screening for younger women. Since then the controversy has continued, with groups reaching opposing conclusions based on the same evidence. As you will see in Chapter 14, the evaluation of screening programmes is not simple, and in this particular instance it appears that we are still a long way from complete agreement.

Consensus conferences and working groups

Consensus conferences on many topics, often similar in format to the IARC working parties, are convened on an ad-hoc basis to evaluate the evidence in a specific area. Independent experts are usually invited to submit papers in advance and these are then discussed at a face-to-face meeting. These conferences may be conducted at an international level or on a smaller scale to provide specific information to inform local planning and practice.

The end result

Policy makers invariably want a black-and-white answer to any question – does this cause/prevent/improve treatment of the condition in question? Unfortunately, as you will have gathered, this yearning for certainty can rarely be fulfilled. Nothing is absolute and, as we discussed in Chapter 10, it is impossible to prove something definitively. As a result you will find that the conclusions of many systematic reviews are couched in fairly cautious terms, but policy makers and planners have to act despite this and make the best of what is available. We will end with a question that is still causing controversy in 2004: should we recommend widespread mammographic screening for women under the age of 50 years (Box 11.3)? (Or, some would argue, should we recommend it at all? Various (2004).)

REFERENCES

AHRQ. (2004). *Guide to Clinical Preventive Services, Third Edition: Periodic Updates*. AHRQ Publication No. 04-IP003, January 2004. Rockville, MD: Agency for Healthcare Research and Quality. (http://www.ahrq.gov/clinic/periodorder.htm.)

Black, N. (1996). Why we need observational studies to evaluate the effectiveness of health care. *British Medical Journal*, **312**: 1215–1218.

Britton, A., McKee, M., Black, N. *et al.* (1998). Choosing between randomised and non-randomised studies: a systematic review. *Health Technology Assessment*, **2** (No. 13): 1–124.

Collaborative Group on Hormonal Factors in Breast Cancer. (1996). Breast cancer and hormonal contraceptives: collaborative reanalysis of individual data on 53 297 women with breast cancer and 100 239 women without breast cancer from 54 epidemiological studies. *The Lancet*, **347**: 1713–1727.

Delgado-Rodriguez, M., Ruiz-Canela, M., De Irala-Estevez, J., Llorica, J. and Martinez-Gonzalez, A. (2001). Participation of epidemiologists and/or biostatisticians and methodological quality of published controlled clinical trials. *Journal of Epidemiology and Community Health*, **55**: 569–572.

Glasziou, P., Irwig, L., Bain, C. and Colditz, G. (2001). *Systematic Reviews in Health Care: A Practical Guide*. Cambridge: Cambridge University Press.

Glasziou, P., Vandenbroucke, J. and Chalmers, I. (2004). Assessing the quality of research. *British Medical Journal*, **328**: 39–41.

Harris, R. P., Helfand, M., Woolf, S. H. *et al.* for the Methods Work Group Third U.S. Preventive Services Task Force. (2001). Current methods of the U.S. Preventive Services Task Force: a review of the process. *American Journal of Preventive Medicine*, **20** (3S): 21–35.

Hirst, G. H. L. and Ward, J. E. (2000). Clinical practice guidelines: reality bites. *Medical Journal of Australia*, **172**: 287–291.

McKee, M., Britton, A., Black, N. *et al.* (1999). Interpreting the evidence: choosing between randomised and non-randomised studies *British Medical Journal*, **319**: 312–315.

Moher, D., Cook, D. J., Eastwood, S. *et al.* (1999). Improving the quality of reports of meta-analyses of randomised controlled trials: the QUOROM statement. Quality of reporting of meta-analyses. *Lancet*, **354**: 1896–1900.

Muir Gray, J. A. (1997). *Evidence-Based Health Care – How to Make Health Policy and Management Decisions*. Edinburgh: Churchill Livingstone.

Oxman, A. D., Cook, D. J. and Guyatt, G. H. (1994). Users' guides to the medical literature VI. How to use an overview. *Journal of the American Medical Association*, **272**: 1367–1371.

Pirozzo, S., Summerbell, C., Cameron, C. and Glasziou, P. (2003). Should we recommend low-fat diets for obesity? *Obesity Reviews*, **4**: 83–90.

Purdie, D. M., Bain, C. J., Webb, P. M. *et al.* (2001). Body size and ovarian cancer: case–control study and systematic review (Australia). *Cancer Causes Control*, **12**: 855–863.

Schultz, K. F., Chalmers, I., Hayes, R. J. and Altman, D. G. (1995). Empirical evidence of bias. Dimensions of methodological quality associated with estimates of treatment effects in controlled trials. *Journal of the American Medical Association*, **273**: 408–412.

Various. (2004). Screening for breast cancer: point–counterpoint. *International Journal of Epidemiology*, **33**: 43–74.

WCRF (World Cancer Research Fund) and AICR (American Institute for Cancer Research). (1997). *Food, Nutrition and the Prevention of Cancer: A Global Perspective.* WCRF AICR. (http://www.wcrf.org/research/fnatpoc.lasso)

Weed, D. L. (2000). Interpreting epidemiological evidence: how meta-analysis and causal inference methods are related. *International Journal of Epidemiology*, **29**: 387–390.

Outbreaks, epidemics and clusters

Box 12.1 An unusual epidemic of pneumonia

On the 21st of February 2003, a doctor from southern China visited Hong Kong and stayed one night in a local hotel. Unwell for several days before the trip, he became seriously ill and the next day was admitted to a hospital with severe pneumonia; he died 10 days later. Before admission he had infected numerous people who came into contact with him, including his own family (wife, daughter, sister and brother-in-law) and 16 guests or visitors to the hotel. Some of the hotel guests left Hong Kong for Singapore, Hanoi and Toronto and outbreaks in those areas rapidly followed. Within a month large outbreaks arose in several Hong Kong hospitals, affecting staff, students, patients and visitors. As family members became infected they infected others and the disease began to spread in the community. On the 12th of March 2003, the World Health Organization issued a global alert on atypical pneumonia, called **severe acute respiratory syndrome** (SARS). By late March a huge outbreak in a Hong Kong housing estate was traced back to a patient discharged from one of the affected hospitals. In Hong Kong there were 1,755 cases and 300 deaths (CFR = 17%), including 8 fatalities among the 386 health workers affected. The high-rise housing estate had 329 cases and 42 deaths. Hong Kong health authorities quarantined 493 households with 1,262 people, traced 26,520 contacts, and screened 36.3 million travellers. Globally, public health organisations collaborated to identify the organism, devise diagnostic tests, introduce control measures and stop the epidemic by August 2003 after 8,422 cases and 916 deaths worldwide

(Chan-Yeung and Yu, 2003).

Investigation of disease outbreaks or epidemics such as that described above is part of the core business of epidemiology. A Medline search yields nearly a million references for 'outbreak' and, as you will see, the utility of epidemic investigations is obvious from the wide variety of applications. Many examples earlier in this book focussed on 'chronic' disease. Now we will spotlight infectious diseases (although not exclusively) and use epidemiological principles to explain the occurrence of endemic, epidemic and pandemic infections. Historically, the study of epidemic infections helped develop methods for epidemiology, especially retrospective cohort analysis and case–control studies, and epidemic investigations retain a high profile in public health practice today. Emerging and re-emerging infections have become prominent over the last two to three decades and the threat of global epidemics (pandemics) mobilised resources to detect and combat such catastrophes. Over the same period, growing awareness of environmental pollution and community detection of clusters of rare diseases, especially cancer, increased demand for epidemiological investigation of 'outbreaks' of non-communicable disease. In response, statisticians are developing new methods for spatial analyses and epidemiologists are studying community risk perception and public communication of risk appraisals.

Infectious disease epidemiology is often presented as a different discipline from the epidemiology we have been describing, but in fact the fundamental principles are identical, as are the study designs used: cohort and case–control studies to investigate causality and experiments to evaluate preventive and therapeutic interventions. Causal reasoning is conceptually simpler but still has its own complexities, as we show below. The identity of the two approaches became more obvious as knowledge expanded to include infectious agents as prime causes of a number of conditions generally considered to be 'chronic', a term often used as a synonym for non-infectious. For example, after decades of study, cervical cancer can now be characterised as a sexually transmitted infectious disease caused by strains of the human papillomavirus. The major difference for most infectious conditions, and other outbreaks we discuss here, is the urgency with which investigations take place. This is often extreme (as with SARS), and demands robust, practical methods for subject identification and selection, as well as for data collection.

Outbreaks, epidemics, endemics and clusters

What do we mean by an **epidemic** or **outbreak**? Generally, they involve unexpected increases in incidence of a disease and Benenson (1990, p. 499) defines both as '*the occurrence in a community or region of cases of an illness clearly in excess of that expected*'. Others have defined them slightly differently, for example Last (2001, p. 129) describes an outbreak as an epidemic limited to a localised increase in incidence of a disease such as in a village, town or institution. Outbreak may also be used to refer to a small epidemic arising in an area that has had no cases for a long time – an epidemic with excess frequency compared with an expected frequency of zero. In such a setting a single case would not be considered an outbreak, but two or more cases could be.

You should also be clear on the distinction between epidemic and **endemic** disease. Last (2001, p. 59) defines endemic disease to be '*the constant presence of a disease or infectious agent within a given geographic area or population group*'. Thus 'endemic' describes attributes of a disease, not an area; 'endemic area' is a frequent misuse of the term endemic. For some diseases, notably malaria, the word endemic has been further defined in reference to the degree of endemicity – with holoendemic the most extreme (children intensely infected, most adults immune), followed by hyperendemic (a disease constantly affecting a large proportion of all age groups in the population).

Epidemics thus represent an unexpected increase in incidence of disease whereas endemic describes a constant presence of disease. Parallel terms referring to infections within animal populations are *enzootic* (constant presence in an animal population) and *epizootic* (an unexpected increase in incidence in an animal population). Sometimes an enzootic infection crosses to humans and causes an epidemic (the most likely explanation for SARS, hantavirus and many other infections). Other times an epizootic infection reaches humans and causes an epidemic (as periodically occurs with plague), or fizzles out after causing great alarm but without any eventual human-to-human transmission (as has happened so far with avian influenza). When a disease affects a large number of people and crosses many international boundaries it is called a **pandemic**. Examples of pandemics last century include plague (around 1900), influenza (1918, 1957 and 1968) and cholera (since 1961). Certain pandemics in history caused great loss of human populations, notably plague in the late middle ages and 'Spanish' influenza at the end of World War I. The modern pandemics of HIV and multi-drug-resistant tuberculosis are of great concern.

One more term must be dealt with here – **cluster**. Last (2001, p. 31) defines it as an '*aggregation of relatively uncommon events or diseases in space and/or time in amounts that are believed or perceived to be greater than could be expected by chance*'. The word is usually used to describe a cluster of cases of a rare (usually non-infectious) disease and putative clusters of disease are often suspected to have an environmental cause on the basis of anecdotal evidence. As a result, much effort is often expended in response to public outcry in attempts to determine whether a true cluster exists, but we should note here generically that all epidemics are 'person–place–time clusters' (also called 'space–time clusters') – occurrences of multiple cases in geo-demographically defined populations over defined periods of time. So the 'cluster problem' described above refers only to rare diseases with low and fluctuating occurrence rates that can appear by chance to cluster as 'epidemics' in small areas. In contrast, a typical epidemic cluster of infection cases in a well-defined population or area does not cause such difficulties.

Box 12.2 Some outbreak and cluster investigations

Re-emergence of fatal avian influenza in humans (China)

The first documented instance of avian influenza subtype H5N1 causing severe respiratory illness in humans was in Hong Kong in 1997 when it affected 18 patients, 6 of whom died. In January–February 2003 it re-emerged when a family from Hong Kong visited China. The seven-year-old daughter developed fever and respiratory symptoms two days after arriving and died of a pneumonia-like illness seven days later; her cause of death was not ascertained. The family returned to Hong Kong and the father was admitted on 11 February after four days of fever, sore throat and coughing. He died six days later and H5N1 was detected. On 12 February the eight-year-old son, who reported having close contact with live chickens in China, was also admitted with a flu-like illness. H5N1 was isolated and he recovered (Peiris *et al.*, 2004).

An outbreak of chromium ulcer in a manufacturing plant (Taiwan)

On 23 May 1989, managers of a manufacturing plant in Taiwan requested investigation of an outbreak of hand ulcers among workers. Ten enamel department workers (13.5%) who developed such chromium ulcers were identified between 1 January and 30 June 1988. Workers who handled conveyer hooks were at greatest risk (RR = 12.4; 95% CI 2.90–53.4). Workers with gloves were protected from developing ulcers (RR = 0.08; 95% CI 0.01–0.60). Analysis of hooks that had passed through the oven revealed chromium VI on their surface (Deng *et al.*, 1990).

An epidemic of paediatric traffic injuries (USA)

This study identified specific regional risk factors for the high rate of paediatric pedestrian trauma in Florida. Of the 29 cases studied, 3 (10%) occurred near ice-cream trucks and 13 (45%) involved 'dart-outs'. Recommendations included an engineering change for a dangerous intersection, and a recommendation to equip ice-cream trucks with extending stop signs (Hameed *et al.*, 2004).

An outbreak of piranha attacks on humans (Brazil)

There are many tales describing ferocious schools of piranha attacking humans, but few scientific data supporting such behaviour. These predacious fish do occasionally injure bathers and swimmers in lakes and rivers and an outbreak of piranha bites was reported in a dammed river in south-east Brazil. The report focussed on epidemiological and clinical aspects as well as piranha biology to gain a better understanding of the natural history of such outbreaks (Haddad and Sazima, 2003).

A cluster of Creutzfeldt–Jakob disease (CJD) (Australia)

Six confirmed sporadic cases of CJD were recognized in 13 years in persons who had been long-term residents of a moderate-sized rural city; the expected number was less than one. An extensive investigation could not find any point-source or case-to-case transmission links. This occurrence was highly statistically significant ($p = 0.003$) and remained significant ($p < 0.02$) when only the cases that arose after the cluster had been recognized were taken into account. However, a more conservative analysis suggested that, when the whole country is taken into consideration, such a grouping could have arisen by chance (Collins *et al.*, 2002).

Insurance and epidemics (Switzerland)

Severe acute respiratory syndrome (SARS) is a reminder that disease emergence is a permanent feature of the world and should be anticipated. The unpleasant fact that human activities are increasing the frequency and severity of these emergences presents the global economy with unprecedented new risks, challenges and even opportunities that must be confronted. As a major contributor to economic stability, the insurance industry must follow these trends very closely and develop scenarios to anticipate these events (von Overbeck, 2003).

Rare disease clusters

Clusters of rare diseases, especially cancer, are increasingly being reported by members of the community in many countries and public awareness of environmental hazards has increased demand for public health authorities to investigate them. Any apparently unusual frequency of any disease will now attract attention and this causes great difficulty for health officials who are asked to respond to the problem. Interpreting the data is not straightforward and pitfalls include the fact that cluster analyses are usually done *post hoc*, without prior hypotheses. Rare diseases will inevitably be distributed in small numbers, thus in small areas their frequency will fluctuate widely due to chance. In a country like the USA with a large population and a large area it is inevitable that numerous small-area clusters will arise for rare diseases and it is difficult to determine whether this is due to chance. This is particularly true for investigations prompted by reported clusters of disease because the cases may represent a much larger population than that in the immediate vicinity of the cluster. (Several of the cases that occur in a large state may just happen to occur in one corner of that state by chance.) Community members are likely first to note the cluster, then to look for possible causes, including any nearby environmental contamination, and then they may well attribute the cluster to the potential source. They will draw boundaries around the cluster after noting it, not before, and there is a danger of overestimating the disease rate through 'boundary shrinkage' of the population from which the cases are assumed to have arisen (Olsen *et al.*, 1996).

Investigating such clusters has rarely led to conclusive evidence as to the cause and usually reveals that the cluster is most probably a chance effect due to variation of small expected numbers. This might not be considered a satisfactory answer, especially if people have formed their own hypotheses as to the cause.

Many public health authorities have developed guidelines and education tools to help them address the problem of rare disease clusters. For example the Cancer Information Service of the National Cancer Institute in the USA (http://cis.nci.nih.gov/) has developed a Cancer Clusters fact sheet and the US Centers for Disease Control (CDC) have issued their own guidelines for investigating clusters (http://www.cdc.gov/nceh/clusters). In 1990 a conference on the topic noted the large volume of work these clusters impose on regional health departments (AJE, 1990). More recently the Royal Statistical Society in the UK revisited the topic (Editorial, 2001). Statisticians are developing new methods for analysing space–time clusters and the field continues to evolve. Many epidemiologists remain concerned that the resources consumed by investigation of rare disease clusters, especially if political pressure is applied, may far exceed the benefits gained. Such expenditure may deprive the community of public funds needed for other activities, including environmental clean-ups that should be done anyway.

Epidemiology of infectious diseases

When would we describe a disease as infectious or communicable? In his *Dictionary of Epidemiology*, Last (2001, p. 35), defines it as

An illness due to a specific infectious agent or its toxic products that arises through transmission of that agent or its products from an infected person, animal or reservoir to a susceptible host, either directly or indirectly through an intermediate plant or animal host, vector, or the inanimate environment.

During the last four to five decades, infectious diseases have not generally been considered a major cause of mortality in developed countries. The production of powerful antibiotics (1950s), polio vaccine (1950s) and measles vaccine (late 1960s) were major milestones along the road to this stage of human history. However, it is worth noting that, in the West, most of the fall in death rates from infections such as TB, pneumonia and diphtheria occurred long before specific clinical treatments or vaccinations were available. Nonetheless, there is no doubt these medical interventions helped speed a further decline in mortality,

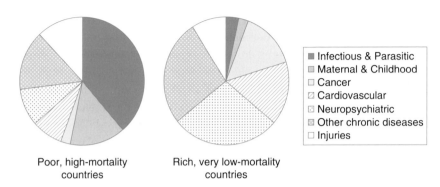

Legend:
- Infectious & Parasitic
- Maternal & Childhood
- Cancer
- Cardiovascular
- Neuropsychiatric
- Other chronic diseases
- Injuries

Poor, high-mortality countries

Rich, very low-mortality countries

Fig. 12.1 The contribution of infectious and chronic conditions to total DALYs in poor, high-mortality versus rich, very-low-mortality countries. (Data source: WHO, 2003.)

lowered morbidity, and have since helped maintain this situation. In some countries, notably in South East Asia and South America, a fall in infection mortality (which is still under way) came later and was greatly accelerated by medical interventions.

In developed countries, mortality due to acute infection is largely restricted to the very young, the elderly and the infirm, but infections remain an important cause of expensive morbidity in these richer nations. Their populations continue to experience considerable sickness and loss of productivity from common infections, notably of the respiratory tract, including influenza, and the gastrointestinal tract, especially food poisoning. Periodically, epidemics of some vaccine-preventable diseases also recur; for example, pertussis (whooping cough), rubella and measles. In addition, there are many infections that have recently emerged or re-emerged and for some we have made little headway with prevention, or treatment. There are also new (or unsolved) problems with the old infections. Worldwide, frequent use and misuse of antibiotics produced resistant bacteria, some now unresponsive to all available drugs. Furthermore, anti-viral drugs remain very expensive, are often toxic, and are of limited utility. They are not yet helpful for transmission control or for treating many viral infections.

Infections still constitute the most important disease group in poor high-mortality countries, where they are responsible for almost half the disease burden (Figure 12.1). In particular, the high incidence of pneumonia, diarrhoeal diseases (including cholera), malaria, tuberculosis and dengue in many poor countries causes much premature mortality and disability. Some populous regions in the tropics have additional problems with environments that are receptive for parasitic infections, notably schistosomiasis, trypanosomiasis, filariasis, onchocerciasis and leishmaniasis. These neglected diseases collectively cause substantial morbidity and premature mortality for a large proportion of the world population.

Infections everywhere may become more important in the future as old, changed or newly encountered microbes pose threats of local or regional epidemics, or even large pandemics. Emerging and re-emerging infections have steadily become more common over the last 30 years. We expect this trend to continue, since it is based on many factors that are sure to persist or increase in the future. These include population growth, expanding trade and travel, mass-produced food, ongoing environmental change, resistance to antimicrobial drugs, human encroachment on wilderness and forest, and global warming. The SARS multi-country epidemic of 2003 was a chilling example of a global threat due to emergence of a new infectious disease. Box 12.1 at the start of this chapter describes its introduction and spread in Hong Kong and beyond. This reveals the problem posed by such lethal fast-moving epidemics of an unknown disease. These important events, and the extraordinary global response, are described more fully in the February 2004 issue of *Emerging Infectious Diseases* (vol. 10, No. 2), which is freely available through the US CDC (www.cdc.gov/ncidod/EID/).

Effective identification and control of outbreaks of infectious disease remains an important and complex component of public health. Epidemics are bad news and bad news is always a valuable commodity for the media, so their investigation and control is often conducted as a health emergency under the public eye. Sometimes epidemic alerts trigger worldwide alarm and politically complex national and international responses, as has been noted over the last decade for cholera in South America, plague in India, avian influenza in Asia, and SARS in Asia and Canada. Increasingly, small or large outbreaks threaten economically important industries, as seen with Hendra virus in Australia (1994, horse racing), Nipah virus in Malaysia (1998–9, pig farming), SARS in Hong Kong (2003, services and tourism) and avian influenza in Asia (1997 and 2003–4, poultry).

Infection **eradication** (removal from all human populations), **elimination** (removal from defined areas) and **control** (reduction below the threshold of public health significance) have made substantial progress over the last 50 years but there is a long way to go. The declaration of smallpox eradication by the WHO in 1980 was probably the most important achievement in terms of global health last century. Ongoing programmes to eradicate polio and leprosy and, in some West African countries, to eliminate onchocerciasis are now being attempted. The global Guinea worm eradication programme is close to final success in East and West Africa but is being impeded by civil wars. There has been moderate success in controlling HIV/AIDS among special risk groups in Australia, New Zealand, North America and Europe over the last decade, and more recently in some other countries (notably Thailand), but elsewhere the global AIDS pandemic, the most lethal in human history, continues to spread at an alarming rate, especially among the general populations of many parts of Asia and Sub-Saharan Africa.

A causal model

Simple models of the 'agent–host–environment' interplay have served infectious disease epidemiology well, providing a neat structure for linking the variety of

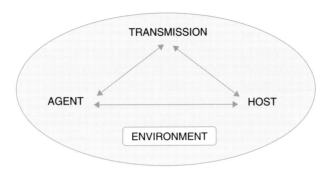

Fig. 12.2 The relationships among agent, host, transmission and environment.

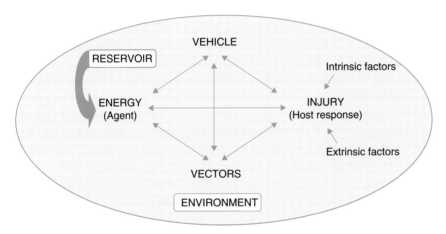

Fig. 12.3 A schematic representation of the epidemiological model of injury. (Adapted from Kraus and Robertson, 1992.)

factors that determine whether disease occurs. Figure 12.2 is a straightforward version that shows the interaction between an infectious agent and its potential host, the transmission process (how the disease is spread) and how all of these may be influenced by the environment. We will use its axes to organise our more detailed examination of the links between exposures to infectious agents and disease occurrence.

Although we did not invoke such a model when dealing with causality in Chapter 10, its relevance to most causal circumstances is readily apparent. The *host* remains the same and mobilises a variety of genetically directed and other adaptive responses against a particular agent; the *agent* can be any infectious or non-infectious risk factor, some of which have a variety of modes of *transmission*; and the *environment* includes the background social, economic and ecological circumstances that surround the host and determine the community risk level. Such models have been used in environmental epidemiology; and a more detailed version (Figure 12.3) has been suggested as a useful tool for explaining pathways to injury.

What influences the spread of infectious diseases?

Before moving to deal with epidemics and their management, it is helpful to consider briefly the biology of infectious agents. Infectious diseases have one distinguishing attribute. They involve one living organism preying on another. Some parasite life cycles even involve two or more hosts and such intersection of biological lifelines is intrinsically complex. Furthermore, within environmental constraints, interacting organisms must evolve elaborate defence or attack mechanisms to maintain their life cycles. Consequently, although infectious diseases may be relatively easy to define (on the basis of presence of the organism and the typical host response), infections are often difficult to understand biologically or epidemiologically. Like many harmful exposures, they have a wide range of host effects, varying from inapparent infection (acute or chronic) to severe disease and death. Also, as environments change, both agents and hosts may be affected, impeding or promoting transmission.

The aims of infectious disease epidemiology reflect those of epidemiology in general: to describe and explain the occurrence and distribution of infections and the relationship of infection to disease. To do this it is necessary to understand the *properties of the agent*, to know (or discover) the *sources of infection* and the existence of any *biological reservoirs* of infection, to clarify the *pathway* or process whereby the agent is transmitted, via the environment, and to know how the *host reacts* to an infectious challenge. Our knowledge of infections has become far more detailed since the development of bacteriology and the germ theory of disease at the end of the nineteenth century, but the agent–host–environment circumstances frequently change and new organisms continually emerge. The relationships are always dynamic and usually extremely complex; it is rarely possible to understand every step of the process, often difficult to assess the probability that infection will occur, and always a battle to keep pace with changes and stay half a step ahead, or even just one step behind.

Exposure variation will often influence the risk of infection. For example, *Mycobacterium tuberculosis* infection is usually contracted by breathing air contaminated with the organism, but crowded, poorly ventilated environments are not always risky for tuberculosis (TB). While there would be a high risk of exposure in a crowded, poorly ventilated area such as a prison in a highly endemic country, the risk in comparable circumstances in a developed country would be much lower. This is one aspect of the crucial role played by the background environment, the population-level influences on individual risk.

Environments also change and this in turn alters infection risks in numerous ways, directly, via effects on humans or agents, or indirectly, via effects on intermediate hosts or infection vectors. This is the basis for recent interest in the effects of global warming on the distribution and incidence of infections. Dengue fever is an example of an infection that will be greatly influenced by climate change if the

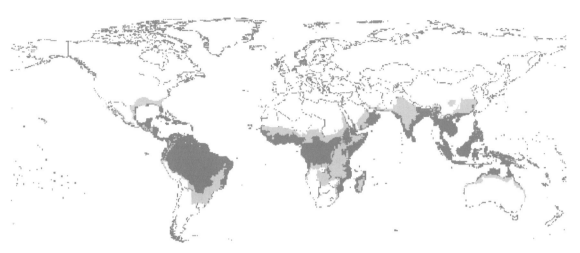

Fig. 12.4 The influence of global warming on the global distribution of dengue fever, dark blue = baseline risk, 1960–1990; light blue = projected risk, 2080. (*Source*: Simon Hales, Australian National University, previously unpublished and reproduced with permission.)

range of the mosquito vector increases (Hales *et al.*, 2002). The minimum period for model estimates is 30 years because climate variability does not allow us to see changes caused by global warming reliably over shorter periods. Accordingly, a long-range forecast is appropriate. It provides a sobering insight into problems we must face if the environment changes substantially (Figure 12.4).

Host factors also come into play. If a person is infected with TB, various personal attributes (such as malnutrition, HIV infection and diabetes) then modulate their risk of developing subsequent *disease*. Such agent–host interactions vary enormously, altering risks of many infectious diseases. In an area highly endemic for malaria, partially immune adults often have detectable blood parasites without becoming ill; but in a less endemic area, or in young children with little or no immunity, detectable parasites in the blood stream would almost always cause symptoms, including fever. This shows how acquired host defences alter clinical manifestations of infection, often affecting the ability of epidemiologists to detect cases accurately.

Finally, the *agent* also varies frequently. As they evolve, microbial agents that appear to be similar may vary considerably over time or place, with powerful or subtle effects on transmission, host responses, treatment and control. Some, such as influenza virus, are constantly changing their structure as part of the quest for survival; TB, and many other bacteria, have evolved to resist antibiotics. Sometimes agent effects are simply a reflection of the intensity of the infection, particularly with multicellular parasites such as hookworms, schistosomes and filaria. Morbidity due to these parasites relates directly to the worm burden – more worms for more time produces more disease.

Overall, whether infection occurs depends on factors influencing the probability and result of contact between an infectious agent and a susceptible host. Some of these factors are described below.

The infectious agent

There are many different types of infectious agent: bacteria, viruses, fungi, protozoa, helminths, etc. In almost every natural habitat there will be agents potentially infectious to humans. Animal contact is particularly important in the genesis of human infections and many (perhaps most) infections afflicting us have been traced back to the beginnings of agriculture and animal farming.

What then is **infection**? It is the entry of a microbial agent into a higher-order host and its multiplication within the host. When a lower organism lives on an external surface of another (usually higher) organism it is called an **infestation** rather than an infection; examples of infestations include lice and scabies. Infections do not necessarily lead to overt disease and the principal characteristics of microbial agents that influence their ability to cause disease are defined below.

Infectivity is the ability of an organism to invade and multiply in a host. It is the proportion of exposures that result in infection. One measure of infectivity is the **secondary attack rate**, which measures the number of cases of infection that develop among the susceptible contacts of an infected case. **Pathogenicity** is the power of an organism to produce overt illness among those infected. It is measured as the proportion of those exposed to infection who develop clinical or overt illness. **Virulence** is the ability of an organism to produce serious disease and is measured by the proportion of those who are infected (determined by immunoassay) who develop severe overt disease. If death is a criterion of severity, this can be measured by the **case–fatality ratio** (CFR, see Chapter 2).

One highly *infectious* agent is the polio virus. If a source of polio infection enters a community of susceptible people, it is likely that the majority will eventually become infected. However, only a small proportion will develop even mild disease; i.e., the polio virus has low *pathogenicity*. An even smaller proportion will develop symptoms of paralysis and only a small percentage of these will have permanent sequelae; i.e., the virus is of relatively low *virulence*. Like polio, measles also has a very high infectivity; secondary attack rates for measles approach 100%, but, unlike polio, the measles virus demonstrates a high degree of pathogenicity because most of those infected will develop symptoms. Typhoid is a disease with variable CFR. Under the best circumstances of early diagnosis and rapid treatment the CFR may be less than 1%, but late presentation, in the absence of high-quality treatment, often results in CFRs of 10%–15%.

Intensity of infection is especially important for helminth infections. Generally a few parasitic worms (such as hookworms or schistosomes) will not cause detectable disease, but when individual worm burdens reach the hundreds (or thousands), serious debility and premature death is often the consequence.

The natural habitat of the agent is known as its **reservoir** and this may be human, animal or environmental. Agents with human reservoirs include the pertussis bacterium, the malarial parasite and the roundworm. With some agents it is not clear where their reservoir is. There is still debate, for instance, about the environmental reservoir of the cholera bacterium – where does it hide between annual epidemics in the Indo-Gangetic delta? We are still searching for the reservoir of the SARS virus, since we do not know whether certain animals found to be infected (such as civet cats) actually acquired it from another source.

The **source** of an infectious agent is the person, animal or object from which the host acquires the infection. The source may be another human who is sick or convalescent. Occasionally infected persons may become long-term carriers of infection without being clinically sick themselves, as with hepatitis B, typhoid and HIV. One of the best-known examples of a long-term carrier is 'Typhoid Mary', who worked as a cook in New York, USA. She is thought to have caused 10 outbreaks of typhoid fever with a total of 51 cases and 3 deaths before her own death in 1938. She was a poor woman and moved from household to household aware that the infection seemed to follow her around but unaware, at least initially, of her own role, and also unaware of the preventive measures needed (scrupulous hygiene).

The host

The host is the human or animal to which an agent acquires entry and in which it multiplies. A host's reaction to infection can be extremely variable, depending on the interplay between the characteristics of the agent, including the dose received, and the specific and non-specific immune status of the host.

The immune response of the very young (especially pre-vaccination) and the old is not as protective as that of a young healthy adult. Most influenza mortality, for example, occurs in the elderly; but this is not always the case and the lethal pandemic of influenza in 1918–19 killed millions of young adults. If the host has been exposed to the agent before, there may be residual natural immunity, or immunity may be induced artificially by vaccination. A person who is susceptible to a particular agent is often referred to simply as a 'susceptible'.

These factors, and others to do with the biology, maturation and replication of the agent, influence the **incubation period**. This is the time between initial infection (entry into host) and the onset of clinical disease (symptoms). For control of infectious diseases it is also important to know the **latent period**; this is defined as the time from entry into the host until the onset of infectiousness and it may be longer or shorter than the incubation period. If it is shorter then infected persons may pass on the infection before they become ill (as with influenza) and if it is longer they will be ill before they are very infectious (like with SARS). This timing is an important determinant of infection dynamics. Infections transmitted before becoming ill (or without becoming ill) are the most difficult to control and the most likely to cause explosive epidemics in susceptible populations. These features are known for the majority of infectious diseases. They are useful tools in the investigation and control of epidemics and are always the focus of attention for new infections such as SARS.

Transmission

Transmission of an agent is its spread from a reservoir or source to a new host by one or more of three possible routes – ***direct***, ***indirect*** or ***airborne***.

Direct transmission
This arises from 'close personal contact' by touching infectious secretions or excreta. This includes touching or inhaling the large (10–100 micrometres) respiratory droplets produced by sneezing, coughing or talking by a person suffering from a patent respiratory infection. These heavy droplets contain mostly water and pass through the air to fall on surrounding objects within 1–2 metres of the source. Examples of direct transmission include sexual, skin, eye, congenital and most respiratory infections, including measles and influenza. Sometimes *vertical transmission* (direct from mother to unborn child) is distinguished from *horizontal transmission* (direct or indirect) among persons already born.

Indirect transmission
This always involves a 'vehicle'. It may be inanimate, such as bedding, clothes or utensils (collectively called 'fomites'), food or water (many intestinal infections), or the soil (a reservoir for many infectious fungi, Legionella and diphtheria, and required to complete the life cycle of Toxoplasma shed by cats and for common human helminths such as ascaris and hookworm). Or the vehicle may be alive and considered a 'vector' (e.g., mosquitoes that transmit malaria and dengue, ticks that transmit lyme disease and lice that transmit typhus) or an obligatory intermediate host (such as snails for schistosomiasis). Most faecal–oral infections, such as polio, typhoid, cholera and many forms of gastroenteritis, are indirectly transmitted (via food or water), but some, such as bacillary dysentery, can also be transmitted via direct contamination of hands and mouth.

Airborne transmission
This became an outmoded concept in the nineteenth century after Snow had shown that London cholera was water-borne, disproving the prevailing theory of

an infectious airborne 'miasma' rising from the river. Later, Pasteur and others demonstrated the existence of germs and showed that they could be transmitted directly. The laboratory production in the 1930s of 'bioaerosols' of tiny infectious droplet nuclei that could be inhaled as well as careful epidemiological studies on TB and Q fever in the 1940s and 1950s eventually resurrected the concept of airborne infection as an important mode of transmission (Langmuir, 1961). Bioaerosols may also be produced in abattoirs when cutting open body cavities of infected animals, in air-conditioning cooling towers, or by germ warfare.

It is important to remember that the type and mode of transmission of an agent are key factors for designing control strategies and that some agents may have several modes of transmission. For example, SARS is usually transmitted by respiratory droplets reaching close contacts, but a few cases spread infection to scores of persons, some of whom had only fleeting contact with cases or no direct contact at all (Li *et al.*, 2004); this raised questions about airborne infection in certain circumstances, such as after intubation and in very confined spaces. The presumed mode of transmission profoundly affects the management of infections, since in hospitals precautions against respiratory droplets (ordinary masks and gloves, clean nearby surfaces) are much less exacting than precautions against airborne infection (special masks, eye shields, negative-pressure ventilation).

The environment

The environment has a strong influence on the transmission of infectious diseases. The physical environment or climate has obvious influences, sometimes for reasons we do not understand well. In temperate zones, influenza and rotavirus appear in the colder winter months, times of close human contact. On the other hand, Ross River fever usually occurs in hot humid months, reflecting the importance of an abundance of mosquitoes for transmission of that disease. Other environmental influences include levels of sanitation, air pollution, water quality, population density, overcrowding, poverty, housing conditions and food availability, to name but a few. The environment affects survival both of arthropod vectors (such as mosquitoes) and of the vertebrate hosts of disease. The environment is, in turn, affected by the agents and, of course, the host. Human behaviour often creates environments suitable for infections. Frequently this is due to imposed ecological circumstances, such as unsanitary households due to lack of clean water and poverty; sometimes it is due to human folly or ignorance, such as creation of mosquito breeding sites in domestic environments of tropical areas and lack of preventive measures to defend against infections such as Q fever in abattoirs. It can also be due to necessity, such as wet-rice farming to produce a crucial food staple that also creates breeding sites for the intermediate host snails of schistosome infections.

Fig. 12.5 The epidemic curve for a point-source epidemic.

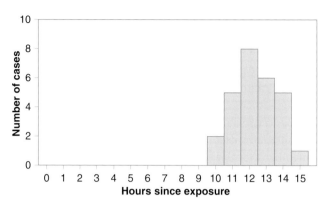

Epidemics or outbreaks

There are two principal types of epidemic. Distinguishing between these can help to narrow an epidemic investigation, leading quickly to the cause of the outbreak and to its control.

Point-source (vehicle) epidemics

This type is sometimes called a common-source, or extended-source, epidemic, the latter implying that the exposure may be spread over a period. This type of epidemic occurs when many people are suddenly exposed to the same source of infection, leading to a clear increase in incidence of disease. We can study the progress of an epidemic by plotting the distribution of cases in relation to the date of onset, producing what is known as an epidemic curve. Figure 12.5 shows the typical shape of the epidemic curve for a point-source outbreak. The number of cases of disease (defined by the onset of symptoms) is plotted against the time (number of hours) since exposure. In this way we can assess the average incubation period, which in this case will be between 12 and 13 hours. This is the typical pattern of an outbreak of food poisoning and shows the distribution of incubation periods in differently susceptible people. Figure 1.3 showed an actual point-source epidemic that you met in Chapter 1.

In practice, the epidemic curve for a common-source outbreak might not be as clear as these examples. A common source like the polluted River Thames in nineteenth-century London could lead to an outbreak of cholera that started at different times in different places, giving a much more complex and drawn-out curve.

Propagative (contagious) epidemics

This type arises from the introduction of an infection into a susceptible population with subsequent transmission from person to person and a progressive

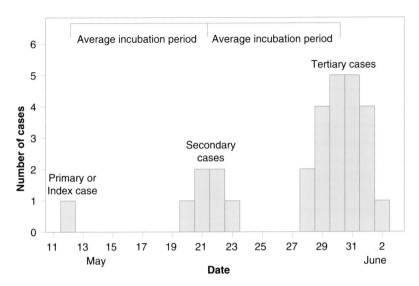

Fig. 12.6 The epidemic curve for a propagative epidemic.

increase in incidence. The pattern in Figure 12.6 is typical of a propagative epidemic. On 12 May there was a single case, referred to as the *index* or primary case (there may be more than one). Eight to eleven days later we see another cluster of cases, sometimes referred to as *secondary* cases, which have arisen from the index case by person-to-person transmission. A further eight to thirteen days later there is a third generation of cases, serially infected by the secondary cases. If the spread of incubation periods is wide, the gaps between the peaks progressively close as long-incubation cases for one generation merge with short-incubation cases for the next generation, producing a fluctuating pattern of continuous cases.

Common conditions for the occurrence (and cessation) of an outbreak

There are numerous agent–host–environment states that might change and precipitate an outbreak. Some of the more common circumstances are

- new appearance of, or sudden increase in, an infectious agent, which may arrive in a human or animal host, a plant, or in an inanimate environment such as soil, and can come from any part of the world by trade, travel or natural spread;
- increase in susceptibles in an environment that has an endemic pathogen (this could be by immigration or birth, or by a drop in immunisation rates in a community); and
- introduction of an effective route of transmission from source to susceptibles (e.g., climatic change bringing a new species of mosquito, or a new process of food preparation or storage).

An epidemic will end or diminish when contrary conditions hold, i.e., anything that leads to a large drop in the number of susceptibles and when each case reproduces on average less than once. This may occur through immunisation (including 'natural' immunisation whereby people actually catch the disease and then become immune) or prophylaxis, by removing the source of infection, or by breaking the transmission cycle (e.g., by spraying mosquito breeding sites to lower vector density, by isolating people while they are infectious, by adopting personal protection measures such as gloves and masks in hospitals, or by treating infectious persons early). We see here another complex causal web with the same demands as for any other disease: the need to identify the most cost-efficient response to the short-term threat together with longer-term planning to lower risk overall.

Investigating outbreaks

As with any epidemiological study, the investigation of an outbreak must be systematic. Going back to first principles, we need to look at the distribution of disease by person, place and time in the early stages of the outbreak, and use those observations together with knowledge of relevant preliminary disease characteristics to formulate rapidly initial hypotheses on which early action can be based.

The 2003 SARS epidemic was a perfect example of the urgent interplay of investigations across many disciplines. The studies were conducted successfully during an epidemic that was killing frontline health system staff and spreading rapidly in many countries. Laboratory scientists quickly defined the organism, its survival in the environment and its susceptibility to antiseptics. Hospital doctors and nurses tested various treatments and instituted exceptional measures to protect hospital staff. Epidemiologists determined the incubation period, the usual mode of transmission, the variable (and usual) infectiousness and the effective control achieved by personal protective measures in hospitals, early isolation of cases and quarantine of contacts. Information managers, computer experts and statistical modellers helped to track the epidemic and analyse control effects. In Hong Kong even the police service played a vital role, collaborating with the Department of Health for contact tracing and identification of high-rise buildings with multiple cases for disinfection teams. This first 'Internet-assisted' global effort for epidemic control led to rapid and complete control of the disease. The overall SARS experience suggests that tools available to combat epidemics are, at least so far, evolving just fast enough to match the increasing demands.

The following series of steps is essential in any outbreak investigation but, with the possible exception of the first three, it is rare to follow them in a neat order as listed below; usually several steps proceed at once.

Provisional case definition. A clear 'working' or 'provisional' case definition is an essential first step. This may be changed or refined – ideally to an aetiological diagnosis – at a later stage in the investigation. For a new or as yet undiagnosed infection a syndromic definition based on some combination of epidemiology (potential exposure), symptoms and signs, and key laboratory information (e.g., elevated white-cell count or radiological evidence of pneumonia) must be developed.

Confirm that the epidemic exists. This will be obvious if there is an abnormally high number of cases of a particular disease concentrated in time or space, or with unique clinical features. With common diseases like influenza or measles you would compare current incidence with background rates in the time before the outbreak, or during the same period or season in previous years. Remember the definition: '. . . clearly in excess of that expected'.

Assess the extent of the outbreak and its essential epidemiological features. Serious cases might not be a problem to identify since they are likely to present to hospital, but the mildly or moderately ill may be hard to find. Inapparent infections can be discovered only afterwards, usually by serology. A rapid initial survey (by phone and/or record searching) of local hospitals, clinics and doctors will give a preliminary estimate of the size. If the outbreak seems to be widespread, a random household telephone survey might be considered. In addition to clinical and sociodemographic data, the person–place–time approach must be tailored to the situation at hand. Depending on the working hypotheses, it may be necessary to collect details from the patients' workplaces or to obtain evidence of current immunisation status, for example, as well as gathering appropriate biological samples for laboratory testing.

Define the population 'at risk' (the denominator). One task is to define those who have been, may have been and have not been exposed to the agent of the particular outbreak. It is sometimes an impossible task, but for other situations it is more straightforward. These data provide us with denominators for calculating *attack rates*.

Formulate working hypotheses. A number of tools can help with the formulation of some initial hypotheses.

- Draw up a list of all potential cases early on, and for each list crucial data, along the lines of Table 12.1. Refine this to include only definite cases as the investigation proceeds.
- Does the case definition need modification? Is there a definitive diagnosis?
- Draw a spot map, looking for clustering of cases or a link to some point source. Maps by site of residence, occupation or education may be informative.
- Draw the epidemic curve, because its shape will reflect both the time distribution of exposure and the distribution of incubation periods and this can lead to hypotheses on the aetiology.
- Note any interesting anomalies. They sometimes hold the key and are worth investigating in detail. (Remember Snow (1855) at the Broad Street pump.)

Table 12.1 An example of a line list used for recording data in an epidemic following a lunch on December 21 2003.

ID	Age	Sex	Time of lunch	Onset of symptoms Date – Time	Sea-food salad	Oysters	Cured ham	Pizza bread	Pavlova	Coffee with milk
01	34	M	1.15	21/12 – 20.30	Y	N	Y	N	Y	Y
02	23	F	1.10	21/12 – 21.15	Y	N	Y	Y	Y	N
03	65	M	1.20	21/12 – 19.30	Y	Y	Y	N	N	Y
04	47	M	1.40	21/12 – 22.00	N	N	Y	N	Y	N
05	61	F	2.10	None	Y	Y	Y	Y	N	Y
06	58	M	1.15	21/12 – 20.10	Y	N	Y	Y	Y	Y
07	39	F	1.00	21/12 – 19.00	Y	N	Y	Y	Y	N
08	43	F	1.30	21/12 – 21.40	Y	Y	Y	Y	Y	Y
09	47	M	1.25	21/12 – 21.15	Y	N	Y	Y	Y	N
10	51	F	2.15	None	Y	Y	Y	Y	N	Y
	etc.									

Test hypotheses. Additional data may be required to test the hypotheses as outlined below. For example, if a meal is suspected to be a common source, it is essential to try to identify which foods are implicated, as in the example in Chapter 1. If one or two specific foods are linked to high attack rates then it is important to attempt to obtain samples of them in order to try to isolate the agent.

Study design and analysis

Most outbreak investigations are carried out retrospectively, although some may be partly prospective. If the source is known or strongly suspected, a retrospective cohort of all people thought to have been exposed, and at least a sample of those not exposed, can be assembled. From the data we can calculate the **attack rate** in those exposed to the source and compare it with the attack rate in those not exposed. Recall that the attack rate is a specific measure of cumulative incidence that is often used for particular groups being observed for a limited period of time and under special circumstances (such as an epidemic). In propagative epidemics it may also be of interest to calculate the **secondary attack rate**. This is the number of cases among the contacts of a primary case that occurred within the likely incubation period following exposure as a proportion of the total number of exposed contacts. The attack rates in the exposed and the unexposed can then be compared to give the **relative risk** (risk ratio) of catching the disease if exposed.

If the source of infection is not known, a case–control study can be used to investigate exposure to a variety of possible events and sources of infection. This allows calculation of an **odds ratio** to estimate the association between the source and disease in the usual way (see Chapter 5).

Epidemic management

Dealing sensibly with the media is always an important element in controlling the wider social effects of a real or perceived outbreak. For alarming and lethal outbreaks, such as SARS in Hong Kong in 2003, the skills required in dealing with the media are very particular: panic can be induced, or prevented; scapegoating is easily aroused and tensions can rise rapidly. In such situations media briefings are best left to senior staff, or those specially trained in media skills. The contrast between media management for SARS in China (initial denial) and Hong Kong (candid accounts) was striking; management within China itself changed enormously towards the end of the emergency when all officials were instructed to disclose the situation. Media problems also arose in other affected areas, not just Asia. Large, lethal and mysterious epidemics are always going to make dealing with the media an unavoidable and vital management issue.

There are several other managerial tasks for public health workers responding to an epidemic. Treatment of cases may need to be organised. This will depend on the type of illness, its severity and the number of cases involved. Can local health facilities cope with additional patient loads or will outside help be required? Are there severe cases who may need to be transferred to a tertiary referral centre? Will cases need to be isolated or staff (including any investigating epidemiologists) protected? It may also be necessary to organise collection, transport and reception of specimens for laboratory investigation. These must be handled carefully and others must not be exposed to any risks. For example, collection of throat specimens from potential SARS cases is a risky procedure unless a protective mask, gown, goggles and gloves are used.

In parallel, control measures, both short- and long-term, need to be initiated, particularly if there are signs of a continuing epidemic. These can be aimed at eliminating or controlling the source of the agent, such as contaminated foods. Alternatively, it may be more efficient to reduce transmission of infection, especially if there is a known vector. It may also be necessary to set up a local surveillance system to monitor further cases of the disease, which may facilitate early prevention measures and avoid a further outbreak. The full investigation of an epidemic may be a protracted affair. Confirmation of diagnoses often depends on serology; vectors may need to be collected and identified and there may be need for further, more formal epidemiological studies.

Finally, it is important to ensure that all aspects of an outbreak are reported accurately. The primary reporting responsibility of an epidemiologist investigating an outbreak is to the health authorities but, as the examples above show, the media and public are also vitally interested in such occurrences and need to be kept informed of the situation as clearly and simply as possible.

Tuberculosis: a case study

The following case study was adapted and condensed with permission from a teaching exercise devised by Dr Donald Hopkins (The Carter Center, USA). It is based on a pioneering report on the transmission and natural history of an outbreak of tuberculosis (TB) at a Danish school in 1942–1943. The approach to the study and the information that emerged remain valid today. The investigation was completed before the availability of anti-TB drugs such as streptomycin (1949) and isoniazid (1952) that would have altered the natural history observed. Few epidemiological studies have had a greater influence on concepts and action for an important infection. The natural histories of primary and post-primary TB were documented, the risks were quantified, and the mode of transmission clarified – all essential information for improving control of the infection.

Background

In the 1940s, the pathogenesis and epidemiology of pulmonary TB was controversial. The mode of spreading was assumed to be prolonged intimate contact but it was not known whether this involved contamination of the environment (e.g., cups or surfaces), direct contact with infectious secretions, or contact via air. Emphasis for control was on contact examination and follow-up, isolation of those with active pulmonary TB and improving home and public hygiene, especially the control of spitting. Use of BCG vaccination was (and remains) of uncertain utility.

The epidemic of tuberculosis in a Danish girls' school, 1942–1943

Between December 1942 and March 1943 an epidemic of an acute febrile disease, first thought to be influenza, occurred in a community public school for girls in Denmark. Over a period of 11 weeks 53 cases occurred among the 368 pupils (Figure 12.7).

During the middle of the epidemic, eight cases of erythema nodosum (small, painful skin nodules) were noted and this suggested a diagnosis of primary pulmonary TB. Investigations included tuberculin skin testing of all apparent non-cases, gastric lavage and culturing of skin-test converters, and the taking of chest X-rays of all the students.

The school was already under observation because one year earlier (October 1941) there had been three cases of pulmonary TB with no further spread.

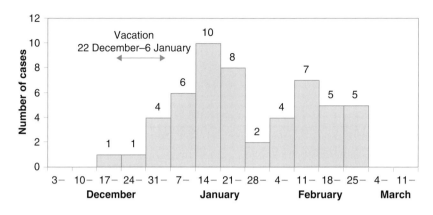

Fig. 12.7 The epidemic curve for the Danish tuberculosis outbreak 1942–1943. (Data source: Hyge, 1947.)

Vaccination (BCG) was offered at the time to those who were skin-test negative. On 7 December 1942 a regular follow-up had revealed that 130 pupils were naturally tuberculin positive, 133 had converted after the BCG and 105 were negative (i.e., overall 71.5% were positive). The negatives included those who had refused BCG and new girls who had entered the school in autumn 1942. Thus, coincidentally, the tuberculin status of the school was surveyed just before the 1942–1943 outbreak.

The source of infection and mode of transmission

Tuberculin tests performed again in March 1943 revealed that 70 (66.7%) of the 105 previously tuberculin-negative pupils had converted to positive. Of these 53 had suffered from a flu-like illness (with or without erythema nodosum) and 17 were apparently asymptomatic.

School classes moved from room to room on a regular schedule throughout the day. The school building was at ground level except for several rooms 'in the basement which were small and dark . . . in particular the physics room of the middle school which also served as the air-raid shelter. This was a permanently blacked out cellar . . . Any ventilation was practically out of the question because of sand bags piled up in front of windows . . .' (Hyge, 1947).

A search for the source of infection begun in March 1943 included X-ray examination of all teachers and employees. Only one teacher showed distinct changes, but the findings were the same as on preceding examinations. She nevertheless became a suspect source of infection.

This female teacher taught a total of nine separate classes in the physics room spending 'all of her hours at the school in these basement rooms'. Four other classes with different teachers were also held in the basement early in the morning before the suspect teacher arrived at the school. Three classes did not normally enter the basement rooms.

The tuberculin conversion rates among the pupils who were negative in December 1942 are shown in Table 12.2, according to their exposure to the suspect teacher.

Table 12.2 Tuberculin conversion rates between December 1942 and March 1943 among known tuberculin-negative pupils by degree of exposure to suspect teacher.

| | | Tuberculin status | | |
| | | Negative | Positive | Per cent |
Group	Degree of exposure	December 1942	March 1943	converted
A	Taught by suspect teacher	53	46	86.8
B	In basement classrooms with other teacher	41	24	58.5
C	In basement classroom prior to arrival of suspect teacher	6	0	0
D	Not in basement	5	0	0
Total		105	70	66.7

(Data source, Hyge, 1947.)

The suspect teacher was placed on leave on 5 March and 'after some objection she was persuaded to submit to gastric lavage on April 6'. (Persons with post-primary infectious pulmonary TB often swallow their sputum and TB organisms may be found in the stomach contents.) The culture revealed four colonies of tubercle bacillus, human type. On careful inquiry 'this teacher stated, as was also confirmed by others, that she had a cold from about the middle of December 1942, when the infection became more aggressive'.

'Very frequent tuberculin tests on the remaining 37 tuberculin-negative pupils who kept attending school' were performed. No new infections appeared after the tuberculin survey in March.

Short-term infection outcomes

All of the 70 converters were repeatedly examined by X-ray and by culturing of gastric lavage specimens. More than half (41) were shown to have a positive culture (5), a positive X-ray (4), or both (32), as evidence of primary pulmonary tuberculosis. The 263 pupils who were found to be tuberculin positive in December 1942 (130 naturally positive and 133 BCG-induced) were also given X-ray examinations in March 1943. 'None was found to show any evidence of active pulmonary tuberculosis.'

Follow-up studies and natural history of TB infection

All 368 pupils in the school were followed at regular intervals over the course of the next 12 years for the development of progressive pulmonary TB. The findings are summarized in Table 12.3. Among the 130 pupils who were naturally positive before the outbreak a total of 9 cases of progressive TB developed. Among the

Table 12.3 The occurrence of progressive pulmonary tuberculosis in a Danish school for girls, 1943–1955.

Tuberculin status	Number of pupils	Total cases of progressive tuberculosis	
		3-Year follow-up	12-Year follow-up
Naturally positive in December 1942	130	4	9
BCG-induced positive in February 1942	133	3[a]	3[a]
Converters between December 1942 and March 1943	70	6	14
Negative[b]	35	0	0
Total	368	13[a]	26[a]

[a] One mild case of tuberculosis developed in a BCG vaccinee whose tuberculin test result had reverted to negative in December 1942.
[b] Those who escaped infection during the epidemic.
(Data source, Hyge, 1957.)

133 who received BCG, 3 cases developed within the first year and none subsequently. Among the 70 who became infected during the epidemic, 6 cases developed within 1 year with a total of 14 cases over the 12-year period (20%).

Implications of the study

Because this study had a defined population and a clear exposure event, we can infer the mode of transmission. In addition, the long follow-up before the advent of specific therapy reveals the natural history of the infection, which is an always important but often elusive component of infectious disease epidemiology. We also note the effectiveness of BCG in that setting, and the 12-year cumulative incidence of progressive (post-primary) TB among four important host categories: recent tuberculin converters, persons naturally infected at an earlier date, BCG vacinees and tuberculin negatives. The information has implications for post-exposure surveillance of TB and for its prevention and control.

The incubation period for primary pulmonary TB had not been defined accurately because point-source outbreaks with single exposures were rare and the dates of onset of first symptoms were often vague because the symptoms are relatively mild (flu-like). This epidemic is one of the few with onsets specified to weeks. Experimental animals take 1–3 months for tuberculin conversion after inoculation. These girls developed acute primary TB after inhaling TB organisms that lodged in their lungs. Primary TB is usually self-healing and the organisms become dormant in the lungs. The usual situation is that, months to years later, post-primary pulmonary TB may develop with chronic coughing and production by some cases of infectious aerosols, usually related to the development of lung cavities connecting to the airway. This is the debilitating and frequently fatal condition generally called 'tuberculosis'.

Conclusion

To conclude this chapter we reiterate that the principles used apply to all disease outbreaks, communicable or otherwise. We have focussed on infectious diseases to introduce their special features which had not been covered by the predominantly chronic disease examples used in other sections of this book.

Questions

The Public Health Training Network of the US Centers for Disease Control and Prevention has developed some excellent computer-based exercises in outbreak investigation. These are freely available from http://www.phppo.cdc.gov/phtn/casestudies/.

The following questions relate to the TB case study described at the end of the chapter.

1. Use the epidemic curve in Figure 12.7 to help estimate the probable time of exposure and the incubation period.
2. Were the initial investigations in March 1943 (Table 12.2) based on a case–control or cohort approach to investigating an epidemic? What sort of study was the subsequent 12-year follow-up (Table 12.3)? What biases or confounders could have arisen?
3. What types of measure (cumulative incidences, prevalence, attack rates or other estimates) are shown in the last column of Table 12.2?
4. Comment on the absence of tuberculin in groups C and D of Table 12.2. Do you think these groups are really different from groups A and B (i.e., is the difference likely to be statistically significant), or are the numbers of students in these two groups too small to warrant confident conclusions?
5. From the information yielded by this outbreak, would you prefer your tuberculin status to be
   • naturally positive, i.e., infected at some unidentified time in the past;
   • BCG-induced, i.e., converted by receiving BCG after a negative test result;
   • recently converted; or
   • tuberculin negative?
6. What has this report shown about the mode of transmission of TB?

REFERENCES

AJE (*American Journal of Epidemiology*). (1990). Volume **132**, supplement.

Benenson, A. S., Ed. (1990). *Control of Communicable Diseases in Man*, 15th edn. Washington: American Public Health Association.

Chan-Yeung, M. and Yu, W. C. (2003). Outbreak of severe acute respiratory syndrome in Hong Kong Special Administrative Region: case report. *British Medical Journal*, **326**: 850–852.

Collins, S., Boyd, A., Fletcher, A. *et al.* (2002). Creutzfeldt–Jakob disease cluster in an Australian rural city. *Annals of Neurology*, **52**: 115–118.

Deng, J. F., Fleeger, A. K. and Sinks, T. (1990). An outbreak of chromium ulcer in a manufacturing plant. *Veterinary and Human Toxicology*, **32**: 142–146.

Editorial. (2001). Disease clusters and ecological studies. *Journal of the Royal Statistical Society*, **164**: 1–2.

Hales, S., de Wet, N., Maindonald, J. and Woodward, A. (2002). Potential effect of population and climate changes on global distribution of dengue fever: an empirical model. *Lancet*, **360**: 830–834.

Haddad, V. and Sazima, I. (2003). Piranha attacks on humans, in southeast Brazil: epidemiology, natural history, and clinical treatment, with description of a bite outbreak. *Wilderness and Environmental Medicine*, **14**: 249–254.

Hameed, S. M., Popkin, C. A., Cohn, S. M. and Johnson, E. W. (2004). The epidemic of pediatric traffic injuries in South Florida: a review of the problem and initial results of a prospective surveillance strategy. *American Journal of Public Health*, **94**: 554–556.

Hyge, T. V. (1947). Epidemic of tuberculosis in a state school. *Acta Tuberculosea Scandinavica*, **XXI**: 1–57.
  (1957). The efficacy of BCG vaccination. Tuberculosis epidemic in a state school with an observation period of 12 years. *Danish Medical Bulletin*, **4**: 13–15.

Kraus, J. and Robertson, L. S. (1992). Injuries and public health. In J. M. Last and R. B. Wallace (Eds.), *Public Health and Preventive Medicine*. Norwalk, N: Appleton and Lange.

Langmuir, A. D. (1961). Keynote address. Epidemiology of airborne infections. *Bacteriological Reviews*, **25**: 173–181.

Last, J. M., Ed. (2001). *A Dictionary of Epidemiology*, 4th edn. New York: Oxford University Press.

Li, Y., Yu, I. T. S., Xu, P. *et al.* (2004). Predicting super spreading events during the 2003 severe acute respiratory syndrome epidemics in Hong Kong and Singapore. *American Journal of Epidemiology*, 160: 719–728.

Olsen, S. F., Martuzzi, M. and Elliott, P. (1996). Cluster analysis and disease mapping – why, when, and how? A step by step guide. *British Medical Journal*, **313**: 863–866.

Peiris, J. S., Yu, W. C., Leung, C. W. *et al.* (2004). Re-emergence of fatal human influenza A subtype H5N1 disease. *Lancet*, **363**: 617–619.

Snow, J. (1855). *On the Mode of Communication of Cholera*, 2nd edn. London: Churchill. (Source: http://www.ph.ucla.edu/epi/snow/snowbook.html.)

von Overbeck, J. (2003). Insurance and epidemics: SARS, West Nile virus and Nipah virus. *Journal of Insurance Medicine*, **35**: 165–173.

WHO (World Health Organization). (2003). *The World Health Report 2003, Shaping the Future*. Geneva: WHO.

Prevention: better than cure?

'Prevention is better than cure' as the saying goes. Or, more poetically, according to T. Adams (1618) 'Prevention is so much better than healing, because it saves the labour of being sick.'

With the exception of a few areas of medicine – obstetrics for example – the primary role of a clinician is to treat people who are sick. In population health we would prefer that people did not become ill in the first place (although we acknowledge that disease control also requires more effective treatments). So prevention stands as our ideal, and epidemiology underpins much of our work in this area. In particular, it provides quantitative measures of relative and absolute risk that help direct preventive action; and it plays a major role in evaluating whether preventive programmes actually work in practice. Additionally, what we might term the 'epidemiological perspective' is helpful in conceptualising both the practical and the ethical elements of prevention.

Disease prevention in public health

When we speak of prevention, we usually mean **primary prevention**, which aims to prevent disease from occurring in the first place, i.e., to reduce the incidence of disease. Vaccination against childhood infectious diseases is a good example of primary prevention, as is the use of sunscreen to prevent the development of skin cancer. Figure 13.1 shows tuberculosis (TB) mortality over time in England and Wales. This is a disease that had all but disappeared from developed countries but is now re-emerging elsewhere as a worldwide scourge.

How important were the BCG vaccine and new therapy in terms of the decline in TB mortality?

Figure 13.1 and other historical trends make it clear that major health gains were made before the advent of sophisticated medical therapies and preventive measures. Social and cultural changes such as improved housing, sanitation, general hygiene and nutrition have had the major influence on TB mortality,

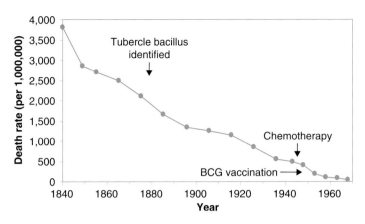

Fig. 13.1 Age-standardised death rates from tuberculosis in England and Wales, 1840–1968. (From McKeown, *The Role of Medicine. Dream, Mirage or Nemesis?* (1979), with permission from Blackwell Publishing.)

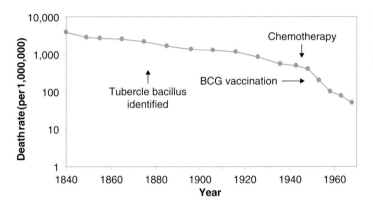

Fig. 13.2 Age-standardised death rates from tuberculosis in England and Wales, 1840–1968, plotted on a logarithmic scale.

presumably both by reducing incidence and by increasing survival. The effects of such 'upstream' effects on disease incidence are sometimes termed *primordial prevention*, because they stem from influences further removed from the more proximal causes that medicine and public health usually deal with. Our view is that the upstream and proximal causes are inter-related and in practice it can be difficult to distinguish the two; any intervention that lowers incidence is thus sensibly termed *primary* prevention.

So, should we dismiss the value of the proximal strategies for TB control? (Note that BCG vaccination was introduced later in the UK than in Denmark, as shown in the example at the end of the previous chapter.) Certainly, on the absolute scale of Figure 13.1, their contribution seems marginal. Would mortality have declined any less quickly if there had been no BCG vaccine and no chemotherapy? Consider Figure 13.2, which shows the same information plotted on a log scale so that a 50% reduction in mortality looks the same regardless of whether the drop is from a death rate of 4,000 to 2,000 per million or from 40 to 20 per million. By graphing the rates logarithmically, Figure 13.2 depicts the *rate of change*.

We now see a slow and steady fall in mortality across the first 80 years that quickens slightly around 1920. The slope steepens just after the introduction of chemotherapy and continues to fall following the introduction of BCG vaccination. These are hardly definitive evaluations of the benefits of these advances, but the acceleration of the fall in mortality around 1950 implies that something has changed and the introductions of vaccination and treatment are the best candidates.

While the principal goal of public health should first and foremost be primary prevention, for many diseases we do not have enough information (biological and/or epidemiological) to mount such a programme effectively (or cost-effectively). Even when we do have sufficient information, the barriers to implementation may be substantial (e.g., financial, cultural, social, ethical). For example, we know already that ensuring everyone has access to clean water would prevent a large proportion of infectious disease, but the practical and financial implications are enormous. Similarly, by persuading people to stop smoking, stay out of the sun, drive safely, exercise more and eat better we could prevent much chronic disease, but changing behaviour remains a major challenge.

Additional strategies are therefore required in order to enhance disease control and, rather confusingly, some of these have also been labelled as prevention. So-called *secondary prevention* is directed towards reducing morbidity and mortality by improving the outcome of disease that has already developed. Generally this means early diagnosis by screening, thereby allowing earlier (and presumably more effective) intervention, which we cover in more detail in Chapter 14. *Tertiary prevention* is even more remote from the everyday concept of disease avoidance, usually implying better rehabilitation or quality of life in the longer term.

In terms of *disease control* it is more useful to distinguish between preventive interventions (primary prevention) and actions that lead to improved clinical outcomes once disease occurs. The former act through lowering incidence of disease and hence limiting clinical burden from that disease, while the latter, e.g., screening, can actually lead to large increases in clinical activity.

Decisions as to the most appropriate approach for disease control are disease-specific: less disease is most desirable, but might not be attainable if causal knowledge is limited. Screening may be a good second choice in some circumstances if advancing diagnosis really does produce better outcomes. Finally, improvements in treatment remain an important avenue for enhancing quality of life for affected individuals. Table 13.1 contrasts two cancers with markedly different control profiles, showing epidemiological and other research findings.

The solution to the lung cancer epidemic is obvious, and concerted multi-level efforts (ranging from targeting individual behaviours to banning advertising and legislating for smoke-free public space) have made big inroads on lung cancer rates in many countries (see Figure 6.2). Nonetheless, it remains a common disease, so efforts to improve clinical outcomes through early detection and better treatments are also important, although their yield to date has been slight.

Table 13.1 The role of epidemiological knowledge in disease control: a case of two cancers.

	Accepted utility for widescale use	
Intervention	Lung cancer	Breast cancer
Prevention	YES. Smoking cigarettes is *the* strong risk factor; and exposure is modifiable by actions at personal and community levels.	NO. Many weak risk factors, most not readily modifiable.
Screening	NO. Even the newest tests (computed-tomography lung scans) yield very limited survival benefits.	YES. Substantial good evidence (from RCTs) of lower mortality due to population screening programmes for over 50s.
Improved treatment	NO. Minor survival improvements only with newer treatments.	YES. Results from RCTs show that a survival advantage can be achieved with appropriate chemotherapy/radiotherapy.

Fig. 13.3 Age-adjusted breast cancer mortality rates per 100,000/year, for Whites in the USA, 1980–2001. (*Data source:* Health, United States, 2003 spreadsheet for Table 40 from www.cdc/nchs/hus.htm, accessed 31 March 2004.)

With breast cancer we see the reverse situation. Quite a lot is known about its aetiology, but no established causal factor offers a basis for widespread intervention. Instead, dual approaches to decreasing morbidity and mortality, namely population screening by mammography to detect early lesions along with more effective non-surgical treatments, have paid off. There have been downturns in mortality from breast cancer in a number of countries from the early 1990s

(Figure 13.3). This suggests that the improved outcomes predicted by tightly controlled clinical trials have transferred reasonably effectively to the community
setting. It is salutary to note the crudeness of the tool commonly used to evaluate
the effects of interventions in the community (i.e., routine descriptive data) and
also that this cannot separate out the relative contributions of early diagnosis and
improved treatment.

We will not consider clinical contributions to disease control any further
here – rather our discussion will focus largely on the applications of both
epidemiological data and epidemiological thinking to disease prevention and
screening. For the former we will concentrate on the conceptual underpinnings
of the preventive approach and some current practical concerns and challenges.
In Chapter 14 we will consider screening in terms of its underlying logic, and
the major challenges to evaluating its contributions to the control of any given
disease.

Box 13.1 Choosing a preventive strategy: the whole story

An important aside to the lung cancer story is that anti-smoking campaigns
have also greatly reduced incidence of other respiratory disease and heart
disease. While causal research is primarily disease-specific, preventive
interventions manipulate exposures that may have many consequences.
Thus we need good information on the full array of effects of any exposure
we plan on modifying: a strong association with one disease is generally
insufficient in itself. Immunisation campaigns against infectious diseases
would seem an obvious exception to this, but they have lowered incidence
so dramatically that fewer lives are now saved and the occasional severe
side-effects of immunisation start to take a more prominent place on the
balance sheet. Although virtually every consequence of decreased exposure
to cigarettes is positive and thus the total benefit-to-cost ratio is huge,
counter-examples for which complexity is the rule abound. For example,
moderate alcohol consumption is linked to *lower* heart disease but *higher*
breast cancer rates and, at high intakes, it is associated with an array of other
health and social problems.

How do we combine the different effects on morbidity and mortality for
various diseases? Does the benefit of avoiding one non-fatal stroke obtained
by long-term aspirin use outweigh the risk of three new life-threatening
gastric bleeds? Measures such as DALYs and HALYs now provide a qualitative
method of doing this, but these are rarely used in primary research
publications. (Note: there are many guides available to aid decision making
in the clinical setting; see, e.g., Hunink *et al.* (2001).)

The scope for preventive medicine

Our earlier examples of disease variation by person, place and time have shown that there are large differences between groups, suggesting that much disease should be preventable if only we could lower everyone's risk to that of the lower-risk populations. Another striking example comes from an investigation seeking an explanation for the three-fold excess of cardiovascular disease (CVD) mortality in Finland compared with China. Contemporaneous surveys carried out in rural villages in the two countries revealed quite different profiles of CVD risk factors (Table 13.2). The first three factors, all more prevalent in Finland, could be taken as related to over-nutrition, and possibly to the fat content of the diet. Given China's history of major famines in the mid twentieth century it is not surprising that differences remain so profound, at least in a rural population. Countries undergoing the health transition (away from a predominance of infectious diseases and problems of marginal nutrition) are, in principle, ripe for intervention to prevent the emergence of Western lifestyle diseases, many of which are related to over-consumption and inactivity. However, social engineering is challenging, and the pace of development and industrialisation in Chinese cities suggests that the risk-factor profiles there are already less favourable than those in rural China. Table 13.2 also reflects the different attitudes to control of smoking, with predictable negative consequences for China that are already emerging in the rising lung cancer and CVD rates there.

Population versus individual risk

There is a tendency in medicine and epidemiology to try to divide people into two groups – those who have a high risk of developing a particular disease and those at low risk. For instance, a woman of child-bearing age with high blood pressure, who

Table 13.2 A comparison of prevalence of CVD risk factors between Finnish and Chinese village populations aged 20–64 years.[a]

Risk factor	Men		Women	
	Finns (%)	Chinese (%)	Finns (%)	Chinese (%)
Being overweight	63	21	61	24
Obesity	19	2	24	5
Hypercholesterolaemia	34	3	28	6
Hypertension	49	32	35	28
Smoking	26	73	7	37

[a]All differences were statistically significant ($p < 0.001$, except $p < 0.05$ for hypertension among women). (Hu *et al.*, 2001.)

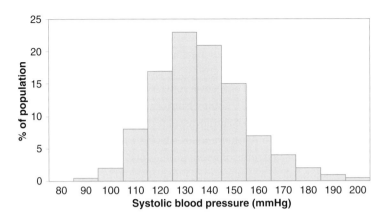

Fig. 13.4 Distribution of systolic blood pressure in a population of middle-aged men. (Adapted from Figure 2.1, *The Strategy of Preventive Medicine*, G. Rose (1992), by permission of Oxford University Press.)

smokes and has a family history of blood clotting would be considered at high risk of complications if she took the oral contraceptive pill and this would not be prescribed. In population terms, however, the benefits of the pill are well recognised to outweigh harms, and it is widely prescribed – not, of course, primarily for prevention of disease (although it does prevent ovarian and endometrial cancers).

So, how should we think about our approaches to preventing ill-health? Should we devote most of our attention to the high-risk groups? This has been the basis of the vast improvements in occupational health and safety since the industrial revolution, and remains an appropriate approach for other specifically disadvantaged or exposed groups, including many indigenous peoples. However, risk of disease is not a simple high–low phenomenon and there are few well-defined natural borders between clearly different levels of risk. As an example, consider the relationship between blood pressure and risk of fatal CVD. Figure 13.4 shows the wide range of 'usual' blood pressure levels in a population. Individuals do not clearly fall into two separate groups with low and high blood pressure and do not, therefore, have a clear-cut 'low' or 'high' risk of heart disease.

As discussed by Rose (1992), the Whitehall cohort study of British public servants showed that the age-adjusted risk of dying from CVD over the 18-year follow-up period increased with increasing blood pressure. The results are shown in Figure 13.5.

In Figure 13.5, is there any level of systolic blood pressure that is not 'riskier' than the one below it?

Looking at Figures 13.4 and 13.5, how many men in a population of 10,000 would have a systolic blood pressure of 150 mm Hg? What is the risk (cumulative incidence) of dying from CVD in this group?

So how many men with a blood pressure of 150 mm Hg will die from CVD? What about those with a blood pressure of 170 mm Hg?

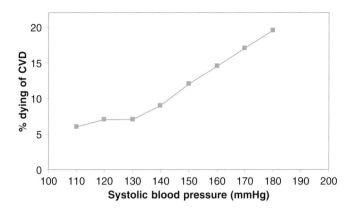

Fig. 13.5 The relationship between systolic blood pressure and risk of fatal coronary heart disease or stroke over 18 years of follow-up. (From Figure 2.2, *The Strategy of Preventive Medicine*, G. Rose (1992), by permission of Oxford University Press.)

Box 13.2 A clinical perspective

The example in the text shows the population perspective on prevention: at the community level more CVD deaths would be prevented by focussing on the larger numbers of people at intermediate risk than on the few at high risk. But let us focus on the individual for a moment: lowering an individual's blood pressure from 150 to 120 mm Hg would reduce their risk of CVD from 12% to about 7%, an absolute risk reduction of 5%. This then translates to a 'number needed to treat' (NNT) of 20 (1 ÷ 0.05) in order to prevent one CVD death. Similarly, lowering an individual's blood pressure from 170 to 120 mm Hg would reduce their risk of CVD from 17% to about 7%, an absolute risk reduction of 10%, which gives an NNT of 10. At the individual level, therefore, the benefits are greatest for those at highest risk. This highlights that what is best for the individual is not necessarily best for the population and vice versa.

From Figure 13.5 we can infer that the risk of dying from CVD at any level of blood pressure is greater than that at the level below. The risk increases slowly up to 140 mm Hg and then increases more sharply. From Figure 13.4 we can estimate that 15% or 1,500 of a population of 10,000 men would have a blood pressure around 150 mm Hg, and from Figure 13.5 the risk of dying of CVD in this group is 12% over the 18 years of follow-up. We would, therefore, expect about 12% $\times$ 1,500 = 180 CVD deaths in this group. Similarly, 4% or 400 of the population would have a blood pressure of 170 mm Hg and they have a 17% risk of dying of CVD. We would therefore expect about 17% $\times$ 400 = 68 CVD deaths in this group. Thus, although the risk of dying of CVD is greater for those with higher blood pressure, many more CVD deaths will actually occur among the much larger number of people with intermediate blood pressure. Targeting prevention at only those with very high blood pressure will not, therefore, address the majority of deaths (Box 13.2).

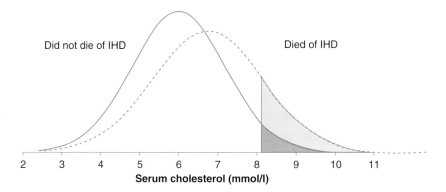

Fig. 13.6 Relative distributions of serum cholesterol levels in men who subsequently died of ischaemic heart disease and men who did not. (From Wald and Law, *BMJ*, 2003; **326**: 1419–1425, reproduced with permission from BMJ Publishing Group.)

Figure 13.6 shows a concrete example of the close overlap in risk-factor distributions (in this case serum cholesterol level) between those who did and did not subsequently die from ischaemic heart disease (IHD). The whole curve for those who died from IHD is clearly shifted to the right, but the two overlap considerably and the cut-off point identifying the extreme upper 5% of the 'healthy' cohort identifies only 15% of those who will develop IHD. Again screening for high-risk individuals is not a good preventive strategy.

Strategies for prevention

Choosing the best way to intervene in order to lower disease risk in a specific population will often be a challenge. We present below some brief comments on the theoretical extremes of practice, the *high-risk* and the *mass* or population strategies. Although we have seen why the mass strategy is widely considered to be preferable, it might not always be practical. To borrow from the old definition of politics, skill in the art of identifying the possible is needed.

The high-risk strategy

Classically, preventive medicine takes the high-risk approach, a targeted rescue operation for vulnerable individuals. First, those individuals in special need are identified (e.g., intravenous drug users). The preventive process then takes the form of controlling the level of exposure to a cause (e.g., introduction of a needle-exchange programme) or providing protection against the consequences of the exposure to forestall complications (e.g., vaccination against hepatitis B) in this high-risk group.

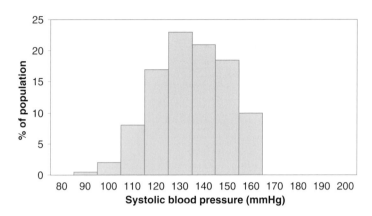

Fig. 13.7 The hypothetical distribution of systolic blood pressure in middle-aged men after applying a 'high-risk' screening strategy. (Adapted from Figure 4.1, *The Strategy of Preventive Medicine*, G. Rose (1992), by permission of Oxford University Press.)

Another example can be found in the blood pressure problem we discussed earlier. We might decide that the high-risk patients are those with a systolic blood pressure over 160 mm Hg. The high-risk strategy would then involve screening out those individuals with high blood pressure, followed by intervention to ensure that their blood pressure is brought below this level. This remains a common approach in clinical practice and, if fully applied, might lead to a population blood pressure distribution like that in Figure 13.7. If we compare this graph with Figure 13.4, we can see that those who were in the upper tail have lowered their blood pressure, and thus presumably their CVD risk, but the main group among whom most cases will occur is unaffected.

High-risk strategies appeal for a number of reasons. The intervention is well matched to individuals and their concerns (e.g., a needle-exchange programme is a specific and tailored response to a tightly defined group), and thus should also improve the benefit-to-risk and benefit-to-cost ratios. Furthermore, avoiding interference with the non-needy group and adopting a 'magic bullet' approach to the target group are readily accommodated within the ethos of the medical care system.

So, can the high-risk strategy play a useful preventive role? Of course, it remains highly appropriate and desirable in clinical practice. If, at the community level, a problem is confined to an identifiable minority and can be successfully controlled in isolation, then the high-risk approach can also be appropriate. However, on its own it is an inadequate response to a common disease or a widespread cause and we need to be very cautious in claiming that a risk really is sufficiently limited to the so-called high-risk group. For example, screening only older pregnant women, who are known to be at highest risk of conceiving a child with Down's syndrome, will miss the majority of afflicted fetuses, which are conceived by younger women in whom most pregnancies occur.

Fig. 13.8 The distribution of systolic blood pressure in a population of middle-aged men before and after a hypothetical intervention. (From Figure 6.5, *The Strategy of Preventive Medicine*, G. Rose (1992), by permission of Oxford University Press.)

The mass strategy

In the case of a common disease or widespread cause, the alternative approach is the mass or population strategy. This starts with the recognition that the occurrence of common diseases and exposures reflects the behaviour and circumstances of society as a whole. The mass strategy thus aims to reduce the health risks of the entire population.

Using the blood pressure data again, we can illustrate a mass-strategy approach to this problem. Instead of targeting only those people with the highest blood pressure, we would aim to reduce everybody's blood pressure by a smaller amount. This would shift both the blood pressure and the CVD risk of the population to a lower level (Figure 13.8). This is a much healthier situation for the whole group (although perhaps not for some highest-risk individuals) than the truncated distribution we saw in Figure 13.7.

Other examples of the mass strategy are immunisation programmes and water fluoridation, as is the legislated use of seat belts for the entire population rather than simply for male drivers under the age of 25 years who are at the greatest risk of dying in a motor-vehicle accident. (Imagine the problems of implementing a 'high-risk' approach to seat-belt use.) Other background and personal aspects of the causal web for motor-vehicle-related deaths and injuries (see Figure 12.3) have also been targeted effectively in many countries, including better road and barrier engineering, car structural safety and legislation backed by enforcement to curb speeding and drink-driving.

Prevention in practice

Box 13.3 describes an innovative population-wide suicide-prevention programme that was developed explicitly from Rose's ideal model of population change.

Box 13.3 Flying higher: the US Air Force suicide prevention programme

Suicide rates in the US Air Force increased notably in the early 1990s, leading to a concerted effort by senior staff to halt and reverse this trend. After piloting, a multilayered population-based prevention programme was introduced in 1996 to reduce risk factors and enhance protective factors among the more than 5 million personnel. The intervention focussed on removing the stigma from mental health problems, enhancing understanding of mental health, and changing policies and social norms. Strong and continuing endorsement of the initiative by senior leaders was a critical element. The approach adopted was explicitly a population-oriented risk-reduction approach. Its effectiveness was measured by comparison of suicide rates before and after the intervention: overall suicide was reduced by 33% (Figure 13.9) (Knox *et al.*, 2003).

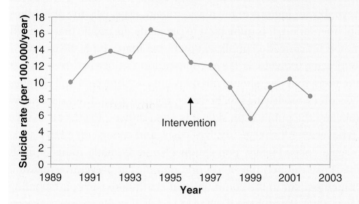

Fig. 13.9 Suicide rates in the US Air Force before and after the population-based intervention in 1996–1997. (*Data source:* Knox *et al.*, 2003.)

How highly would you rate this study design for evaluating such a programme?

How easily can we generalise from these findings to, say, the US population as a whole?

The actual study design used is a simple pre–post-intervention comparison of suicide rates (i.e., descriptive data). It would be nice to have RCT data on this issue but, for pretty obvious reasons, it is very difficult to conduct such a trial on this scale. Furthermore, since the interventions have to be applied to an entire community, not just to individuals, it would have to be a cluster randomised trial with only a few large groups and so would miss out on the core benefits of randomisation.

A trial would, however, avoid the possible confounding of pre–post studies when there are underlying time trends in suicide rates that are independent of any intervention. (In this particular situation the unexposed and exposed cohorts, pre- and post-intervention, are likely to have been quite similar with regard to 'internal' confounders.) While the summary figures indicate the programme's likely benefit, we can see from Figure 13.9 that the pattern of change for suicide is not simple to interpret. It would be helpful to see the longer-term pattern before 1990, and the future rates will be telling.

Generalising the specific findings to the whole population is more problematic, but the underlying theories may well apply more generally. Taken at face value, these results show that the mass strategy is capable of addressing the underlying social, economic and political determinants of ill-health in a population, and need not be restricted to immediate causes. It is also a desirable approach to intervention because it aims to change not only the risk factors, but also the context in which they are embedded: it is easier to seek help for a problem, or give up smoking, for example, if the rest of the population is supportive.

There are inevitably limitations to the mass strategy, especially the difficulties of effective implementation. It is quite hard to persuade the public that a health problem is a matter for concerted public action rather than simply the responsibility of the few affected individuals. If everyone wants to smoke or drive cars fast then persuading them that they should not do is not easy (the enforced changes in society's views on drink-driving are, however, encouraging). Even if we know what is desirable and the public is on side, it is often difficult to effect a change (e.g., to reduce poverty). All change involves costs, and change on a large scale involves large-scale costs. Finally, population change is made more difficult because of what Rose dubbed the *prevention paradox*: 'a preventive measure which brings much benefit to the community offers little to each participating individual' (Rose, 1981). We all have to change our risk profile (by wearing seat belts, changing our behaviour, etc.), but the only people who really benefit are the unidentifiable minority among us whose seat belt will save them in an accident or who would have died from CVD if they had not reduced their blood pressure. In practice we often fall short of fully informing the populace of the very limited individual benefits that result from mass prevention programmes (and screening programmes; see Chapter 14).

Let us end this chapter on a more upbeat note. The editor of the *British Medical Journal* speculated that the 28 June 2003 edition might be 'The most important *BMJ* for 50 years' (Smith, 2003). He referred to an article by Wald and Law (2003) proposing the 'Polypill', a six-drugs-in-one cardiovascular panacea that might prevent 80% of all vascular morbidity and mortality beyond the age of 55 by reducing blood pressure (a three-drug cocktail), serum levels of LDL cholesterol (a statin) and homocysteine (folate), and clotting tendency (aspirin). Their quantification of the benefits and risks of such a pill is based on combining

Frank and Ernest

© 2003 Thaves. Reprinted with permission. Newspaper dist. by NEA, Inc.

relevant evidence from RCTs and long-term cohort studies drawn from a series of systematic reviews and meta-analyses. They recommend implementing a population strategy aimed to shift the whole cardiovascular 'risk curve' well to the left, exactly the sort of outcome of which Rose would have approved. This achieves the same preventive end as the Air Force suicide intervention programme by moderating whole-of-population risk, but the onus on achieving the goal is shifted from society to the individual, from primary structural and behavioural change to life-long pill taking (and if compliance is not high the benefits shrink rapidly). Whether this 'medicalisation' of a society is desirable or acceptable is contentious, and the paper has engendered debate.

REFERENCES

Adams, T. (1618). *Happiness of Church*; p. 146.

Hu, G., Pekkarinen, H., Halonen, P. *et al.* (2001). Different worlds, different tasks for health promotion: comparisons of health risk profiles in Chinese and Finnish rural people. *Health Promotion International,* **16**: 315–320.

Hunink, M., Glasziou, P., Siegel, J. *et al.* (2001). *Decision Making in Health and Medicine.* Cambridge: Cambridge University Press.

Knox, K. L., Litts, D. A., Talcott, G. W., Feig, J. C. and Caine, E. D. (2003). Risk of suicide and related adverse outcomes after exposure to a suicide prevention programme in the US Air Force: a cohort study. *British Medical Journal,* **327**: 1376–1380.

McKeown, T. (1979). *The Role of Medicine. Dream, Mirage or Nemesis?* Oxford: Blackwell Publishing.

Rose, G. (1981). Strategy of prevention: lessons from cardiovascular disease. *British Medical Journal,* **282**: 1847–1851.

(1992). *The Strategy of Preventive Medicine.* London: Oxford University Press.

Smith, R. (2003). The most important BMJ for 50 years? *British Medical Journal,* **326**: un-numbered pages at the beginning of issue 7404.

Wald, N. J. and Law, M. R. (2003). A strategy to reduce cardiovascular disease by more than 80%. *British Medical Journal,* **326**: 1419–1425.

Early detection: what benefits at what cost?

The major public health value of screening is the potential for earlier detection of disease to give improved health outcomes (with an emphasis on improved outcomes – see Box 14.1 above). Here we will introduce you to the requirements of a successful screening programme and to some of the problems that we encounter when trying to determine whether such a programme is actually beneficial in practice.

Why screen?

The aim of screening is to detect disease before the usual time of diagnosis. When used as a public health measure for disease control, screening implies the widespread use of a simple test for disease in an apparently healthy (asymptomatic) population. A screening test will often not diagnose the presence of disease directly but will instead separate people who are more likely to have the disease from those who are less likely to have it. Those who may have the disease (i.e., those who screen positive) can then undergo further diagnostic tests and treatment if necessary.

The improved public health outcomes we seek through screening are reduced morbidity, mortality and/or disability. The benefits of public health screening are primarily for those who are actually screened, and generally even among them only very few will benefit directly, but it may also lead to wider social benefits if overall health costs are reduced.

Screening is also used, in a slightly different fashion, to protect the general population from exposure to disease. As an example, immigrants to a number of countries are screened for HIV and hepatitis B infection. This is not done primarily for the benefit of the individual who is screened, but to protect the local population from these viruses. Similarly, some occupations require regular screening; for example airline pilots have regular medical checks in an attempt to ensure that they will not have a heart attack while flying. Insurance companies often require people to undergo health checks and screening before they offer them a life insurance policy. Here the 'screening' is done for purely financial reasons, because insurance companies charge higher premiums for people at higher risk.

The disease process

The first we know of the existence of disease in a person is when it is diagnosed. This is usually some time after it first produces the symptoms which cause the person to seek medical care. The actual onset of disease will naturally be earlier than this – how much earlier depends on the disease concerned. Figure 14.1 illustrates this point.

At some stage between the onset of disease and the time of usual diagnosis there may come a time when early signs of disease are there, if only we could detect them. The position of this point will vary depending on the disease, perhaps occurring many years before the appearance of clinical disease (e.g., high blood pressure, some cancers), or it may occur only shortly before symptoms appear (e.g., acute infectious diseases).

At some stage during the disease process there is also likely to be a *critical point*, after which the disease process is irreversible and treatment will confer little or no benefit. An example might be the point at which a cancer starts spreading to other tissues (metastasis). If this 'point of no return' occurs before it is possible to detect the disease (CP1 in Figure 14.1) then advancing the time of detection will simply mean that the person knows about their disease for longer

Fig. 14.1 The natural history of a disease (adapted from Sackett *et al.*, 1991).

but their outcome will not be improved. Similarly, if this point occurs after the usual time of diagnosis (CP3) there is no need to detect the disease any earlier, given that treatment following usual diagnosis will be effective.

Screening is, then, of greatest potential benefit when such a critical point occurs at CP2 – between the time of first possible detection and the usual time of diagnosis. It may then be possible to improve outcome by picking up the disease early, and this is the aim of a screening programme. Unfortunately, we currently have too little knowledge of the progress of most diseases for this to have much practical value in planning screening programmes.

Screening versus case-finding

Debate about the best way to implement early detection of disease continues. Should the focus be on large-scale mass population screening, or are we better off pursuing opportunistic early detection (case-finding) when someone comes into contact with the health system for another reason? There are some parallels here with the mass versus high-risk approach to primary prevention, but they are not exact. The terms 'screening' and 'case-finding' can also have quite different meanings to different practitioners. We think it is most useful, and best accepted, to use the term 'screening' for organised population-wide approaches and 'case-finding' for more opportunistic attempts at early detection. If systematically applied, the latter approach can nonetheless form the basis for quite good population coverage. If a large proportion of the people visit a primary care physician within the desired screening interval, this contact could permit early detection of risks (e.g., cigarette smoking, high blood pressure) in a setting that allows good follow-up.

The requirements of a screening programme

Screening differs from diagnostic testing in that it is performed *before* the development of clinical disease. Those who undergo screening are thus free, or appear to be free, of the disease of interest. They are not seeking care because they are sick, but are instead persuaded to be screened by the health services. The requirements of a screening test are, therefore, quite distinct from those of a diagnostic test, which is performed only when someone is suspected to have a disease. The suitability of a *disease* for screening has to be considered explicitly; the quality and acceptability of the *screening test* must be demonstrated; and the whole *programme* must be shown to confer a net benefit to the community.

The disease

We need to consider the following characteristics of a disease before deciding whether screening for it is desirable.

- The disease should be severe, relatively common and perceived as a public health problem by the community.
- We must understand the natural history of the disease sufficiently well that we can be reasonably sure that earlier detection will give a better outcome. Prostate cancer shows us the importance of this. It appears to occur in a number of biological forms that we cannot tell apart, and it is probable that many men in whom a cancer could be detected by screening (e.g., with a PSA test) would never develop symptoms or suffer from the disease (and therefore would not otherwise be diagnosed). To detect and treat these men would be wholly harmful and, largely for this reason, screening for prostate cancer is generally not recommended, even though there are tests that could be used. Research is under way in a number of countries in an attempt to shed light on this dilemma and allow a more informed judgement to be made.
- In general, there should be a high prevalence of pre-clinical (early-stage) disease. This criterion becomes less important as the severity of the disease increases. For example, it may be of benefit to screen for a fairly uncommon disease if not treating it has severe consequences – an example is the use of screening for phenylketonuria (PKU) in new-borns. Babies born with this condition lack an enzyme that metabolises the amino acid phenylalanine. When they eat proteins containing this amino acid the end-products accumulate in the brain, leading to severe mental retardation. By simply restricting the phenylalanine in their diet this can be prevented. Although only about one in 15,000 babies is born with this condition, the availability of a simple, accurate and inexpensive test makes it worthwhile to screen all new-born babies (Wilcken *et al.*, 2003).
- Screening is likely to be more effective if there is a long period between the first detectable signs of disease and the overt symptoms that normally lead to

diagnosis (the *lead time*). If a disease progresses rapidly from the pre-clinical to clinical stages then early intervention is less likely to be of benefit, and it is much harder to catch the disease in the more benign phase. (Clearly metabolic conditions of early life, such as PKU, are exceptions to this).

The screening test

The next requirement for a worthwhile screening programme is that we have a test that will enable us to detect the disease before the usual time of diagnosis. Any such test that we use must meet the following criteria.

- It should be both *accurate* and *reliable*. Accuracy reflects the degree to which the results of the test correspond to the true state of the phenomenon being measured and most of the following discussion deals with test accuracy. In terms of reliability, suffice it to say that it is usually related either to the standardisation or calibration of the testing apparatus or to the skill and expertise of the persons interpreting the test. So what should we expect of a screening test? We would expect it to be

  sensitive – ideally it would identify *all* people with the disease; in practice, it should identify *most* of these people.

  specific – ideally it would identify *only* those with that particular disease; in practice, *most* of those identified should have the disease.

- It must be *safe* and *acceptable* to the population being screened. Since we are advising apparently well people to undergo screening, we should not offer them a test that might adversely affect their health. The only exception might be for those at very high risk of developing a serious disease, when a slight risk from screening might be outweighed by a large benefit of early diagnosis (e.g., regular colonoscopy for people with ulcerative colitis, who develop large bowel cancer at a high rate). Social and cultural acceptability is a separate issue and is seldom related to the safety of the screening test. For example, cervical cancer screening is not immediately appealing in many societies and in some it may be prohibited, particularly if the health professional is male. Likewise, persuading people to take a sample of their faeces to test for blood as an early indicator of colon cancer is unpalatable to many.

- It should be *simple* and *cheap*. If we wish to screen a large proportion of the population any test used should be relatively cheap to administer and simple to perform or it would be too costly to perform large-scale screening.

Mammography is neither simple nor cheap. Why then do you think that mammographic screening to detect early breast cancer is recommended?

Although mammography is neither simple nor cheap, breast cancer is a severe disease of substantial concern to many communities. It occurs relatively commonly and, if detected early, is usually highly treatable.

Table 14.1 Hypothetical results from a school hearing test programme.

School hearing test	True hearing status		
	Hearing problem	Normal	Total
Fail (positive test result)	45	30	75
Pass (negative test result)	5	420	425
Total	50	450	500

Fig. 14.2 Possible outcomes from a screening test.

Test performance

We can evaluate the performance of a test by comparing the results with a 'gold standard' method that ideally would give 100% correct results (but more commonly is the best test available). This standard might be a more costly or time-consuming test, or perhaps a combination of investigations performed in hospital that is reliable for diagnosis but unsuitable for routine use in screening.

For example, children in many countries undergo a simple hearing test in their first year at school. Any who fail this screening test are retested at a later date and/or referred to a hearing clinic for further, more extensive tests to identify whether they have a real hearing problem. Imagine that, in a group of 500 children, 50 have a genuine hearing problem. Of these, 45 fail the school hearing test, as do 30 of the children with normal hearing (perhaps they had a cold on the day of the test). We could summarise the results of the test as in Table 14.1.

There are four possible outcomes for a child, as shown in Figure 14.2. A child with a real hearing problem may either fail the screening test (**true positive**; group 'a' in Figure 14.2) or pass the test, suggesting falsely that they do not have a problem (**false negative**; group 'c'). Similarly, a child without a problem may pass the test (**true negative**; group 'd') or fail, falsely implying that they do have a problem (**false positive**; group 'b').

For a test to be accurate it should produce few false-positive and false-negative results. So how good is the school hearing test? There are two issues to consider: how well has the test identified the children who do have a problem; and how well has it classified the normal children as normal? We can quantify these as follows.

What percentage of children with a real hearing problem failed the school test?

What percentage of children with normal hearing passed the school test?

Looking at Table 14.1, we see that 90% (45 ÷ 50) of children with a hearing problem failed the school test and 93% (420 ÷ 450) of children with normal hearing passed the test. These measures of a test are known respectively as its **sensitivity** and **specificity**.

Sensitivity

This measures how well a test classifies people with the disease as sick. It is the *percentage of people with the disease who test positive* (90% in the example above). It is calculated by dividing the number of true-positive results (a) by the total number of people with disease ($a + c$) from Figure 14.2:

$$\text{Sensitivity (\%)} = \frac{\text{True positives}}{\text{All with disease}} \times 100$$

$$= \frac{a}{a + c} \times 100 \qquad (14.1)$$

Specificity

This measures how well the test classifies people without the disease as healthy. It is the *percentage of people without disease who test negative* (93% in the above example). To calculate it, divide the number of true negative results (d) by the total number of people without disease ($b + d$):

$$\text{Specificity (\%)} = \frac{\text{True negatives}}{\text{All without disease}} \times 100$$

$$= \frac{d}{b + d} \times 100 \qquad (14.2)$$

A combination of high sensitivity and high specificity is essential for a good screening test – in this regard the school hearing test works quite well.

Note that it is necessary to do a special study, as discussed in 'Diagnostic studies' in Chapter 6, to assess the sensitivity and specificity of a test. In the usual service setting only those who test positive (groups a and b from Figure 14.2) will

HARDIN

"Now relax and the Doctor will begin your hearing test in just a moment."

be followed up with formal diagnostic testing to determine the true positives. Unless there is a specific plan to do so (which usually is possible only in a research setting), those who test negative are usually not followed up, so the proportion of false negatives is not known and we cannot measure either the sensitivity or the specificity of the test.

Two other measures, the **positive** and **negative predictive values**, are sometimes given as test criteria, but they really measure how well a test performs in a given population. However, it is helpful to look at how they are calculated together with sensitivity and specificity.

In practice we would not know whether a child did have a real hearing problem – we have to predict this from the screening test result. We need, therefore, to know how well a positive test result (fail) predicts that a child does have a hearing problem and, conversely, how well a negative test result (pass) predicts that their hearing is normal.

What percentage of children who failed the school hearing test had a real hearing problem?

What percentage of children who passed the school hearing test really did have normal hearing?

Out of 75 children who failed the school hearing test, 45 (60%) had a real hearing problem. Out of 425 children who passed the school test, 420 (99%) really did have normal hearing. These measures are known as the **positive** and **negative predictive values (PPV** and **NPV)** of the test in that situation. Unlike the sensitivity and specificity, they are not fixed properties of the test but instead tell us how well the test is performing in a particular population.

Positive predictive value (PPV)

This tells us how likely it is that a positive test result indicates the presence of disease. It is the *percentage of all people who test positive who really have the disease* (60% in the example). It is calculated by dividing the number of true-positive results (*a*) by the total number of positive results (*a* + *b*):

$$\text{Positive predictive value (\%)} = \frac{\text{True positives}}{\text{All positives}} \times 100$$

$$= \frac{a}{a+b} \times 100 \qquad (14.3)$$

Negative predictive value (NPV)

This is the *percentage of all people who test negative who really do not have the disease* (99% in the example). To calculate it, divide the number of true-negative results (*d*) by the total number of negative results (*c* + *d*):

$$\text{Negative predictive value (\%)} = \frac{\text{True negatives}}{\text{All negatives}} \times 100$$

$$= \frac{d}{c+d} = 100 \qquad (14.4)$$

These measures of test performance are best thought of as operational measures of the overall programme. They reflect both the *validity of the test* (sensitivity and specificity) and *disease prevalence* in the population tested. Even a superb test (very high sensitivity and specificity) will yield a low positive predictive value if the disease is rare.

An example – testing blood donors for HIV/AIDS

It is routine practice in most countries to screen all blood donors for HIV, but what is the probability that someone who tests positive really does have HIV?

To answer this we must calculate the positive predictive value of the test. Assume that we are using the test to screen a high-risk population of intravenous drug users in New York City who have an HIV prevalence of 5,500 per 10,000.

How many of a group of 10,000 intravenous drug users would you expect to have HIV infection?

Of these, how many would test positive if the test had a sensitivity of 99.5%, and how many would falsely test negative?

How many of the drug users will not be HIV-positive and, of them, how many would test negative if the test had a specificity of 99.5%? How many would falsely test positive?

What proportion of the people who test HIV-positive would truly have HIV infection?

Table 14.2 Positive and negative predictive values of an HIV test in high- and low-risk populations.

| Test | True HIV status | | | |
	Positive	Negative	Total	
Intravenous drug users				
Positive	5,473	22	5,495	PPV = 5,473 ÷ 5,495 = 99.6%
Negative	27	4,478	4,505	NPV = 4,478 ÷ 4,505 = 99.4%
Total	5,500	4,500	10,000	
New blood donors				
Positive	4	50	54	PPV = 4 ÷ 54 = 7.4%
Negative	0	9,946	9,946	NPV = 9,946 ÷ 9,946 = 100%
Total	4	9,996	10,000	

We would expect 5,500 of a group of 10,000 intravenous drug users to be HIV-positive and the remaining 4,500 would be HIV-negative. Of the HIV-positive group, 99.5% or 5,473 would correctly test positive and the remaining 27 would falsely test negative (Table 14.2). Among the HIV-negative group 99.5% or 4,478 would correctly test negative and the remaining 22 would falsely test positive. This means that we would expect a total of 5,495 positive test results and, of these, 5,473 or 99.6% would be true positives. Similarly, of the 4,505 negative test results, 4,478 or 99.4% would be true negatives. The test therefore performs very well in this high-risk population.

Repeat the calculations for a population of new blood donors where the prevalence of HIV is only 4 per 10,000.

Among the blood donors we would expect only about 4 out of 10,000 people to be HIV-positive and the remaining 9,996 would be HIV-negative. All four of the HIV-positive people should correctly test positive (Table 14.2). Among the HIV-negative group 99.5% or 9,946 would correctly test negative and the remaining 50 would falsely test positive. This means that we now have a total of 54 positive test results but, of these, only 4 or 7.4% are true positives. This means that 93% or more than 9 of every 10 positive test results would be false positives! Thus, even with a very high sensitivity and specificity, the same test performs badly in this low-risk population. The influence of changes in disease prevalence and test accuracy on the positive predictive value of a test is shown in Table 14.3.

Table 14.3 Variation in the positive predictive value of a test with prevalence of disease and accuracy of test.

Prevalence (%)	Sensitivity and specificity[a]			
	99%	95%	90%	80%
20	96.1%	82.1%	69.2%	50.0%
10	91.7%	67.9%	50.0%	30.8%
5	83.9%	50.0%	32.1%	17.4%
1	50.0%	16.1%	8.3%	3.9%
0.1	9.0%	1.9%	0.9%	0.4%

[a] Assuming that sensitivity and specificity have the same value.

The prevalence of prostate cancer in 60-year-old men is approximately 1%. Using Table 14.3, how accurate would you want a screening test to be before you would consider starting a screening programme to detect early prostate cancer?

With such a low prevalence, even a test with 99% sensitivity and specificity would give a positive predictive value of only 50%; i.e., 50% of all positive test results would be false positives. While this is less than ideal, in practice this is not necessarily the sole consideration in initiating a screening programme. For example, most studies of screening mammography have demonstrated that it achieves a positive predictive value in the range of only 10%–20% for women aged between 50 and 69 years. However, the reduction in breast cancer mortality associated with screening women over the age of 50 is deemed to outweigh the consequences of the large number of false positives that inevitably result.

The trade-off between sensitivity and specificity

Let us assume that we have developed a new blood test that will screen people for a debilitating but treatable disease. The test involves measuring blood levels of a marker X and is far less invasive than the 'gold standard' test. To evaluate the new test, X levels were measured in 225 people believed to be at moderately high risk for the disease and the results were compared with a reference ('gold standard') test, which each person underwent independently of the blood test. For the blood test, the 'criterion of positivity' was set at an X level of 20 mg/l or more; i.e., those with X levels at or above this were said to have the disease. Figure 14.3 shows the distribution of X levels in people with and without the disease as diagnosed by the 'gold standard' test. The light bars on the left represent the 99 people who truly do not have the disease and the dark bars on the right represent the 126 people who truly do. When compared with the 'gold standard' results, 115 of 126 with disease tested positive (X levels $\geq$20 mg/l) as did 10 of 99 without

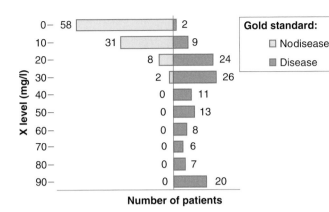

Fig. 14.3 Distribution of X levels by disease status according to the 'gold standard' test.

Table 14.4 A summary 2 × 2 table for the X test with a cut-off point of 20 mg/l.

| X test result | True disease status | | |
	Positive	Negative	Total
⩾20 mg/l (positive)	115	10	125
<20 mg/l (negative)	11	89	100
Total	126	99	225

disease; the remaining 11 with disease and 89 without had negative test results. We can summarise the data as shown in Table 14.4.

How accurate is the X test? *(i.e., what are the sensitivity and specificity?)*

How well has the test performed in this population? *(Here we can extract some useful information from the predictive values of the test.)*

Using a cut-off of 20 mg/l to classify people as positive or negative we can calculate the following:

$$\text{Sensitivity} = \frac{115}{126} \times 100 = 91.3\%$$

$$\text{Specificity} = \frac{89}{99} \times 100 = 89.9\%$$

$$\text{PPV} = \frac{115}{125} \times 100 = 92.0\%$$

$$\text{NPV} = \frac{89}{100} \times 100 = 89.0\%$$

These look pretty good but ideally we would like to have all of these values as close to 100% as possible. The X test has, for instance, incorrectly diagnosed 11 people who truly had the disease as not having it because their X values were less than 20 mg/l. So what if we were to lower the cut-off point to 10 mg/l? Looking again at Figure 14.3, this would mean that 9 of the 11 false-negative people would now be correctly diagnosed as having the disease, but it would also mean that an extra 31 people without the disease would be included in the diseased group.

Calculate the sensitivity, specificity and PPV for this new cut-off point. (Hint: first use Figure 14.3 to lay out a 2 × 2 table for the new cut-off point)

How do the values compare with those obtained using the higher cut-off point (20 mg/l).

If we change the cut-off point to 10 mg/l the results now look like Table 14.5. We can calculate the new sensitivity, specificity and PPV as we did above:

$$\text{Sensitivity} = \frac{124}{126} \times 100 = 98.4\%$$

$$\text{Specificity} = \frac{58}{99} \times 100 = 58.6\%$$

$$\text{PPV} = \frac{124}{165} \times 100 = 75.2\%$$

$$\text{NPV} = \frac{58}{60} \times 100 = 96.7\%$$

On changing the *criterion for positivity* to ⩾10 mg/l the sensitivity has increased but the specificity has markedly decreased. With the drop in specificity, the PPV of the test has fallen from 92% to 75% because there are now far more false positives (41 instead of 10).

Looking at the distribution of X levels in the two groups of people (Figure 14.3), we find that, although they are clearly different, there is some overlap between the two. Where we decide to make the cut-off to try to differentiate

Table 14.5 Results of the X test using a cut-off point of 10 mg/l.

X test result	True disease status		
	Positive	Negative	Total
⩾10 mg/l (positive)	124	41	165
<10 mg/l (negative)	2	58	60
Total	126	99	225

Box 14.2 Accuracy and predictive values of clinical characteristics

The aspects of accuracy and predictive values discussed in relation to screening also apply to all **diagnostic tests**. For example, a red tympanic membrane is generally considered a good predictor of acute otitis media (AOM) or middle-ear infection in children. However, in a study conducted to determine the accuracy of this sign compared with the results of the 'gold standard' test, myringotomy (incising the tympanic membrane), the sensitivity and specificity were found to be only 18% and 84%, respectively (Karma *et al.*, 1989). If we assume a **pre-test probability*** or prevalence of AOM of 50%, this means that only 53% of children with a red tympanic membrane will actually have AOM (the PPV or **post-test probability**), the other positive test results will be false positives. Similarly, 49% of those who do not have a red tympanic membrane will have AOM (false negatives). On its own, then, this is not a very accurate marker of AOM, but if seen together with other signs such as bulging and reduced mobility of the tympanic membrane the accuracy of diagnosis improves. Clinical decision rules based on the presence or absence of several known clinical features of a condition are useful tools to enhance diagnostic accuracy.

* Note that this is another situation in which clinical epidemiologists tend to use different terms to describe the same things. In clinical epidemiology the term '*pre-test probability*' is often used synonymously with *prevalence*. It represents the probability that the patient had the condition on the basis of information available before the test was undertaken, i.e., the prevalence of the condition and the patient's clinical picture. Similarly, the predictive values, which represent the probability that the patient has (or does not have) disease on the basis of test results, are often called '*post-test probabilities*'.

between 'disease' and 'no disease' determines how many false-positive and false-negative test results we find. *There is, therefore, a trade-off between sensitivity and specificity.* For any disease, the optimum point has to be selected depending on the consequences of missing a few positives if the cut-off point is set higher or falsely classifying more negatives as positive if the cut-off point is set lower. If early detection greatly reduced mortality from the disease and if false positives could be identified fairly quickly and cheaply, then clearly we would set the criterion for positivity lower than if the reverse were the case.

The screening programme

Although a disease appears suitable for screening and there is a valid and acceptable test, this does not ensure that the public will benefit from a screening programme. Some major concerns beyond predictive values should be that

- the programme is demonstrably effective in practice, i.e., all its elements work near enough to plan that lives are saved or morbidity reduced and the cost is acceptable; and
- the healthcare system can cope with the flood of extra diagnostic testing and treatment due to finding prevalent disease as well as false positives.

We thus have to measure the practical outcomes of a screening programme, and consider the facilities and resources required to maintain it.

Facilities required

Before embarking on a screening programme it is important to assess the infrastructure that will be required to support it. Facilities are obviously required for the screening process but, equally importantly, are also needed for the subsequent confirmatory testing and diagnosis, treatment and follow-up of those who test positive. Estimates are needed as to the likely uptake of screening, the total number of positive test results (including false positives) expected (on the basis of the prevalence of the disease and the sensitivity and specificity of the test) and the likely effect that this will have on the demand for medical services. *It is of no use, and is indeed unethical, to initiate a screening programme if the resources required in order to act upon the results are not available.*

Treatment

The proposed treatment must be effective and early initiation of treatment must improve the disease outcome. If it does not, then by diagnosing the disease earlier we will simply lengthen the time a person is aware of, and worrying about, the disease.

Cost

The cost of introducing a screening programme, in terms of the financial and also emotional cost of the screening and of the treatment of those who test positive, must be considered in relation to the costs of treating those who develop disease later. A balance between the costs of screening and the consequences of not screening is required.

Evaluation of a screening programme

The fact that a programme ought to work does not mean that it will in practice (see Box 14.1 at the start of the chapter). No mass screening should be introduced without convincing evidence of its likely effectiveness and it is imperative that the programme be evaluated *in practice*. We emphasise here approaches to the initial research that should precede the introduction of any full-scale population screening, with some subsequent comment on practical in-service monitoring.

It can be difficult to assess whether a programme will work. There are some relatively simple early process measures that can give an idea of how things are going, but finally we also have to show that the programme delivers improved outcomes.

To see whether we have succeeded in detecting disease earlier than usual, we can compare the *stage of disease* in patients whose disease was detected at screening with the stage in those in whom it was detected in the normal way. If cases identified at screening are less advanced, then at least the potential for benefit has been demonstrated. If this is not so, then the programme can be abandoned without any need for outcome evaluation.

Another simple check on the process is the *positive predictive value* (PPV) of the screening test in the programme. A high PPV reflects a good combination of an accurate test and an appropriate population (reasonably high prevalence); a low PPV implies that the programme may be in trouble. Why is this so? A low PPV indicates that, of all the positive test results, only a few reflect true instances of disease among those screened, and the large number of false positives will lead to unnecessary concern. Since virtually all diseases considered serious enough for screening in the general population will have a fairly low prevalence, the PPV of any test will be less than optimal however high its sensitivity and specificity (refer back to Table 14.3). Health authorities and the general public need to agree explicitly on what level of false positives is acceptable, in the light of what these people will suffer. The community should also be given the chance to declare that they believe that a large benefit for a small minority (some of the 'true positives') outweighs the smaller losses (and the costs) suffered by a much larger number (the 'false positives').

There are three areas we need to address when considering the outcome evaluation of screening programmes:

- target outcomes to be considered,
- potential sources of bias in the evaluation of a screening programme and
- the design of an evaluation study.

Target outcomes to be considered

Reductions in mortality are the most important outcomes to be gained from screening programmes for fatal conditions such as cancers. However, mere prolongation of life might not adequately justify screening if the quality of life is poor. Thus we should also consider absence or reduction of serious morbidity and improvement in quality of life as essential target outcomes. Other sensible endpoints need to be set for other conditions: for example, we would want to know that detecting impaired hearing in school children led to some measurable benefits of consequence – perhaps improved performance at school.

Potential sources of bias in the evaluation of a screening programme

The best way to evaluate the effectiveness of screening is by following up people who have and have not been screened to see what effects the screening has on their subsequent morbidity and mortality. However, the presence of bias is a major problem in this area, making simple cohort comparisons unreliable, implying the need for evidence from randomised trials.

Volunteer bias

People who attend for screening are likely to be different from those who do not. They tend to be of higher socioeconomic status, to be more health-conscious and to comply better with prescribed advice. Thus better results for a screening programme of volunteers compared with disease outcomes in non-volunteers may relate to factors associated with the 'volunteerism', rather than benefits of treatment following earlier diagnosis. (This is the same volunteer bias as that which you saw in Chapter 7.)

In the HIP trial of mammographic screening (see Box 14.3), only about two thirds of the 31,000 women randomly allocated to the mammography group actually took up the initial offer to be screened and less than half received all four annual examinations. After 5 years of follow-up, both the all-cause mortality rate and mortality from cardiovascular disease were much higher in women who had refused breast screening than in those who had been screened (Table 14.6). Since the screening was directed just at breast cancer, why would women who came for screening have lower mortality rates for causes other than breast cancer? The most likely reason is 'volunteer bias' – the women who took up the offer of screening were different in important ways from those who did not.

The only way to avoid this type of bias is to recruit a pool of volunteers and *then* assign them randomly to receive screening or no screening as they did in

Table 14.6 Volunteerism among women randomly allocated to the mammography group in the HIP study, showing that mortality was lower among women who took up the offer of mammography than among those who did not.

Women randomly allocated to mammography	Deaths per 10,000 women per year	
	All causes	Cardiovascular
Women who underwent mammography	42	17
Women who refused the offer of mammography	77	38
Total	54	24

(Shapiro *et al.*, 1985.)

Box 14.3 Mammographic screening for breast cancer – still generating controversy

Mammographic (X-ray) screening for breast cancer has been evaluated in a number of different countries. One of the first randomised trials conducted to determine its efficacy was the Health Insurance Plan (HIP) study in New York – an inspired initiative that linked the introduction of breast screening to the offerings of a health insurance scheme. In this large-scale trial, 62,000 women aged 50–64 who were members of this insurance plan were invited to participate in the early 1960s. About 31,000 women were randomly allocated to the intervention group and offered an initial mammographic (and physical) screening examination followed by three additional examinations at yearly intervals. Another 31,000 women were randomly allocated to the control group and were not offered the screening programme. After 18 years of follow-up, breast cancer mortality was 23% lower in the group offered screening (Shapiro *et al.*, 1985). These promising first results were the basis for many countries to consider mammography as a valuable public health tool, particularly in 50–64-year-old women.

   However, there are still controversial issues to be resolved.

- Results of most studies have not shown a benefit of screening women aged under 50 years.
- There have been criticisms of the core mammographic screening trials and, although these have generally been rebutted, they indicate that there are complex issues involved, both in conducting the studies and in interpreting the results.
- The ability to implement programmes in routine public health practice at the same high standard as those shown to be of benefit in the well-funded research projects is still a matter of concern for many countries.

However, recent evidence shows that there has been a persisting downturn in deaths from breast cancer in a number of countries (Figure 13.3). Although the reasons for this downturn have been a subject of heated debate, it is likely that both better treatment (particularly chemotherapy) and screening have played their part (Webb *et al.*, 2004).

the HIP trial. It is also important to ensure that as many as possible of those assigned to screening are actually screened (as will be true of public health practice). The correct analysis is then by *intention to treat*, i.e., comparing the groups as they were originally randomised, regardless of whether women were actually screened. If only those who actually received the screening are compared with the rest, we lose all the benefits of the randomisation in terms of controlling for

Fig. 14.4 The lead-time associated with screening in two individuals. The shaded area represents the lead-time.

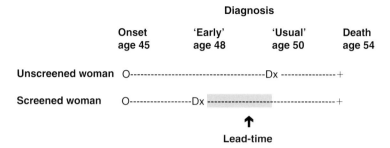

confounding and avoidance of selection bias. (As you saw in Table 14.6, those who do take up screening are likely to have inherently better health outcomes than those who do not, regardless of the screening.) This analysis is not only theoretically correct, but also reflects the reality of public health practice, because not all of us will eagerly take up each preventive opportunity.

Lead-time bias

Lead-time is the period between when disease is detected by screening and when it would have become symptomatic and been diagnosed in the usual way. Consider a situation in which breast cancer starts to develop (disease onset) in two women at age 45. One attends for mammography and the tumour is detected at age 48, while the other is diagnosed at the age of 50 when she notices a lump in her breast. Both women die of their cancer at age 54 (Figure 14.4). The first woman has survived for 6 years following the discovery of the tumour while the second has lived for only 4 years following diagnosis.

Without knowledge of the time of onset of disease, the screening process appears to have increased the survival time by 2 years for the woman who was screened when in fact their disease courses were identical. Both women have lived for 9 years following the initial development of the tumour. The first woman has just known and worried about her disease, and perhaps been without one breast, for 2 years longer. This is known as 'lead-time bias' and, if ignored, it would distort a direct comparison of the case–fatality ratio (CFR) in screened and unscreened groups. Conventionally, the CFR is calculated for a 5-year period after diagnosis of cancer: in this example the woman diagnosed clinically (unscreened) who died 4 years after diagnosis would be in the numerator of the CFR, but her exact counterpart in the screened group who died 6 years after diagnosis would not. If lead-time bias is ignored, therefore, the CFR among women who were screened would appear to be lower than that among women diagnosed clinically, even if their disease courses were identical.

Unless we have some idea of the actual lead-time, perhaps from previous studies, we cannot use survival time from diagnosis to evaluate the effectiveness

Table 14.7 Detection of new breast cancers and mortality from breast cancer, all causes other than breast cancer and cardiovascular disease in the HIP study.

| Study group | Breast cancer cases in the first 10 years (per 1,000 person-years[a]) | Deaths (per 10,000 women per year[a]) | | | | |
| | | Breast cancer | | | | |
		Age 40–49	Age 50–59	Age 60–69	All other causes	Cardiovascular disease
Control	2.1	2.4	5.0	5.0	54	25
Mammography	2.1	2.5	2.3	3.4	54	24
Change	—	+4%	−54%	−32%	—	−4%

[a] Units as reported.
(Shapiro, 1989; Sackett *et al.*, 1991.)

of a screening programme. Instead, we should consider the effects on age-specific morbidity or mortality rates of the disease. These rates are less likely to be affected by early diagnosis than CFRs and should therefore reflect the benefits of early treatment. (Note that, in terms of morbidity, there is likely to be an initial *increase* in the incidence of disease in a screened group because some prevalent cases will be diagnosed earlier than usual.) Table 14.7 shows the results from the HIP study evaluating the effectiveness of mammography, in which they did just this.

Would you implement a breast-screening programme on the basis of the data shown in Table 14.7?

Table 14.7 compares breast cancer detection rates and breast cancer mortality rates (separately for three age groups) among the group randomly allocated to mammography (regardless of whether they actually underwent mammography) and the control group. It also shows the mortality rates for cardiovascular disease and for all causes other than breast cancer. Cardiovascular and 'all-other-cause' mortality rates were similar for the two groups (suggesting that the randomisation process had created two equivalent groups of women), but breast cancer mortality rates in women aged 50–59 and 60–69 years were lower in the group randomly allocated to screening. (Note that the breast cancer detection rates in the two groups were very similar – screening does not alter the incidence of disease but simply improves the outcome after diagnosis.) On the basis of these data alone it would appear that a breast cancer screening programme for women between the ages of 50 and 70 should certainly be considered. In practice it would also be important to consider other aspects of this study, to ensure that the results were valid, as well as the results of other studies in this area.

Length-time bias

When we screen for disease we are more likely to detect cases where the disease is progressing slowly. This is because rapidly developing disease will come to clinical attention sooner and so be more likely to be diagnosed outside a screening programme. The 'slower' cases that are more likely to be detected by screening are likely to have an inherently more favourable outcome, and the effect of this will again tend to make screening appear more favourable than it really is. **Length-time bias** refers to the over-representation of slowly progressing disease among cases detected by screening. Randomisation should give an even balance of each type of case in screened and unscreened groups, again eliminating this as a problem for comparison of age-specific mortality.

Design of a screening evaluation study

Randomised studies

Secure long-term benefits of a screening programme must be documented before it can be adopted for widescale use. Ideally, this demands a number of randomised trials with persons assigned to be offered screening or not, and then followed for some time (usually many years) to assess their health. Inevitably more disease will be found among those screened in the short term, so the real issue is whether their survival or quality of life is enhanced in the long term. The HIP study mentioned above was a landmark in this respect, showing great foresight in realising the need for very large-scale and long-term trials to answer these questions. It included over 60,000 women and the length of follow-up was 18 years, but even so, from the point of view of obtaining reliable results, the numbers of deaths from breast cancer were not very great in the earlier years of the study. A smaller study, or one that was conducted for only a short period of time, would not have been sufficient to show with any certainty (i.e., precision) whether breast cancer screening was of benefit.

Non-randomised studies

Ecological studies have been used to evaluate the impact of cervical screening on rates of cervix cancer and, as an example, Figure 14.5 shows changes in cervical cancer mortality rates over time in Scandinavia. Perhaps the most conspicuous feature of the graph is the fact that, until about 1975, cervical cancer mortality rates in Denmark were double those elsewhere in Scandinavia. Leaving Denmark aside for the moment, we can see that, between 1965 and 1980, mortality fell more rapidly in Finland and Sweden, where nationwide screening programmes had been introduced in the early 1960s, than it did in Norway, where, at that time, only 5% of the population was covered by screening (nationwide screening was not introduced until 1995). This visual impression is reinforced by a more formal analysis that suggested that, between 1965 and

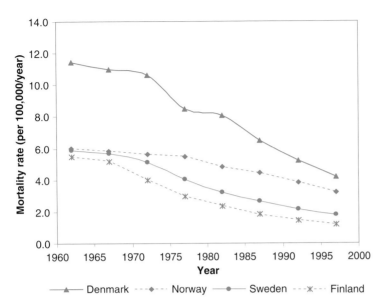

Fig. 14.5 Cervical cancer mortality rates (standardised relative to the world population) from 1950–1998 in the Nordic countries. (Data source: WHO Statistical Information System, accessed via http://www-depdb.iarc.fr/who/menu.htm, March 2004.).

1982, cumulative cervical cancer mortality rates fell by 50% in Finland and 34% in Sweden compared with a drop of only 10% in Norway (Laara *et al.*, 1987). Since 1980 the rates have continued to fall in all three countries.

So what about Denmark? Mortality has also fallen there, but, although the *absolute* drop is quite dramatic, the *relative* fall between 1965 and 1982 was only 25%, i.e., somewhere between that in Sweden and that in Norway, and this fits with the intermediate level of screening in Denmark – about 40% coverage of the population by 1980. Thus the data appear to support the hypothesis that screening does reduce mortality from cervical cancer, but, as you have seen, the results of an ecological study can be hard to interpret. For example, it has been pointed out that the fall in cervical cancer rates in some of these countries actually began before the introduction of screening, emphasising the problems of separating out other temporal effects, such as social change. It is difficult from these data to say how much of an impact the screening really had, although other evidence now supports the claim that cervical cancer screening confers a real benefit in terms of saving life.

Case–control studies have also been used to compare those with and without disease with respect to their history of screening. For example, case–control studies of bowel cancer have shown that screening sigmoidoscopy is associated with 50%–70% lower mortality from cancers in the parts of the bowel that are within reach of the sigmoidoscope, but with no difference in mortality from tumours in parts of the bowel that cannot be reached (Selby *et al.*, 1992). Although non-randomised studies are much more prone to biases, as discussed previously, sometimes they will provide the only evidence available.

The negative consequences of a screening programme

The negative effects or harm that can result from screening are different for those people with positive test results and those with negative test results. Potential harm for those with a positive test result includes the possibilities of

- complications arising from investigation,
- adverse effects of treatment,
- unnecessary treatment of persons with true-positive test results who have inconsequential disease,
- adverse effects of labelling or early diagnosis,
- anxiety generated by the investigations and treatment and
- costs and inconvenience incurred during investigations and treatment.

For example, it has been estimated (Kerlikowske *et al.*, 1993) that, of 1,000 women aged less than 50 years screened by mammography, 53 women will have an abnormal mammogram. This group will then undergo a total of 102 additional procedures, including 13 excisional biopsies, and only 2 women will finally be diagnosed as having cancer and 1 of these will have ductal carcinoma *in situ*, a pre-cancerous lesion for which the benefit of surgical and medical intervention remains uncertain. This represents a positive predictive value for mammography of about 4% for all cancers and 2% for invasive cancer; the other 51 women whose mammograms were abnormal will have undergone the stress of follow-up testing for no clear benefit. The corresponding PPVs for women over the age of 50 are 11% and 7%, i.e., approximately three times higher. (Improvements in technology may improve the situation somewhat, but the fundamental problem of very low prevalence remains.)

Potential harm for those with a negative test result includes the possibilities of

- anxiety generated by the screening test and waiting for the result,
- false reassurance if the result turns out to be a false negative and there is delayed presentation of symptomatic disease later and
- costs and inconvenience incurred during the screening test.

Harm from screening programmes can therefore include the following.

(1) *Physical harm* from complications, invasive tests and/or treatments, delayed presentation if falsely negative.

(2) *Psychological harm* from anxiety, anger or depression from waiting, distress from invasive tests or procedures, knowing a serious diagnosis earlier without improved prognosis, and from falsely negative or positive test results.

(3) *Financial harm* from the costs of tests, medical appointments, possible hospitalisation and treatments.

We detail these negatives to emphasise the need for taking a balanced view of what we are really offering the public when we introduce a screening programme. If we over-emphasise the potential benefits, and neglect seriously considering how a community might view the harms, we do everyone a disservice.

Summary

Screening is an inherently attractive public health strategy for controlling some diseases, particularly when no or few feasible avenues for primary prevention exist. Nonetheless, its present vogue amongst some segments of the public and the health professions seems to over-represent its capabilities. A cool-headed approach is required, and some simple questions make a good starting point to sum up how close to action we might be:
- is this a disease ripe for screening;
- do we have a truly valid test; and
- how well could a screening programme work in our community?

   Points to look for include the stage of disease in cases detected by screening, a high positive predictive value and, most importantly, demonstrated and worthwhile improvement in outcomes in randomised trials.

   These are the scientific aims. We then have to think practically and ethically. Do we have the resources to mount the campaign, and to deal with the extra clinical and psychological load that will ensue? If we are taking resources from other public health programmes, are we sure that we are improving the overall cost–benefit ratio for the community? Does our community truly understand and accept the inherent trade-off: that there will be a large benefit for only a few and some costs (mostly smaller) for a lot more and that some disease will be missed?

Questions

1. Papanicolau (Pap) smear screening is the accepted method for early detection of cervical cancer and women with an abnormal Pap smear result are referred to a gynaecologist for colposcopy for definitive diagnosis. To see whether repeat Pap screening would reduce the number of unnecessary referrals, 110 women with an abnormal Pap smear were given both a second Pap smear and colposcopy. The colposcopy showed that 13 women had high-grade lesions and 97 did not. The result of the repeat Pap test was abnormal for 12 of the women with and 72 without high-grade lesions.
   (a) Construct a 2 × 2 table comparing repeat Pap test with colposcopy.
   (b) Calculate the sensitivity and specificity of the repeat Pap test.
   (c) What is the positive predictive value of the repeat test?
   (d) What is the probability that a woman whose repeat Pap test gives a negative result actually has a high-grade lesion?
   (e) Could a second Pap smear be used to identify women who should be referred for colposcopy?

2. An experimental screening test for hepatitis B has a sensitivity of 82% and a specificity of 93%. The prevalence of hepatitis B in the population to be screened is estimated to be 3%.

   (a) What is the probability that an individual with a positive test result does not have hepatitis B?

   (b) Using this imperfect test, what proportion of a population free of hepatitis B would falsely test positive?

3. A school physician examined a population of 2,000 school children in an attempt to detect heart disease. Assume that the prevalence of heart disease in this school-age population is known to be 10% and that the sensitivity and specificity of the physician's examination are each 80%. All children who were labelled as 'positive' (i.e., suspected of having heart disease) by the school physician were sent for examination by a cardiologist. The sensitivity and specificity of the cardiologist's examination are each 90%.

   (a) How many children were labelled 'positive' by the school physician?

   (b) How many children were labelled 'positive' by the cardiologisit?

   (c) What is the overall sensitivity of both examinations combined?

   (d) What is the overall specificity of both examinations combined?

   (e) What is the positive predictive value of the school physician's examination?

   (f) What is the positive predictive value of the cardiologist's examination?

   (g) Explain why the positive predictive values of the two tests are so different.

For further questions relating to screening, see an excellent case study, '*Screening for antibody to the human immunodeficiency virus*' from the Epidemiology Program Office of the Centers for Disease Prevention and Control (CDC-EIS, 2003, Case studies in applied epidemiology No. 871–703), which is available from their website: http://www.cdc.gov/eis/casestudies/casestudies.htm.

REFERENCES

Karma, P. H., Penttila, M. A., Sipila, M. M., and Katajs, M. J. (1989). Otoscopic diagnosis of middle ear effusion in acute and non-acute otitis media. I. The value of otoscopic findings. *International Journal of Pediatric Otorhinolaryngology*, **17**: 37–49.

Kerlikowske, K., Grady, D., Barclay, J. *et al.* (1993). Positive predictive value of screening mammography by age and family history of breast cancer. *Journal of the American Medical Association*, **270**: 2444–2450.

Laara, E., Day, N. E., and Hakama, M. (1987). Trends in mortality from cervical cancer in the Nordic countries: association with organised screening programmes. *Lancet*, **1**: 1247–1249.

Sackett, D. L., Haynes, R. B., Guyatt, G. H., and Tugwell, P. (1991). *Clinical Epidemiology. A Basic Science for Clinical Medicine*, 2nd edn. Boston, MA: Little Brown and Co.

Selby, J. V., Friedman, G. D., Quesenberry Jr, C. P., and Weiss, N. S. (1992). A case–control study of screening sigmoidoscopy and mortality from colorectal cancer. *New England Journal of Medicine*, **326**: 653–657.

Shapiro, S., Venet, W., Strax, P., Venet, L., and Roeser, R. (1985). Selection, follow-up, and analysis in the Health Insurance Plan Study: a randomized trial with breast cancer screening. *National Cancer Institute Monograph,* **67**: 65–74.

Shapiro S. (1989) Determining the efficacy of breast cancer screening. *Cancer,* **63**: 1873–1880.

The South-East London Screening Group. (1977). A controlled trial of multiphasic screening in middle-age: results of the South-East London Screening Study. *International Journal of Epidemiology,* **6**: 357–363; reprinted in 2001; *International Journal of Epidemiology,* **30**: 935–940.

Various. (2001). Commentaries on the South-East London Screening Study. *International Journal of Epidemiology,* **30**: 940–947.

Webb, P. M., Cummings, M. C., Bain, C. J. and Furnival, C. M. (2004). Changes in survival after breast cancer: improvements in diagnosis or treatment? *Breast,* **13**: 7–14.

Wilcken, B., Wiley, V., Hammond, J., and Carpenter, K. (2003). Screening newborns for inborn errors of metabolism by tandem mass spectrometry. *New England Journal of Medicine,* **348**: 2304–2312.

A final word . . .

Up to this point we have dwelt mostly on the core principles and methods of epidemiology as well as outlining some ways in which epidemiological evidence is used in practice to underpin policy and planning. You will also have gained a sense of the breadth and depth of the subject from the various examples throughout the book. We would like to leave you with some further thoughts in relation to the modern world and its health concerns.

We might start by exploring the boundaries of epidemiology. The definitions given in Chapter 1 are not limiting and imply wide engagement with all influences on health – epidemiology is a 'big-picture' discipline. The proximal causes of disease (e.g., infectious agents, industrial toxins, smoking, diet) are inextricably intertwined with the social, economic and physical environments, so epidemiology must give due attention to these upstream drivers of a population's health.

In 1848, a year of political revolution in Germany and elsewhere in Europe, the great German medical scientist Rudolph Virchow was sent by the Prussian government to investigate an epidemic fever raging among the destitute Polish weavers of Silesia. He diagnosed it as typhus or relapsing fever, noting that such mass phenomena have mass causes (Virchow, 1985, cited by Drotman, 1998; Azar, 1997). He stunned the establishment by recommending political freedom and sweeping educational and economic reforms as the only solutions to the health problem. Although he could not then know the undiscovered proximal bacterial cause, he correctly perceived the upstream social and environmental causes: poor hygiene, malnutrition, poverty, lack of opportunity and oppression. However, without methods to establish such links, his opinion was easily dismissed as political activism rather than science, an accusation still sometimes levelled at epidemiologists who focus on socio-political causes of disease.

Virchow's epidemiological insight was ignored, but a few years later John Snow's epidemiological studies on water pollution and cholera led to sanitary reforms that swept across northern Europe to combat environmental causes of infectious disease. Social causes of disease came back on to the agenda with the pioneering field studies of Goldberger and others in the first two decades of twentieth-century America (Buck *et al.*, 1988). Their work shone the epidemiological torch on pellagra, once thought to be an infectious disease but now known to be a consequence of dietary niacin deficiency. They gathered meticulous data on numerous social factors, including family income, diet, food supply and food habits, and showed that there was a strong relationship between pellagra and poverty with its consequent lack of fresh meat and milk (the major dietary contributors of niacin).

The nineteenth- and early-twentieth-century health activists, like Rudolph Virchow, John Snow and Louis Pasteur, to name but a few, were not 'epidemiologists' but they were giants of medical science and most played a prominent role in health policy later in their lives. Much of their logic and the other tools they used are clearly recognisable as epidemiological and they broke the ground that now connects epidemiology to the allied fields of biology, natural and environmental science, economics and social and political science. Today, many of those confronting the excess burdens of the developing world and Eastern Europe *are* epidemiologists, but to be effective all must operate in the wider spheres of public health and public policy. Within this partnership epidemiology provides some of the keys to causation, prevention and, particularly, health evaluation.

At the other end of the scale, the new potential for genetic mapping and dawning understanding of the functional variations of particular alleles of the genes which control metabolism have opened a new avenue of 'micro-epidemiology' for studying interactions between risk factors and genes. Smoking is strongly associated with lung cancer, but nevertheless many heavy smokers do not develop lung cancer – perhaps because of a beneficial combination of genetically controlled metabolic and/or immunological responses to tobacco carcinogens. Understanding these interactions could help in predicting and modifying future disease burdens with changing patterns of smoking (although in this case we should not lose sight of the main game: dealing with smoking itself will remove most of the problem of lung cancer and a large fraction of other respiratory and cardiovascular diseases).

In more privileged settings such as Western Europe and North America, the explosive growth of epidemiology in recent decades has spawned negative perceptions of a developing industry in 'risk-factor epidemiology', sometimes being done more for its own sake rather than with clear and useful public health goals in mind. So is this true? Certainly the multivariable and often hard-to-measure causes of many chronic diseases, for which relevant exposures may have occurred in the distant past, do not readily yield their secrets. It may also be that the 'easier' work on chronic disease epidemiology has been done and we now confront diminishing returns – a problem that some think affects many areas of science (Horgan, 1996). As a result, studies are finding weak effects and different studies find different effects. The end result is a flow of contradictory headlines and journal articles depicting new panaceas or 'lifestyle' risks (although some of this information overload stems more from the economic imperatives of publicity and circulation than from flawed research). No wonder members of the public (and some epidemiologists) are becoming disillusioned.

The answer? Think smarter. We have discussed the main hurdles to be overcome when interpreting the results of epidemiological research – our old friends chance, bias and confounding (Chapters 7 and 8). We can never eliminate the play of *chance* from research but can ensure that studies are big enough to reduce it to acceptable levels, and should also view the results of any individual study in the context of what others have found. One result might be due to chance but similar results from different studies are unlikely to be. We also know about *confounding* – how to look for it and how to control it, always assuming that we can measure the confounders with sufficient accuracy.

Which brings us to *measurement error* – in exposure and outcome but also for confounders (we cannot control for them if they are not measured well). Even a moderate amount of non-differential random misclassification can completely mask an association, so if the associations we are looking for today are better hidden than those discovered previously then we need to sharpen our tools to find them (Michels, 2001). New technologies now allow more sophisticated measurement both of exposure (e.g., serum biomarkers, DNA damage in cells) and of outcome (e.g., early cellular changes, molecular subtypes of disease based on genetic profiles). Increasing the precision and accuracy of our measurement is paramount but we also need to be more specific about what we mean by exposure and outcome. A single infectious agent may have a number of different strains, cigarettes have different levels of tar, hormone replacement therapy comes in a number of different formulations and doses and so on. Duration, intensity, pattern and timing of exposure (for example childhood versus adult) may also be important. Is someone who drinks a glass or two of wine each night the same as their neighbour who drinks only on Friday nights but then drinks a bottle or two? Is diet in childhood more important than recent diet?

Similarly, we need to be more precise about our definition of 'outcome'. Pathologists have known for years that cancers at one site can take many different forms, yet until recently epidemiologists would often treat them as a single disease. Different subtypes of cancer may have different aetiologies and, if we lump them all together in a single analysis, it is no wonder that clear patterns of risk don't fall out at our feet. This was certainly the case for uterine cancer until the mid twentieth century when cancers of the body of the uterus were separated from those of the cervix (or neck of the uterus) and they were found to have diametrically opposite sets of risk factors.

A dramatic example of the effects of clearly defining both exposure and outcome comes from studies of the relation between human papillomavirus (HPV) infection and cervical cancer. In early studies HPV was detected in 30%–60% of cases – improved detection methods mean that it is now identified in 99% of cases. As a result of both improvement in detection and a focus on individual types of HPV and cervical cancer, we now see odds ratios of 100–900 for the specific associations between HPV-16 and squamous cell cancers and between HPV-18 and adenocarcinomas of the cervix (Bosch *et al.*, 2002).

The debate over the perils of pure risk-factor epidemiology has been valuable in forcing a re-evaluation of perspectives (McMichael, 1999; Rothman *et al.*, 1998; Susser, 1998). In addition to improving measurement, the key to maximising the discipline's future contributions to understanding and enhancing health lies with integration across levels (from macro to micro), across lives (from birth to death) and over time. The tools and related issues that we have covered in this book are central to some of these dimensions and relevant to all of them, although other perspectives from sociology, social history, anthropology and economics may dominate on some of the larger scales. Thus both macro-level ecoepidemiology (ranging from studying the health effects of climate change to the toxic sequelae of a local chemical hazard) and micro-level molecular epidemiology (perhaps to inform development of a vaccine against a parasite predicted to spread with global warming) can be relevant to the same specific goal of disease control.

Which brings us back to our ultimate goal of disease control. There is no doubt that Rose's view of prevention (Chapter 13) is right, and that societies should aim for changes that promote community-wide shifts in distributions of risk factors (as with the US Air Force suicide-prevention programme). However, that approach is never easy and is necessarily slow, so the potential for a 'quick fix' as an alternative or an interim measure remains appealing. We need to remove just one weak link in a causal chain for effective prevention, so seeking this at any point, proximal or upstream, makes sense. Of course trade-offs may need to be made in relation to the net balance of benefits and harms from removing a particular component cause when this affects multiple different health outcomes.

The public health argument for using vaccines against common, important infections is strongly supported by the very high population attributable fraction of these causal agents – by definition this must be 100%. However, vaccines might not be affordable for most of those who need them and many diseases that afflict the poor are neglected by research funding and still have no modern vaccine, or no vaccine at all. Furthermore, when large numbers are vaccinated, the very small risks of adverse effects feature more strongly in the equation. The well-child schedule is already full of injected vaccines, to the alarm of many parents, most children and some epidemiologists concerned about risks of unsafe injections, hepatitis and HIV. Thus the magic-bullet approach to prevention of infectious disease is still far away and there is much to be done now without vaccines – e.g. lessons from the West show the strong influence of an improved social environment (Figure 13.1).

For the majority of non-infectious diseases we have no safe and secure magic bullet to achieve the parallel preventive end. Here population-level change must be the key, linked to removal of harmful habits such as smoking cigarettes via changes to the social environments that promote these habits. Such interplay between the proximal (individual) and upstream (societal) levels is well exemplified by the recent epidemic of obesity in most nations where food supply is ample. Greater relative body weight is in turn closely linked to an elevated risk of type-2 diabetes, hypertension and other conditions. While some of the causal metabolic consequences of obesity are understood, the key intervention is to reverse the pendulum swing towards increasing weight and declining physical activity – population-level phenomena. Causes operating upstream have created a so-called 'obesogenic' environment and this is where we must seek solutions – no easy task, but one being tackled by epidemiologists, nutritionists, psychologists and sociologists. We all know what a challenge this is – the parallel shifts to readily available, energy-rich refined foods and the decreased need and opportunity for physical effort both in the workplace and at home hinder attempts to redress the imbalance. Epidemiology has given us insight into the nature of the problem, but the solutions are not simple.

Having said that, we nonetheless remain seduced by the potential of one-shot interventions such as the Polypill (Chapter 13), which might allow us to improve our health forecast with minimal personal pain (although three decades of pill taking is no light task!). Other single preventive agents have been sought but, to date, most have been found wanting (see Box 15.1).

What does the future hold for epidemiology?

Extensions to analytic epidemiology through time and to levels beyond the individual offer potential to integrate some of the more remote factors into a single causal web. The latter might include linking multiple levels of data in the one analysis:

- information provided by an individual that characterises their direct exposures, their social position (e.g., level of education, income) and their local environment (e.g., distance from health services);
- molecular-level information from, for example, a blood sample provided by the individual; and
- macro-level descriptors that capture attributes of the wider community in which the individual dwells, such as indicators of disadvantage (average income, crime rate, education, accessibility of health services) and environmental challenges (e.g., air or noise pollution).

This would allow the molecular and community contexts to become part of the explanation of individual health states. Inclusion in a single analytic model allows some quantification of interactions over levels, in contrast to the more qualitative assessments that will otherwise prevail. For example the Whitehall II study

Box 15.1 Beta-carotene: an epidemiological tale

The history of nutritional epidemiology is based on the identification and correction of specific deficits in what came to be called vitamins, as well as the need to provide adequate energy for growth. In the second half of the twentieth century, observations from descriptive studies comparing populations with adequate energy intake led to hypotheses that much of the uneven distribution of non-infectious diseases, especially cancers and heart diseases, could be due to dietary differences between populations. This led to a flood of analytic epidemiology and parallel laboratory work as scientists tried to identify specific cancer-causing agents (carcinogens) and possible cancer preventives.

Dietary epidemiology suggested that a number of cancers occurred less commonly among individuals and groups who ate more fruit and vegetables, and laboratory workers found that vitamin A and related compounds (retinoids) were promising anti-carcinogens. The strands were woven together and beta-carotene, the principal dietary precursor of vitamin A, was identified as a substance that might underlie the beneficial effects of fruits and vegetables. Beta-carotene's appeal as a preventive agent was substantial: it combined a number of theoretical anti-cancer properties and appeared to be entirely safe (vitamin A itself being far more toxic at effective anti-cancer doses).

This message was captured most cogently in a paper published in *Nature* (Peto *et al.*, 1981), and several epidemiological groups were stimulated to conduct randomised preventive trials using beta-carotene. (Experiments were required to quantify precisely the 'beta-carotene effect' separately from effects of other inter-related dietary elements.) When put to the test in this way, the hypothesis failed to stand up; and in fact beta-carotene may actually have been harmful to some smokers (ATBC, 1994).

In retrospect we know now that beta-carotene is a good marker of a beneficial diet, but insufficient on its own to provide any protection. Thus knowledge advances. We have learned that dietary epidemiology is more challenging than was perhaps initially appreciated; that we have not yet found our magic bullet for cancer; and that for now our public health message has to be directed towards encouraging a hearty intake of fruit and vegetables.

linked *individual* data on health, and socioeconomic status to a *neighbourhood* deprivation index derived from census data, and showed that both individual and neighbourhood deprivation were associated with poor general and mental health (Stafford and Marmot, 2003).

An emerging and attractive, albeit challenging, approach to temporal integration is found in **lifecourse epidemiology** (Kuh and Ben-Shlomo, 2004). The aim here is explicit in the name; that is, to identify and integrate exposures and other influences during a person's life (back as far as conception) and relate them to the person's state of health. Finding out details of habits, diets and other influences in early life is mostly too much to expect from retrospective questioning in adulthood, but historical record-based data from early surveys, schools, hospitals and other institutions are opening some windows. For example, an innovative group of Bristol epidemiologists has scoured the UK for records of past surveys that might yield early-life exposure information for people who are now adults. They have identified high-quality dietary records from the 1930s for over 4,000 children, more than 85% of whom have been followed for mortality, and a proportion resurveyed six decades later (the Boyd Orr study; Frankel *et al.* (1998)). Detailed early-life data on a number of contemporary pregnancy and birth cohorts are also being collected, with the intention of life-long follow-up of the study participants. As is true for any long-term cohort study, deciding the optimal methods for analysing the mass of data generated remains daunting.

Having implied that it is still uncommon to capture all desirable dimensions in one study, we end with an example in which investigators are attempting to do exactly this. Certain nations are currently undergoing a health transition with a shift away from a predominance of infectious diseases towards an epidemic of chronic disease, in parallel with many of the accompanying social changes that also occurred in the West. Thailand is one such country, with its own unique socio-historical context. In an attempt to capture and understand the drivers of this health transition, a team of Thai and Australian investigators is preparing to embed a conventional-looking cohort study of 100,000 young to middle-aged Thai adults within the context of the existing social structures and short-term changes (A. Sleigh, 2005, personal communication). Information will come both from the participants' own experiences and perceptions across their lives (spanning two generations) and from a contemporary analysis of a number of major Thai social structures and determinants, based on documents, key informants and surveys. A further dimension will be added by a historical 'look-back' survey that will chart changes in the domains of health, work, environment, diet and social structures in Thailand over the last half-century or longer. Describing and interpreting the interplay among these manifold influences should be interesting. Of help will be the broad range of interdisciplinary skills contributed by the team of investigators – epidemiology, community nutrition, ecology, environmental health, anthropology, economics, demography, occupational health, psychology, sociology and statistics. This exemplifies the partnerships that epidemiology needs if it is to make a difference to understanding and influencing mass-scale health phenomena, such as the transitions currently under way in Thailand and many other countries.

REFERENCES

ATBC (The Alpha-Tocopheral Beta Carotene Prevention Study Group). (1994) The effect of vitamin E and beta carotene on the incidence of lung cancer and other cancers in male smokers. *New England Journal of Medicine*, **330**: 1029–1035.

Azar, H. A. (1997) Rudolf Virchow, not just a pathologist: a re-examination of the report on the typhus epidemic in Upper Silesia. *Annals of Diagnostic Pathology*, **1**: 65–71.

Bosch, F. X., Lorincz, A., Muñoz, N., Meijer, C. J. L. M. and Shah, K. J. (2002). The causal relation between human papillomavirus and cervical cancer. *Journal of Clinical Pathology*, **55**: 244–265.

Buck, C., Llopis, A., Najera, E. and Terris, M. (1988). *The Challenge of Epidemiology. Issues and Selected Readings*. New York: Pan American Health Organization.

Drotman, D. P. (1998). Emerging infectious diseases: a brief biographical heritage. *Emerging Infectious Diseases*, **4**: 372–373.

Frankel, S., Gunnell, D. J., Peters, T. J., Maynard, M. and Davey Smith, G. (1998) Childhood energy intake and adult mortality from cancer: the Boyd Orr cohort study. *British Medical Journal*; **316**: 499–504.

Horgan, J. (1996). *The End of Science. Facing the Limits of Knowledge in the Twilight of the Scientific Age*. London: Abacus.

Kuh, D. and Ben-Shlomo, Y., Eds. (2004). *A Life Course Approach to Chronic Disease Epidemiology*, 2nd edn. Oxford: Oxford University Press.

McMichael, A. J. (1999). Prisoners of the proximate: loosening the constraints on epidemiology in an age of change. *American Journal of Epidemiology*, **149**: 887–897.

Michels, K. B. (2001). A renaissance for measurement error. *International Journal of Epidemiology*, **30**: 421–422.

Peto, R., Doll, R., Buckley, J. D. and Sporn, M. B. (1981). Can dietary beta-carotene materially reduce human cancer rates? *Nature*, **290**: 201–208.

Rothman, K. J, Adami, H.-O. and Trichopoulos, D. (1998). Should the mission of epidemiology include the eradication of poverty? *Lancet*, **352**: 810–813.

Stafford, M. and Marmot, M. (2003). Neighbourhood deprivation and health: does it affect us all equally? *International Journal of Epidemiology*, **32**: 357–366.

Susser, M. (1998). Does risk factor epidemiology put epidemiology at risk? Peering into the future. *Journal of Epidemiology and Community Health*, **52**: 608–611.

Virchow, R. L. Report on the typhus epidemic in Upper Silesia. Translated in: Rather, L. J., Ed. (1985). *Rudolf Virchow: Collected Essays on Public Health and Epidemiology*, 2 vols. Canton, MA: Science History Publications.

Answers to questions

Chapter 2

1. Cumulative incidence $= 23 \div 1{,}000 = 2.3\%$ in 10 years

2. Incidence rate $= 36 \div 2{,}000 = 1.8/100$ person-years *or*
$$18/1{,}000 \text{ person-years } or$$
$$1{,}800/10^5 \text{ person-years}$$

3. Incidence rate $= 9 \div 15{,}000 = 60$ per 100,000 per year

4. (a) Prevalence at age 55 $= 100 \div 2{,}000 = 0.05$ or 5%
   Prevalence at age 65 $= 400 \div 2{,}000 = 0.20$ or 20%

   (b) Number of women 'at risk' $= 2{,}000 - 100$ (who already had high blood
   pressure)
   $$= 1{,}900$$

   (c) Cumulative incidence $= 300 \div 1{,}900 = 0.16$ or 16% in 10 years
   It is a measure of cumulative incidence because the same women have
   been followed for the 10-year period.

   (d) We could estimate the total number of person-years at risk by assuming
   that all 1,900 initially healthy women were followed for the whole
   10 years, giving

   $$1{,}900 \times 10 = 19{,}000 \,\text{py}$$

   but 300 of the women developed high blood pressure and so were not
   at risk for the whole period. If we assume that, *on average*, they
   developed it half way through the follow-up period, we can improve our
   estimate of the number of person-years to

   300 women who developed high blood pressure $\times 5$ years $= 1{,}500$
   $+ 1{,}600$ women with no high blood pressure $\times 10$ years $= 16{,}000$

   giving a total of 17,500 py.

   (e) Incidence rate $= 300 \div 17{,}500 = 17.1/1{,}000$ person-years or $1{,}710/10^5$
   person-years (actually 1,714 but we have rounded this off to 1,710).

Chapter 5

1. (a) $\text{Cumulative incidence} = \dfrac{\text{Number of people who develop disease}}{\text{Number of people at risk at the start of the period}}$

So the cumulative incidence in
  (i)   exposed workers = 30 ÷ 2,500 = 1.2% in 10 years
  (ii) unexposed workers = 60 ÷ 7,500 = 0.8% in 10 years
  (iii) all workers = 90 ÷ 10,000 = 0.9% in 10 years

(b) The relative risk $= \dfrac{\text{Incidence in exposed group}}{\text{Incidence in unexposed group}}$

$$= CI_e \div CI_o$$
$$= 1.2 \div 0.8 = 1.5$$

Workers exposed to ionising radiation were one and a half times or 50% more likely to develop the disease than those not exposed.

(c) The attributable risk
  = Incidence in exposed group − Incidence in unexposed group
  $= CI_e - CI_o$
  = 1.2 − 0.8 = 0.4% in 10 years

An additional 0.4 cases of disease will occur in every 100 men exposed to ionising radiation for 10 years (over and above the background rate of disease in the unexposed group). This is the amount of disease that can be said to be *attributable to the radiation* assuming that we believe that the ionising radiation is actually causing the disease.
  Note: the attributable fraction would be 0.4 ÷ 1.2 = 33%

(d) The population attributable fraction $= (CI_T - CI_o) \div CI_T$
$$= (0.9 - 0.8) \div 0.9$$
$$= 0.11 \text{ or } 11\%$$

This tells us that *if radiation exposure is a cause of the disease* then 11% of all cases occurring among the workers (regardless of whether they were exposed to radiation) could be attributed to radiation exposure.
  Note: the population attributable risk would be 0.9 − 0.8 = 0.1% in 10 years. The difference between the *population attributable fraction* (PAF) and the *attributable fraction* (AF) depends on the prevalence of the exposure. An exposure with a high AF may have a low PAF if the exposure is very rare (very few of the cases in the whole population could be attributed to the exposure). Conversely, an exposure with a lower AF may have almost as high a PAF if the exposure is very common.

2. (a) Relative risk = $IR_e \div IR_o$ = 53 ÷ 6 = 8.8
   (b) RR for low dose versus never used = 39 ÷ 6 = 6.5
       RR for high dose versus never used = 62 ÷ 6 = 10.3

Results such as these are often presented as follows:

OC use	Incidence rate	Relative risk (versus never/past user)
Never/past user	6	1.0
Low-dose user	39	6.5
High-dose user	62	10.3

(Note: the relative risk in never/past users is set as 1.0 because this is the reference to which we are comparing the other groups; $IR_o \div IR_o = 1.0$.)

(c) The results suggests that, compared with women who have never used OCs, users of low-dose oestrogen OCs have a 6.5 times higher risk of thromboembolism and users of high-dose oestrogen OCs have a 10.3 times higher risk of thromboembolism. The risk of thromboembolism therefore increases with increasing level of oestrogen. This pattern is called a 'dose–response' relationship.

3. (a)

A case–control study of smoking and lung cancer

	Cases	Controls	Total
Ever smokers	647	622	1269
Never smokers	2	27	29
Total	649	649	1,298

(b) To answer this question you need to calculate the *odds ratio*:

$$\text{Odds ratio} = \frac{a \times d}{b \times c} = \frac{647 \times 27}{622 \times 2} = 14.0$$

(c) and (d) You need to calculate first the *attributable fraction* and then the *population attributable fraction*:

$$\text{Attributable fraction} = \frac{\text{OR} - 1}{\text{OR}} = \frac{14 - 1}{14} \times 100 = 92.9\%$$

If smoking is a cause of lung cancer then 93% of lung cancers *among smokers* can be attributed to their smoking and, theoretically, would not have occurred if the men had never smoked.

$$\text{Population attributable fraction} = \frac{P_e(\text{OR} - 1)}{P_e(\text{OR} - 1) + 1}$$

$$= \frac{0.958 \times 13}{(0.958 \times 13) + 1} \times 100 = 92.6\%$$

where P_e = prevalence of exposure among controls = 622 ÷ 649 = 0.958.

While the AF told us the proportion of lung cancers *among smokers* that could be attributed to smoking, the PAF tells us the proportion of *all* lung cancers attributable to smoking. In this particular example the prevalence of exposure is so high that the AF and PAF are almost identical.

4. (a) The incidence rates can be calculated as follows:

	Cases	Person-years (py)	Incidence rate (per 100,000 py)	Rate ratio
7–8 hours sleep	541	451,393	120	1.0
6 hours sleep	267	175,629	152	1.27
⩽5 hours sleep	67	30,115	222	1.85
All women	875	657,137	133	

(b) The rate of CHD increases as the length of time a woman sleeps decreases. A woman who sleeps for 6 hours is 27% more likely, and a woman who sleeps for 5 hours or less is 85% more likely, to develop CHD than a woman who sleeps for 7–8 hours.

(c) To answer this you need to calculate the *population attributable fraction*:

$$PAF = (CI_T - CI_0) ÷ CI_T$$
$$= (133 - 120) ÷ 133$$
$$= 0.098 \text{ or } 9.8\%$$

The PAF is quite low because most women, or at least most of the person-time, is for women who sleep for 7–8 hours.

Chapter 7

1. Women who read health magazines obviously have an interest in health and so are probably more likely to be vegetarian than women who do not read such magazines. On top of this, the vegetarian readers may also be more likely to respond to the questionnaire. Both of these biases would mean that the percentage of vegetarians in the community would be overestimated. Note also that the study would provide information just about women and men might be very different.

2. (a) People with high alcohol intake are probably less likely to agree to take part.

(b) Alcohol consumption in the control group is, therefore, likely to be lower than in the whole community.

(c) Assuming that patients with liver disease tend to have a higher than average alcohol consumption, the difference between the cases and controls would be exaggerated because of the falsely low level of consumption among the controls. This would make the association between alcohol consumption and liver disease look stronger than it really was.

3. The results from the first study suggest that alcohol is associated with an 80% increase in risk of the cancer. The confidence interval is quite narrow, suggesting that the study was fairly large and the estimate of the RR is quite precise. The results of the second study suggest that caffeine may also be associated with an 80% increase in risk of the cancer, but in this case the confidence interval is very wide, implying that it was a small study and hence that the estimate of the OR is very imprecise. It is possible that the association seen in the second study could simply represent the play of chance since the confidence interval includes the no-effect value of 1. Overall, the data suggest that there is a moderately strong association between alcohol and the cancer (although we would still like to see additional data to support this), but they tell us little about the risks of caffeine other than to flag a possible association that needs evaluating in a larger study.

4. (a) The misclassification is *systematic* (because cases have systematically underestimated their exposure) and *differential* (because it has occurred only among cases).

   (b) The best way to answer this is to draw up a 2 × 2 table showing the results that would have been obtained:

	Cases	Controls
Exposed	300 − 60 = 240	250
Unexposed	100 + 60 = 160	150
Total	400	400

$$OR = \frac{240 \times 150}{250 \times 160} = 0.9$$

   The observed OR is therefore much lower than the true OR of 1.8 (the bias is so great that the observed OR is less than 1.0 when the true OR was greater than 1.0).

   (c) This contrasts with the situation in Table 7.10, where cases systematically *overestimated* their exposure to the same extent and the OR was biased *upwards* to 2.4.

Chapter 8

1. Odds ratio $= \dfrac{a \times d}{b \times c} = \dfrac{20{,}921 \times 94{,}183}{64{,}422 \times 7{,}827} = 3.9$

2. (i) Moped drivers:

$$\text{Odds ratio} = \frac{17,869 \times 86,212}{51,900 \times 7,342} = 4.0$$

(ii) Moped passengers:

$$\text{Odds ratio} = \frac{3,052 \times 7,971}{12,522 \times 485} = 4.0$$

3. The crude and stratum-specific odds ratios are almost identical, suggesting that position on the moped does not confound the association between not wearing a helmet and head injury.

4. The crude association between rider position (drivers versus passengers) and head injury is given by

$$\text{Crude odds ratio} = \frac{25,211 \times 20,493}{138,112 \times 3,537} = 1.1$$

(i) No helmet:

$$\text{Odds ratio} = \frac{17,869 \times 12,522}{51,900 \times 3,052} = 1.4$$

(ii) Helmet:

$$\text{Odds ratio} = \frac{7,342 \times 7,971}{86,212 \times 485} = 1.4$$

The crude odds ratio suggests that rider position does not affect their risk of head injury (OR = 1.1) but when we stratify by helmet use we see that moped drivers have a 40% higher risk of head injury (OR = 1.4) than moped passengers regardless of whether they wear a helmet. The crude association was therefore confounded by helmet wearing.

Chapter 12

1. There are two clear clusters of cases, one starting in late December and the other about a month later. The girls in the first cluster must have been infected before the holiday and those in the second peak must have been infected when they returned to school. The occurrence of the second peak 4–8 weeks after the girls had returned to school on 7 January 1943 gives the clearest indication of the incubation period. Some girls infected early in the first cluster must have been exposed in November; i.e., the teacher must have been infectious then but became much more so when she developed the cold in mid December.

2. Overall this was an informative 'natural experiment', comparing children with different exposure categories for the *agent* (produced by the teacher), *environment* (the basement classroom) and *host* (different immune states, including that conferred by BCG vaccine). The March 1943 analysis was a *retrospective cohort study* of the 105 girls who were skin-test negative in December 1942. This enabled calculation of the cumulative incidence of infection (skin-test conversion) according to the four exposure categories (Table 12.2).

    The 12-year follow-up was a *prospective cohort study* of the incidence of progressive post-primary pulmonary tuberculosis among 368 girls attending the school in March 1943. The exposures measured at the start were the initial immunological states (skin test, BCG) and evidence of recent infection (Table 12.3).

    The incidence of infection (skin-test conversion) among those taught by the positive teacher was very high (86.6%). Environmental conditions in the basement were suitable for transmission (no ultraviolet light, probably high humidity and no ventilation) and the high infection rate among those entering the basement after the teacher was there (58.5%) supports this.

    This study revealed the natural history of primary TB. A high proportion (20%) of the epidemic-infected girls developed post-primary TB over 12 years, nearly half within the first three years. The risk attenuated over time, but continued. Several features should be noted. The study involved adolescent girls; after infection, they are known to have higher rates of post-primary TB than boys. Also, the girls may have been malnourished due to wartime food shortages. This would boost post-infection disease rates even higher than usual.

    The classification of skin-test positives is likely to have some inaccuracy; it is a difficult test to standardise and the old tuberculin used then was more heterogeneous than the equivalent used today. Those negative in December 1942 included children whose parents had refused to have them vaccinated with BCG. These girls may have been socioeconomically distinct (poorer or richer) and this (via nutrition) could influence the course of events after infection – confounding the comparison of disease rates among skin-test positives in Table 12.3.

3. They are attack rates or measures of cumulative incidence (the proportion of girls who converted from negative to positive between December and March).

4. The numbers in groups C and D are small, but the percentage conversion rates in the other groups were very high (60%–85%), so we would have expected to see some converters if they really did have the same rates as groups A and B. (Note: formal statistical tests give the following results: C versus A, $p = 0.03$; D versus A, $p = 0.06$; and C + D versus A, $p = 0.002$, suggesting that the results are not likely to be due to chance.)

5. Preferences: (1) tuberculin negative (0% risk); (2) BCG-induced positive (2.2% risk); (3) 'naturally' positive (6.9% risk); (4) recent converters (20% risk).

6. Tuberculosis (TB) was transmitted in the basement classroom with highest risk to those actually taught by the infected teacher, next highest to those who occupied the room after she had used it that day (the air took time to clear after she had left the room), but not affecting those taught in the morning before she arrived (infected air settled overnight). This defines airborne transmission due to infectious droplet nuclei, respiratory droplets (10–100 micrometres in diameter) containing viable TB organisms from which water molecules evaporated until they reach a size of 1–5 micrometres. Droplet nuclei are small enough to stay suspended in the air for many hours and are easily inhaled to reach the lung alveoli and cause TB infection. The fluctuating infectiousness of the teacher is not unusual with pulmonary tuberculosis.

Chapter 14

1. (a) The 2×2 table for repeat Pap smear:

| | Colposcopy | | |
Pap smear	Positive	Negative	Total
Positive	12	72	84
Negative	1	25	26
Total	13	97	110

   (b) Sensitivity and specificity for Pap smear:
       Sensitivity = 12 ÷ 13 = 0.923 or 92%
       Specificity = 25 ÷ 97 = 0.258 or 26%
   (c) Positive predictive value = 12 ÷ 84 = 14%
   (d) Probability of high-grade disease in women testing negative by Pap smear
       = 1 ÷ 26 = 0.038 or 4%
   (e) The repeat Pap smear had low specificity. In this population with a prevalence of 11.8% (pre-test probability), the positive predictive value is low, and all women testing positive would still have to go on to colposcopy. So, although only 8% of higher-grade lesions would have been missed, this is not a very helpful extra step to add to the diagnostic process.

2. The first thing to do is complete a 2×2 table based on an artificial population of, say, 1,000 people. We know that 3% or 30 will be hepatitis B-positive and that the test will detect 82% or about 25 of them, leaving 5 false negatives.

With a specificity of 93%, 902 of the 970 who are truly hepatitis B negative will correctly test negative, leaving 68 false positives:

	True status		
Hepatitis B test	Positive	Negative	Total
Positive	25	68	93
Negative	5	902	907
Total	30	970	1,000

(a) The probability that an individual with a positive test result does not have hepatitis B is thus $68 \div 93 = 73\%$.

(b) In a population free of hepatitis B, 7% ($68 \div 970$) of people would falsely test positive.

3. The first thing to do is draw up a 2×2 table for the physician as follows.

(i) The physician examines a total of 2,000 children.

(ii) The prevalence of heart disease is 10%; therefore, 200 children will have heart disease and 1,800 (i.e., $2,000 - 200$) will not.

(iii) The sensitivity of the physician's examination is 80%; therefore, 80% or 160 of the 200 children with disease will be labelled 'positive' and the remaining 40 (i.e., $200 - 160$) will be labelled 'negative'.

(iv) The specificity of the physician's examination is 80%; therefore, 80% or 1,440 of the 1,800 children without disease will be labelled 'negative' and the remaining 360 (i.e., $1800 - 1440$) will be labelled 'positive'.

Result of examination by physician	Actual heart disease		
	Positive	Negative	Total
Positive	160	360	520
Negative	40	1,440	1,480
Total	200	1,800	2,000

(a) A total of 520 ($160 + 360$) children will be labelled as positive by the physician and so will go for testing by the cardiologist.

The next step is to draw up a 2×2 table for the cardiologist.

(v) The cardiologist will see the 520 children who were positive on the physician's test, 160 who truly have heart disease and 360 who do not.

(vi) The sensitivity of the cardiologist's examination is 90%; therefore, 90% or 144 of the 160 children with disease will be labelled positive and the remaining 16 will be labelled negative.

(vii) The specificity of the cardiologist's examination is 90%; therefore, 90% or 324 of the 360 children without disease will be labelled negative and the remaining 36 will be labelled positive.

Result of examination by cardiologist	Actual heart disease		Total
	Positive	Negative	
Positive	144	36	180
Negative	16	324	340
Total	160	360	520

(b) A total of 180 (144 + 36) children will be labelled as positive by the cardiologist.

   We then need to combine the results of both tests by including those who were labelled as negative by the school physician and so did not go on to see the cardiologist.

Combined examination	Actual heart disease		Total
	Positive	Negative	
Positive	144	36	180
Negative	56 (40 + 16)	1,764 (1,440 + 324)	1,820
Total	200	1,800	2,000

(c) The overall sensitivity of both examinations combined is
    $144 \div 200 = 72\%$.

(d) The overall specificity of both examinations combined is
    $1,764 \div 1,800 = 98\%$.

(e) The PPV of the school physician's examination is $160 \div 520 = 31\%$.

(f) The PPV of the cardiologist's examination is $144 \div 180 = 80\%$.

(g) One reason why the PPV of the cardiologist's examination is higher is because this test is more sensitive and specific. In addition, he or she sees only those children who have already been classified as having heart disease by the school test. The prevalence of heart disease in this group (31%) is much higher than in the original group (10%), so the PPV is inevitably higher.

Appendix 1: Direct standardisation

To use direct standardisation you need to know:
(1) the age-specific disease rates in your study population and
(2) the age distribution of the standard population.

An example: standardising the IHD mortality rate for males in Germany to the World Standard Population

See Table 1. You first multiply each age-specific rate (column D) by the number of people in that age group in the standard population (column E) to calculate the number of events that you would expect to see in the standard population if it had the same rates as your study population (column F).

You then divide the total number of events expected (the total of column F) by the total number of people in the standard population (the total of column E) to calculate the standardised rate.

Crude mortality rate = Total deaths ÷ Total population
= 211 per 100,000 per year

Standardised mortality rate = Expected deaths ÷ Standard population
= 121 per 100,000 per year

Table 1 Standardising the IHD mortality rate for males in Germany to the world standard population.

A Age group (years)	B Number of IHD deaths (males) in Germany	C Number of males in Germany	D Mortality rate in Germany (per 100,000) $(B \div C)$	E World standard population	F Cases expected in standard population $(D \times E)$
0–4	0	2,032,000	0.00	12,000	0.00
5–9	0	2,296,000	0.00	10,000	0.00
10–14	0	2,362,000	0.00	9,000	0.00
15–19	11	2,353,000	0.47	9,000	0.04
20–24	15	2,283,000	0.66	8,000	0.05
25–29	42	2,990,000	1.40	8,000	0.11
30–34	142	3,722,000	3.82	6,000	0.23
35–39	407	3,548,000	11.47	6,000	0.69
40–44	839	3,061,000	27.41	6,000	1.64
45–49	1,484	2,801,000	52.98	6,000	3.18
50–54	2,396	2,295,000	104.40	5,000	5.22
55–59	5,352	2,903,000	184.36	4,000	7.37
60–64	8,080	2,505,000	322.55	4,000	12.90
65–69	11,562	1,844,000	627.01	3,000	18.81
70–74	12,605	1,350,000	933.70	2,000	18.67
75–79	12,700	869,000	1,461.45	1,000	14.61
80–84	12,727	403,000	3,158.06	500	15.79
85+	16,213	376,000	4,311.97	500	21.56
Total	84,575	39,993,000	211.47	100,000	120.89

(*Source for raw data:* Global Cardiovascular Infobase, www.cvdinfobase.ca, accessed 23 September 2003.)

Appendix 2: Standard populations

Table 2 Examples of some commonly used standard populations.

Age (years)	World standard[a]	African standard[a]	European standard[a]	New WHO world standard[b]
0–4	12,000	10,000	8,000	8,860
5–9	10,000	10,000	7,000	8,690
10–14	9,000	10,000	7,000	8,600
15–19	9,000	10,000	7,000	8,470
20–24	8,000	10,000	7,000	8,220
25–29	8,000	10,000	7,000	7,930
30–34	6,000	10,000	7,000	7,610
35–39	6,000	10,000	7,000	7,150
40–44	6,000	5,000	7,000	6,590
45–49	6,000	5,000	7,000	6,040
50–54	5,000	3,000	7,000	5,370
55–59	4,000	2,000	6,000	4,550
60–64	4,000	2,000	5,000	3,720
65–69	3,000	1,000	4,000	2,960
70–74	2,000	1,000	3,000	2,210
75–79	1,000	500	2,000	1,520
80–84	500	300	1,000	910
85+	500	200	1,000	635
Total	100,000	100,000	100,000	100,000[c]

[a] From Waterhouse *et al.* (1976); [b] From Ahmad *et al.* (2002); [c] The numbers do not sum to exactly 100,000 because of rounding.

REFERENCES

Ahmad, O., Boschi-Pinto, C., Lopez, A. *et al.* (2002). *Age Standardization of Rates: A New WHO Standard*. EIP/GPE/EBD World Health Organization. Report No.: GPE Discussion Paper Series: No. 31. Geneva: World Health Organization.

Waterhouse, J., Muir, C., Correa, P. and Powell, J., Eds (1976). *Cancer Incidence in Five Continents*, Volume III. IARC Scientific Publication No. 15. Lyon: International Agency for Research on Cancer.

Appendix 3: Calculating cumulative incidence and lifetime risk from routine data

The 'quick and dirty' method

If a disease is rare, it is possible to make a rough estimate of the cumulative incidence by adding up the incidence rates for *each year* of life from 0 to 74. Since incidence rates are usually presented for 5-year age groups, e.g., 0–4 years, 5–9 years, etc., the rate at age 0 is the same as that at ages 1, 2, 3 and 4 years; similarly the rate at age 5 is the same as that at ages 6, 7, 8 and 9 years; and so on for each 5-year age-group. This means that, if the incidence in a 5-year band is 3/100,000, the chance a person develops disease during one of the 5 years is 3/100,000 and it is 15/100,000 for the whole 5-year period. One way to add up all the incidence rates to age 74 is therefore to multiply each of the age-specific rates by 5 (assuming that they are for 5-year age groups) and then to add them up. Or, to save time, you can do it the other way around and add up the 5-year rates and then multiply by 5 to obtain the same answer. This is then usually presented as a percentage:

$$\text{Cumulative incidence (CI)} \approx 5 \times (\text{sum of rates from 0 to 74}) \times 100 \qquad \text{(A3.1)}$$

As an example, consider the age-specific IHD mortality rates in Germany shown in Appendix 1. If we add up the rates from ages 0–4 up to 70–74, we find a total of $2{,}270/100{,}000 = 0.0227$, so

$$\text{Cumulative incidence (CI)} \approx 5 \times 0.0227 \times 100 = 11.4\%$$

The proper method

Technically, the measure above is called the 'cumulative rate' because it is just the incidence rates summed or 'accumulated' for all ages from 0 to 74 years.

To calculate a more accurate estimate of the cumulative incidence you have to use a slightly more complicated formula:

Cumulative incidence (CI) = 1 − exp(−cumulative rate)   (A3.2)

where exp(x) means e^x, where e = 2.7183, the base for *natural* logarithms (as opposed to 10, which is the base for standard logarithms).

   So, if the cumulative rate of IHD mortality is 11.4% (=0.114) then the cumulative incidence is

Cumulative incidence (CI) = 1 − $e^{-0.114}$ = 1 − 0.892 = 0.108 or 10.8%

Note that this figure of 10.8% is slightly lower than the 'quick and dirty' value of 11.4% we calculated above. This difference arises because IHD is quite common. The rarer the disease and, therefore, the lower the cumulative incidence, the closer the answers from the two methods will be.

Lifetime risk

Lifetime risk can then be calculated by dividing 1 (or 100% if the cumulative incidence is expressed as a percentage) by the cumulative incidence:

Lifetime risk = 1 in (1 ÷ cumulative incidence)   (A3.3)

So the lifetime risk of IHD mortality in Germany is

1 in (1 ÷ 0.108) = 1 in 9

   It is important to note that, in this context, the cumulative incidence and lifetime risk are artificial measures. They assume that people do not die of any other causes along the way and they are also based on the current rates of disease without taking into account the fact that these may change over time. However, despite these limitations they can be a useful measure for comparing the burdens of various diseases within a population or for comparing the same disease across different populations.

Appendix 4: Indirect standardisation

To use indirect standardisation you need to know
(1) the age distribution of your study population and
(2) the age-specific disease rates in the standard population.

An example: calculating the SMR for IHD in males in Brazil compared with Germany

See Table 3. You first multiply each age-specific rate in the standard population (column C) by the number of people in that age group in the study population (column B) to calculate the number of events you would expect to see in the study population *if* it had the same rates as the standard population (column D). You then divide the total number of events actually *observed* in the study population by the number of events *expected* (the total of column D) if the study population had had the same rates as the standard population. This gives you the *standardised mortality ratio* (SMR), or *standardised incidence ratio* (SIR) if you are using incidence rates.

Observed number of deaths in Brazil = 39,437
Expected number if Brazil had same mortality rates as Germany = 70,979
∴ Standardised mortality ratio (SMR) = $O \div E$ = 39,437 ÷ 70,979 = 0.56

The *crude* mortality rate from IHD in Brazilian men was less than one-quarter of that in Germany (47 versus 211/100,000 per year) but the average age of the population is much lower in Brazil than in Germany. When we standardise for age, the SMR = 0.56 suggests that IHD mortality in Brazil is about half that in Germany.

Table 3 Calculating the SMR for IHD in males in Brazil compared with Germany.

A Age group (years)	B Male population in Brazil ($\times$1000)	C Mortality rate (males) in Germany (per 100,000)	D Expected deaths in Brazil ($C \times B$)
0–4	9,025	0.00	0.00
5–9	8,703	0.00	0.00
10–14	8,604	0.00	0.00
15–19	8,109	0.47	38.11
20–24	7,360	0.66	48.58
25–29	6,841	1.40	95.77
30–34	6,642	3.82	253.72
35–39	5,622	11.47	644.84
40–44	4,707	27.41	1,290.19
45–49	3,745	52.98	1,984.10
50–54	2,912	104.40	3,040.13
55–59	2,454	184.36	4,524.19
60–64	1,957	322.55	6,312.30
65–69	1,583	627.01	9,925.57
70–74	1,138	933.70	10,625.51
75–79	721	1461.45	10,537.05
80+	583	3715.02	21,658.57
Total	80,706	211.47	70,978.64

(*Source for raw data:* Global Cardiovascular Infobase, www.cvdinfobase.ca, accessed 23 September 2003.)

Appendix 5: the Mantel–Haenszel method for calculating pooled odds ratios

When you do a stratified analysis to control for confounding you end up with a number of different odds ratios – one for each stratum. If these are all fairly similar, the next stage is to combine them into a single **adjusted odds ratio** that summarises the effect of the exposure *adjusted* for the confounder. Note that it is practical to do this only when you have a fairly small number of strata; once you need to adjust for more than one or two confounders it is better to use multivariable modelling techniques.

An adjusted odds ratio is essentially a *weighted average* of the stratum-specific odds ratios. We calculate a weighted average rather than a straight average so that strata with more people (and therefore greater precision) have a bigger influence on the final result than small strata. To calculate a weighted average, each individual value is multiplied by its weight and these new values are then added up and divided by the sum of the weights. Various sets of weights can be used for pooling odds ratios, but those proposed by Mantel and Haenszel (1959) are commonly used.

Imagine a case–control study with a total of T people in each stratum (T may be different for each stratum) as follows:

	Cases	Controls
Exposed	a	b
Unexposed	c	d

$T = a + b + c + d$

The odds ratio in each stratum is

$$OR = \frac{a \times d}{b \times c}$$

The weight for each stratum is

$$w = \frac{b \times c}{T} \tag{A5.1}$$

So for each stratum we calculate

$$OR \times w = \frac{a \times d}{b \times c} \times \frac{b \times c}{T} = \frac{a \times d}{T} \qquad (A5.2)$$

We then add these values up for each stratum ($=\Sigma[(a \times d) \div T]$, where Σ (sigma) means summed over all strata), and divide by the sum of the weights ($=\Sigma[(b \times c) \div T]$), so

$$\text{Mantel–Haensel pooled OR} = \frac{\Sigma[(a \times d) \div T]}{\Sigma[(b \times c) \div T]}$$

As an example, imagine a case–control study in which we are concerned about possible confounding by socioeconomic status (SES) because high SES is associated with a lower risk of disease but an increased risk of exposure:

Table 4 A hypothetical case–control study, stratified by SES.

	High SES		Low SES		Total	
	Cases	Controls	Cases	Controls	Cases	Controls
Exposed	460	490	90	45	550	535
Unexposed	60	150	70	95	130	245
Total	520	640	160	140	680	780
Odds ratio	2.35		2.71		1.94	

To calculate the Mantel–Haenszel adjusted odds ratio;
(1) first calculate *for each stratum separately* $(a \times d) \div T$ and add these up for all of the strata,
(2) then calculate *for each stratum separately* $(b \times c) \div T$ and add these up for all of the strata, and
(3) then divide the result from (1) by the result from (2).

Table 5 Calculation of the Mantel–Haenszel adjusted odds ratio.

	High SES	Low SES	Total
(1) $(a \times d) \div T$	$(460 \times 150) \div 1{,}160 = 59.48$	$(90 \times 95) \div 300 = 28.50$	$59.48 + 28.50 = 87.98$
(2) $(b \times c) \div T$	$(60 \times 490) \div 1{,}160 = 25.34$	$(70 \times 45) \div 300 = 10.50$	$25.34 + 10.50 = 35.84$
(3) $\dfrac{\Sigma[(a \times d) \div T]}{\Sigma[(b \times c) \div T]}$			$87.98 \div 35.84 = 2.45$

In this example the pooled or adjusted OR of 2.45 is higher than the crude OR of 1.94, confirming that there was some confounding by SES. The adjusted OR is much closer to the OR in the low-SES group (2.35) than it is to the OR in the high-SES group (2.71) because the low-SES group is much larger.

Meta-analysis

Exactly the same method can also be used to pool odds ratios from different studies in a meta-analysis.

REFERENCE

Mantel, N. and Haenszel, W. (1959). Statistical aspects of the analysis of data from retrospective studies of disease. *Journal of the National Cancer Institute*, **22**: 719–748.

Index